The Men with Broken Faces

CULTURAL HISTORY AND LITERARY IMAGINATION

EDITED BY CHRISTIAN J. EMDEN & DAVID MIDGLEY

VOL. 25

PETER LANG
Oxford · Bern · Berlin · Bruxelles · Frankfurt am Main · New York · Wien

The Men with Broken Faces

Gueules Cassées of the First World War

Marjorie Gehrhardt

PETER LANG
Oxford · Bern · Berlin · Bruxelles · Frankfurt am Main · New York · Wien

Bibliographic information published by Die Deutsche Nationalbibliothek
Die Deutsche Nationalbibliothek lists this publication in the Deutsche Nationalbibliografie; detailed bibliographic data is available on the Internet at http://dnb.d-nb.de.

A catalogue record for this book is available from the British Library.

Library of Congress Control Number: 2015952171

france (manche channel) england interreg

European Regional Development Fund
The European Union, investing in your future

Fonds européen de développement régional
L'Union européenne investit dans votre avenir

Cover image: John Hodgson Lobley, *The Queen's Hospital for Facial Injuries, Frognal, Sidcup: The Toy-makers' Shop* © IWM (Art.IWM ART 3756). Reproduced with permission.

ISSN 1660-6205
ISBN 978-3-0343-1869-3 (print)
ISBN 978-3-0353-0773-3 (eBook)

This publication has been peer reviewed.

Contents

Illustrations

Preface

Gueules cassées, 'broken faces': this is how facially disfigured veterans came to be known in France after the First World War. While the work of their surgeons such as Harold Gillies and Jacques Joseph still influences surgical practices today, historians have largely overlooked the destinies of the many combatants who suffered from these wounds. This book delves into the experiences and representations of such First World War combatants who suffered injuries to their faces. The subject matter may not seem easy at first; indeed, not only is the sight of facial disfigurement challenging, but the idea itself confronts the researcher or reader with their own fears of 'losing face', both literally and metaphorically. Unlike the dark, often over-simplified portrayal of people with disfigurement still found in popular culture today – see, for example, the character played by Jack Huston in *Boardwalk Empire*, a TV series set during the Prohibition era – the analysis of facially wounded soldiers and disfigured veterans reveals a multitude of complex reactions to what is both a very personal and an extremely public mutilation. Beyond the specific cases of 'men with broken faces', then, this study sheds new light on the effects of the First World War in different European countries and questions what we remember about, and how we remember, the conflict.

The Men with Broken Faces: Gueules Cassées *of the First World War* finds its origins in a conversation about the terms used in different countries to refer to First World War disfigured veterans. The observation of linguistic differences sparked my interest in the destinies and perceptions of *gueules cassées*, literally the 'broken mugs', as they came to be known in France. For starting this stimulating exchange I want to thank Professor Ulrike Zitzlsperger, who went on to become my PhD supervisor, mentor, colleague, proof-reader and unfailing supporter. Without her help and encouragement this book would not have been written, let alone published, and the example she sets in her teaching, research and supervision is one I can only hope to emulate in my own career.

While writing this book I was privileged enough to come into contact with individuals whose close relatives suffered from facial injury in the Great

War, and with organizations supporting people with facial disfigurement in France and Great Britain. Their testimonies have reinforced my conviction of the relevance of this book in today's society. Indeed, looking at how combatants – who were more often than not civilians-in-uniform – coped with their wounds one hundred years ago provides a 'safe' approach to the topic of the reintegration of people with facial difference today. Through uncovering the diverse destinies of the 'men with broken faces' it has been my aim to challenge conventional depictions of soldiers and veterans as monolithic figures, be they heroic embodiments of patriotism or examples of ultimate victimhood.

The structure adopted in this book allows for the exploration of the implications of facial injuries from the point of view of the wounded, and of the onlooker. The introductory section stresses the transgressive dimension of facial wounds as well as interrogating the status of disfigured veterans as walking reminders of the war. The second section follows the soldiers' journey from the moment of their injury, to their treatment, and their return to civilian life (for those of them who survived). The focus here is not on medical aspects but on how the wounded and the people around them coped with disfigurement. Relationships amongst the wounded and between the patients and the medical staff, their relatives and society at large, are examined. Questions concerning the perceptions of and responses to disfigurement are central in this part of the book. In contrast, the third section explores images of facially wounded combatants in visual arts and literature; these representations suggest variations in the ways in which different societies perceived *gueules cassées*. Several other publications on this topic preceded the current volume in which I have explored related aspects that are here only mentioned in passing.[1]

1 Marjorie Gehrhardt, '*Gueules Cassées*: The Men Behind the Masks', *Journal of War and Culture Studies*, Special Issue on Veterans' Identities, 6 (2013), 267–81; 'Walking Reminders of the War: The Case of Facially Disfigured Veterans', in Jozef Niznik, ed., *Twentieth Century Wars in European Memory* (Oxford: Peter Lang, 2013), pp. 103–15; 'World War One *Gueules Cassées* and the Ambiguity of Violence', in Ulrike Zitzlsperger, ed., *Gender, Violence and Agency* (Cambridge: Cambridge Scholars Publishing, 2013), pp. 151–63.

The present book is the fruit of five years of doctoral and post-doctoral research at the University of Exeter, supported by the University and the EU INTERREG IVa-funded project 1914FACES2014, as well as small grants from the Association for the Study of Modern and Contemporary France and from EdmissionUK. Thanks to this generous support I was able to carry out research in archive repositories in Great Britain and abroad, and to meet people whose expertise and, on occasion, personal connection with disfigured veterans, helped me better understand the impact of facial wounds on combatants and their loved ones.

Thanks are also due to Professor David Houston Jones for his patient and careful reading of my chapters, and for being such a great project lead when working together on the FACES project. The fruitful collaboration with my colleagues and friends Cristina Burke-Trees and Suzanne Steele in the course of 1914FACES2014 would not have been possible without David's inspiring leadership. I am also indebted to Professor David Midgley and Professor Katharine Hodgson for their careful reading of an earlier version of this book and for the stimulating conversation they engaged in during my PhD viva. Their helpful comments and their kindness gave me the confidence to submit a proposal for this book. I am grateful to Professor Midgley and the team at Peter Lang for believing in this book and in me; their help throughout the publication process has been invaluable. Many other people have generously shared ideas and resources with me; these include Andrew Bamji, Suzannah Biernoff, Sophie Delaporte, Bernard Devauchelle and the team at the *Institut Faire Faces*, the *Association des Gueules Cassées*, the Musée du Val-de-Grâce, the Royal College of Surgeons, the Staatliche Museen zu Berlin-Preußischer Kulturbesitz, BAPRAS and many other institutions who have kindly given me permission to use their images in this book. Thanks are also due to Louise Adams, whose friendship and proof-reading skills have been a great help. Finally, friends and family in Exeter and France have faithfully stood by me and provided an endless supply of joy, prayer and much-needed relaxation time. I simply want to thank them, and David in particular, for their love and friendship.

Introduction
Gueules Cassées: The Face of War

On 28 June 1919, participants in the Paris Conference gathered to sign the peace treaty that officially marked the end of the First World War. In the dramatic setting of the Hall of Mirrors in Versailles, delegates made their way to the table where the document was displayed. Before reaching it, they had to walk past five facially injured French soldiers invited there by the French Prime Minister Georges Clemenceau. Although they remained silent during the ceremony, they did not go unnoticed by the attendees.

Despite the place of the five disfigured combatants on centre stage at this symbolic event, the presence of these men and the role they played in the war and the interwar period are not often talked about or studied. This is not because *gueules cassées* [broken faces], as the disfigured combatants came to be known in France, were very few, or because they did not mix with civilians, on the contrary. The silence surrounding disfigured soldiers and veterans can be accounted for by the painful memories evoked by their faces, and by the fact that they themselves often wished to blend in, not to stand out.

The experiences and representations of facially injured soldiers during and after the First World War reveal some of the individual and collective challenges faced by the people who lived through wartime. This book highlights the visibility of facially injured men and explores different responses to their presence, whilst also interrogating their role and representation in wartime and interwar societies. It underlines the often paradoxical situation of men who sought to lead ordinary lives and yet also became symbols of the war.

The place facially injured men were given, or that they made for themselves, differed notably depending on their country of residence. Through a discussion of the fates and representations of *gueules cassées*, this book shows their cultural significance and their varied perception in France,

Germany and Great Britain.[1] This is best understood through a study of their journey from the hospital to their return to civilian life, analysed here with special emphasis on the relationships established or maintained by wounded combatants. Using a variety of primary sources, ranging from medical accounts to contemporary press reports and artistic representations, this account explores society's responses to facial injury as well as the experiences of disfigurement narrated by *gueules cassées* themselves.

Facial injuries in the First World War: Traditional attitudes and new developments

Facial disfigurement was nothing new in 1914. It could be observed in peacetime as a consequence of accidents, malformation or diseases such as smallpox and syphilis. In particular, a missing nose was often interpreted as shameful, a sign of immorality for the person concerned who had either fought in a duel or lost it due to a venereal disease. Soldiers had also suffered facial injuries in previous wars. French combatants who sustained such wounds during the Napoleonic Wars were in fact for the most part killed by their comrades to spare them further misery.[2]

A similar prejudice could still be observed during the First World War, on the part of stretcher-bearers and of the combatants themselves, for whom facial injuries were a particular fear. Wounds to the face were horrifying, and it was commonly thought that they would lead to death. Thus the British soldier Percy Clare describes how the first two rescue parties who found him on the battlefield refused to take him, convinced that it was

1 The French term *gueules cassées* will be frequently used throughout this book as a concise way of referring to the general phenomenon.

2 François-Xavier Long, 'Les Blessés de la Face durant la Grande Guerre: Les Origines de la Chirurgie Maxillo-Faciale', *Histoire des Sciences Médicales*, 36 (2002), 175–83.

not worth carrying him to the casualty clearing station.[3] Likewise, Albert Jugon, who was later to become one of the founders of the French organization for facially injured soldiers *Union des Blessés de la Face* (Organization for Facially Injured Soldiers) was given absolution on the battlefield. He himself requested, 'Look after the other wounded first, and if there is still time when you have finished, remember that I am here'.[4] Wounded on 16 September 1914, Jugon expected to die from his injuries. But between the time Jugon was injured and the end of the war, the survival prospects of the facially wounded improved dramatically.

Destruction and reconstruction

When taking stock of the material and psychological changes concerning facial injury during the Great War, two trends must be considered: the unprecedented number of disfigured men and the advances in medical practice that took place in the period. If the war was a pivotal moment in the development of reconstructive maxillofacial surgery, it is partly the huge number of facially wounded combatants that permitted these ground-breaking medical advances.

Different reasons account for the high number of casualties. The length and intensity of combat are one explanatory factor, although it should be noted that the influx of wounded men was irregular, months of stalemate following intense battles. Trench warfare and new weaponry (in particular shells and machine guns), as well as the slow development of protective helmets, increased the proportion of injuries to the head and face. The

3 Percy Clare, *Private papers of P. Clare*, 3 vols, III, 06/48/1, London Imperial War Museum [no pagination]. This manuscript was written in 1918, revised in 1920 and recopied in 1932 and 1935.

4 'Emportez les autres, après seulement, si vous avez le temps, souvenez-vous que je suis ici', Raymond Noël Bréhamet and Noëlle Roubaud, *Le Colonel Picot et 'Les Gueules Cassées'* (Rennes: Nouvelles Editions Latines, 1960), p. 19. All translations are by the author.

American surgeon Fred Albee commented on the soldiers' lack of awareness of the danger:

> French soldiers failed to understand the menace of the machine gun. They seemed to think they could pop their heads over a trench and move quickly enough to dodge the hail of machine-gun bullets. By the time they found out that this was the wrong idea, head-wound cases were filling the hospitals of France.[5]

Determining the exact number of combatants who suffered facial injuries is difficult. Sophie Delaporte estimates that 11 to 14 per cent of the wounds sustained by French soldiers affected the face, which would make a total of over 500,000 victims; Martin Monestier gives a similar figure.[6] On the German side, Michael Hagner suggests 300,000 as a likely number.[7] Pinning down figures for Great Britain is no easier despite the fact that one central structure, the Queen's Hospital at Frognal, Sidcup, emerged in 1917 under the leadership of surgeon Harold Gillies and 8,000 patients were treated there between 1917 and 1921. Joanna Bourke estimates the total number of British soldiers who suffered head or eye injuries to be around 60,500, a figure that is very low compared with other countries.[8] The statistics raise a question of definition regarding who was considered to be facially disfigured. This book is concerned with veterans who were sent to specialized hospitals, and whose appearance was fundamentally changed as a consequence of their injury, whether accompanied or not by functional disability. Jay Winter posits that 'at least 12 per cent of all men

5 Frederick H. Albee, *A Surgeon's Fight to Rebuild Men: An Autobiography* (London: Robert Hale Ltd, 1950), p. 108.

6 Sophie Delaporte, *Les Gueules Cassées: Les Blessés de la Face de la Grande Guerre* (Paris: Noêsis, 1996), p. 30. Martin Monestier, *Les Gueules Cassées: Les Médecins de l'Impossible, 1914–1918* (Paris: le cherche midi, 2009), p. 55.

7 Michael Hagner, 'Verwundete Gesichter, verletzte Gehirne: Zur Deformation des Kopfes im Ersten Weltkrieg' in *Gesichter der Weimarer Republik: Eine physiognomische Kulturgeschichte*, ed. by Claudia Schmölders and Sander Gilman (Köln: DuMont Buchverlag, 2000), pp. 78–95 (p. 78).

8 Joanna Bourke, *Dismembering the Male: Men's Bodies, Britain and the Great War* (London: Reaktion, 1996), p. 33.

wounded suffered from facial wounds' and gives an overall estimate of 280,000 soldiers who remained disfigured in France, Germany and Great Britain.[9] Delaporte argues that 10,000 to 15,000 men remained severely disfigured in the French case, which is the best-documented to date.[10]

Although the provision of care for facially injured soldiers was very limited in 1914, if it existed at all, the creation of medical units specializing in maxillofacial surgery during the course of the conflict bears testimony not only to the great number of cases, but also to the development of 'plastic surgery of the face'.[11] If the Queen's Hospital was the largest of its kind, other maxillofacial hospitals remained in activity across Great Britain, in Manchester and in London, for example. Specialized centres in France included Paris (Val-de-Grâce and Lariboisière hospitals) and Lyon (Albéric Pont's unit); in Germany soldiers could be directed, for example, to the Charité (Berlin) or the Westdeutscher Kieferklinik (Düsseldorf). Many wounded servicemen sustained multiple injuries and were treated first outside maxillofacial wards. This occasioned delays in the treatment of facial wounds, about which maxillofacial surgeons repeatedly complained. When patients were finally referred to specialized units, their damaged tissue had started to heal, leaving unsightly scars and rendering facial reconstruction more complex. Before they were able to start reconstructive surgery procedures, Harold Gillies and his peers' first task was often to reopen improperly healed wounds.

The changing terminology of facial injury highlights the different ways in which it has been perceived. Several telling phrases have been used to refer to surgical procedures and related medical specialty that aims to repair maimed faces. In his cultural history of aesthetic surgery, Sander Gilman defines the activity as 'the opposite of "reconstructive" surgery, which is

9 Jay Winter, 'Forms of kinship and remembrance in the aftermath of the Great War' in *War and Remembrance in the Twentieth Century*, ed. by Jay Winter and Emmanuel Sivan (Cambridge: Cambridge University Press, 1999), pp. 40–60 (p. 48).

10 Delaporte, *Les Gueules Cassées*, p. 30.

11 Harold Gillies, *Plastic Surgery of the Face Based on Selected Cases of War Injuries of the Face Including Burns, with Original Illustrations* (London: Frowde, 1920).

understood as restoring function'.[12] According to him, the term 'plastic surgery' started to be used more often in the nineteenth century, at a time when facial surgery was associated with 'beauty' surgery. This preoccupation, or even obsession, with beautiful bodies increased again in the interwar years. In contrast, wartime practitioners were performing *reconstructive* surgery. The adjectives 'aesthetic' and 'reconstructive' help to clarify the aim, i.e. restoring or increasing beauty or functions, but Gillies and his contemporaries seem to have rarely used them. Their preferred periphrases are indicative of anatomical localization, such as 'plastic surgery of the face' (Gillies), 'facial surgery' (Pickerill), 'blessures de la face' (Morestin), 'blessures de la face et du cou' (Dufourmentel and Bonnet-Roy), 'chirurgie cranio-maxillo-faciale' (Lebedinsky and Virenque), 'Kieferverletzungen' (Bruhn) and 'Gesichtsplastik'.[13] Specifying the affected part of the body makes it possible to move away from the stigma which had started to be associated with 'beauty' surgery in previous decades. Whilst the cause of the damage is often mentioned (wounds as opposed to illness), the fact that it was war-induced is terminologically ignored.

Plastic surgeons were keen to establish that every injury affecting the face (and sometimes also the head and neck), fell within their remit, as

12 Sander Gilman, *Making the Body Beautiful: A Cultural History of Aesthetic Surgery* (Princeton: Princeton University Press, 1999), p. 8.

13 Henry Percy Pickerill, *Facial Surgery* (Edinburgh: E. & S. Livingstone, 1924); Hippolyte Morestin, 'Les blessures de la face', *Science et Dévouement*: *Le Service de Santé de la Croix-Rouge, Les Œuvres de Solidarité* (Paris: Editions d'Art Aristide Quillet, 1918), pp. 137–59; Léon Dufourmentel and Flavien Bonnet-Roy, *Chirurgie d'urgence des blessures de la face et du cou* (Paris: Maloine et fils, 1918); J. Lebedinsky and Maurice Virenque, *Prothèse et chirurgie cranio-maxillo-faciale* (Paris: Baillière et fils, 1918); *Die gegenwärtigen Behandlungswege der Kieferschussverletzungen*, ed. by Christian Bruhn (Wiesbaden: Bergmann, 1916); Jacques Joseph, *Nasenplastik und sonstige Gesichtsplastik: nebst einem Anhang über Mammaplastik und einige weitere Operationen aus dem Gebiete der äusseren Körperplastik: ein Atlas und Lehrbuch* (Leipzig: Curt Kabitzsch, 1931). The term *Kieferoperationen* is also used, for instance, in Georg Hermann, *November 18* (Berlin: Das neue Berlin, 2000), p. 32. The original date of publication (1930) suggests that German society, not only medical specialists, were familiar with the term.

shown in Hippolyte Morestin's declaration that 'Everything that contributes to facial expression, everything in the face, belongs to us'.[14] Maxillofacial surgery was simultaneously developing in intimate connection with other specialties such as dental surgery and prosthetics, and striving to assert its singularity. Advances in general medicine – in anaesthetic and antiseptic measures, for example – also significantly increased the patients' chances of recovery. Skin and bone grafts developed significantly during the First World War, pioneers in this field being plastic surgeons Bruhn, Lindemann and Lexer in Germany, Morestin and Delagenière in France.[15] Likewise, procedures originally developed in the field of plastic surgery of the face found applications in other medical specialties during and after the war.

The growing attention given by the medical world to facial wounds is demonstrated by the publication of related articles in medical journals and by the prominent place this topic was given at the 1916 Inter-Allied Dental Congress.[16] If, at the beginning of the conflict, wounded soldiers were still regarded as doomed, recommendations made by specialized surgeons regarding the immediate care of facially injured men (for instance, the position in which they should be transported, half sitting), contributed to improving chances of survival. The delays with which wounded men reached maxillofacial centres remained a bone of contention between plastic surgeons and the medical staff on the front. In order to be sure that 'facial' cases would be sent to him as quickly as possible, Gillies had tags printed and distributed in field hospitals.[17] But the number of casualties meant that in military hospitals, as in the trenches, soldiers were viewed simply as medical

14 'Tout ce qui contribue à l'expression faciale, tout le visage, nous appartient', Morestin, *Science et Dévouement*, p. 137.

15 The history of plastic surgery and its developments during the First World War have been well-researched, such as by Delaporte, *Les Gueules Cassées*, Gilman, *Making the Body Beautiful*, and Antony F. Wallace, *The Progress of Plastic Surgery: An Introductory History* (Oxford: Willem A. Meeuws, 1982).

16 In France a specialized journal, *La Restauration Maxillo-Faciale*, was created in 1917.

17 The New Zealand surgeon spent £10 on these labels at the time when he was working at Aldershot hospital; this initiative proved to be a success. Andrew Bamji, *Queen Mary's Sidcup, 1974–1994: A Commemoration* (1994), p. 13.

cases rather than individual men with complex needs. This dehumanizing dimension of war on the battlefield could also be observed in hospitals, and Jay Winter even compares the latter to a mechanical assembly line.[18]

These two developments – the growing number of maimed men and the progress in medicine – go hand in hand. The former speaks of large-scale destruction, whilst the latter points to new possibilities in the reconstruction of bodies; yet despite this seeming disparity, the massive damage created the need for progress in reconstructive surgery as well as providing the 'raw material' on which new techniques could be experimented and perfected. Thirty years before Archibald McIndoe's burnt airmen became the Guinea Pig Club, facially injured soldiers of the First World War acted as guinea pigs for new reconstructive techniques. The advances achieved during the Great War had a lasting impact on individual men, on society and on plastic surgery. As a consequence of these advances, a great number of disfigured men returned to civilian life. The novelty of this phenomenon, as well as its long-term repercussions on ways of thinking, makes the interwar years a particularly interesting period to study disfigured veterans.

The many facets of the study of facially injured soldiers

The multiple implications of facial injuries, for the people who sustained them and also for the onlookers, call for an interdisciplinary approach to their study. Traditionally, this group of veterans and their role in wartime and interwar societies have been little explored. Considering the number and the role played by disfigured veterans, it is surprising that they seldom appear as a focus of attention amongst the plentiful studies of the First World War and its aftermath. But if no comprehensive comparative studies have yet been published on the topic, research on specific aspects of the fates and representations of *gueules cassées* has been carried out in intersecting

18 Jay Winter, 'Hospitals', in *Capital Cities at War: Paris, London, Berlin 1914–1919*, ed. by Jay Winter and Jean-Louis Robert, 3 vols (Cambridge: Cambridge University Press, 2007), II: *A Cultural History*, pp. 354–82 (p. 360).

fields of scholarship, including the history of medicine, psychology, disability, war, gender and visual culture studies, as well as the cultural history of the Great War. However, facially disfigured combatants have often been reduced simply to their faces, and the emphasis has been mainly upon the positive steps taken (usually by others) to alleviate their conditions.

Medicine, and medical history in particular, stands out as the area of study in which the greatest attention has been paid to the subject. First World War surgeons were aware of the significance of their work and attempted to keep records of cases for dissemination amongst their peers. Decades later, other publications were prompted by the rediscovery of these medical treatises and of patients' records.[19]

Approaching facial injuries from the medical angle has enabled scholars to emphasize the positive consequences of wounds on science: doctors can repair the damage caused by war. Doctors, whose lives are better documented than those of the *gueules cassées* themselves, have been integrated in a wider narrative about the Great War: they symbolize a nation's capability to bring good out of evil.[20] This literature is therefore inscribed within an interpretative trend that emerged during the conflict in France, Great Britain and Germany, a trend that highlights the progress achieved rather than dwelling upon the destruction brought about by the war.

Sander Gilman's cultural history of aesthetic surgery also touches upon the First World War as an agent of change in the understanding and practice of this specialty. Of particular interest is his reflection on the

19 Andrew Bamji, 'The Macalister Archive: Records from the Queen's Hospital, Sidcup, 1917–1921', *Journal of Audiovisual Media and Medicine*, 16 (1993), 76–84, and Andrew Bamji, 'Facial Surgery: the Patient's Experience' in *Facing Armageddon: The First World War Experienced*, ed. by Hugh Cecil and Peter H. Liddle (London: Cooper, 1996), pp. 490–501.

20 See, for example, Albee, *A Surgeon's Fight to Rebuild Men*; Xavier Riaud, *Première Guerre mondiale et stomatologie: des hommes d'exception* (Paris: L'Harmattan, 2008); Jean-Pierre Fumex, *Le Docteur Albéric Pont, sa vie, son œuvre* (PhD thesis, Lyon, 1971); Reginald Pound, *Gillies, Surgeon Extraordinary: A Biography* (London: M. Joseph, 1964).

notion of 'passing', which, I argue, is also relevant in the context of First World War *gueules cassées*:

> The pursuit of happiness through aesthetic surgery presupposes decisive categories of inclusion and exclusion. Happiness in this instance exists in crossing the boundary separating one category from another. It is rooted in the necessary creation of arbitrary demarcations between the perceived reality of the self and the ideal category into which one desires to move. It is the frustration or fulfilment of this desire that constitutes 'unhappiness' or 'happiness'. The patient and the surgeon know that there is a group that the patient wants to join, and that the surgeon can help him or her to do so. The surgeon can enable the patient to 'pass' as a member of the desired group.[21]

Rather than achieving a greater degree of beauty, facially wounded soldiers wished to go unnoticed, the desired target group being that of 'ordinary' or 'normal' people. These considerations point to the psychological and social impact of disfigurement and surgery, an element that was already acknowledged in the First World War: it was mentioned by doctors, described in sensationalist terms by journalists, and romanticized in fiction. However, little provision was made for the disfigured combatants and their families and little research was conducted on the topic. In the second half of the century, research on social stigma provides keys to understanding the difficulties faced by disfigured people.[22] The work of Nichola Rumsey since the 1980s has additionally addressed the impact of facial difference, and the work of social psychologists has contributed to enlightening our understanding of the experience and perceptions of 'visible facial differences' (VFDs).[23] If historical evidence suggests that some of the mechanisms at work in the individual and the group observed during and after the First

21 Gilman, *Making the Body Beautiful*, pp. 21–22.

22 See, for example, Erving Goffman, *Stigma: Notes On the Management of the Spoiled Identity* (London: Penguin, 1963).

23 See Ray Bull and Nichola Rumsey, *The Social Psychology of Facial Appearances* (New York: Springer-Verlag, 1988); Eileen Robinson, Nichola Rumsey and James Partridge, 'An Evaluation of the Impact of Social Interaction Skills Training for Facially Disfigured Soldiers', *British Journal of Plastic Surgery*, 49 (1996), 281–89; Richard Lansdown, Nichola Rumsey, Eileen Bradbury et al., *Visibly Different: Coping with Disfigurement* (London: Hodder Arnold, 1997). See also Nicola M. Stock, Katie

World War bear resemblance with the experience of people with facial disfigurement today, it nevertheless remains true that war wounds and the context of the interwar period represent a specific and unique situation, not least in terms of their association with wartime heroism.

Research in this field has revealed that difficult interaction with people with VFDs is often caused by the onlooker's fear of saying or doing something wrong: 'Being uncertain about what to say and how to act around people with VFDs was a commonly reported behavioural response [...] this stemmed from a lack of confidence and a lack of understanding about how to approach and interact with someone who was visibly different.'[24] Feelings of uncertainty or unease may also account for the scholars' reluctance to investigate this category of war veterans before the generation had passed away. The face has an almost sacred dimension and its violation is disturbing on many levels, for according to ethnologist David Le Breton, 'the face is the most human locus in Man. It is perhaps in the face that the feeling of sacred is born.'[25] The turn of the century, which coincided with the death of the last veterans of the First World War, was thus marked by a new wave of scholarly research on the topic, this time not limited to medical aspects or to individual figures such surgeons. In particular, Sophie Delaporte's pioneering essay, *Les Gueules Cassées: Les Blessés de la Face de la Grande Guerre*, was published in 1996. Although the perspective is mostly that of the medical staff, the author follows the wounded men from the battlefield to civilian life, with special emphasis on the impact in terms of identity. Her case study of the Amiens maxillofacial centre clearly explains the workings of these new medical facilities, and her chapter on the disfigured men's organization provides an insight into the creation and role of this group in the lives of its members.

Whale, Elizabeth Jenkinson et al., 'Young People's Perceptions of Visible Difference', *Diversity and Equality in Health and Care*, 10 (2013), 41–51 (p. 46).

24 Stock et al, 'Young People's Perceptions of Visible Difference', p. 47.

25 'Le visage est le lieu le plus humain de l'homme. Le lieu peut-être d'où naît le sentiment du sacré', David Le Breton, *Des Visages: Essai d'Anthropologie* (Paris: Métailié, 2003), p. 14.

The existence of this organization may account for the greater interest in the subject in France. Facially injured soldiers remain marginal in British and German studies of the First World War. Among the works that consider facially disfigured combatants in more detail are Juliet Nicolson's social history *The Great Silence*, which holds disfigured men as examples of acceptance and denial, and a collection of essays, under the co-editorship of Gilman, on the significance of the face in the Weimar Republic.[26] In it, special emphasis is placed upon surgery and visual representations. This last dimension was given further attention in French and English publications, notably in terms of the work of Slade School professor Henry Tonks.[27] The focus on Tonks can be explained by the rediscovery of his pastels and the concerns about their preservation (they were restored between 2008 and 2010, following an appeal). Suzannah Biernoff's recent essays have offered a new insight into the role of visual representations of facially injured soldiers as constructs and rhetorical tools.[28] In Britain as in France, the renewed academic interest in depictions of facially disfigured soldiers in the arts has coincided with an increase in the popular attention paid to *gueules cassées*, as shown in the release of novels and movies narrating their destinies.[29]

26 Juliet Nicolson, *The Great Silence: 1918–1920, Living in the Shadow of the Great War* (London: John Murray, 2009); *Gesichter der Weimarer Republik*, ed. by Schmölders and Gilman.

27 Louis-Paul Fischer et al., 'Les Gueules Cassées Représentées par de Grands Peintres (O. Dix – G. Grosz – R. Freida): La Défiguration en Histoire de l'Art', *Histoire des Sciences Médicales*, 41, 4 (2007), 337–46. Emma Chambers, 'Fragmented Identities: Reading Subjectivity in Henry Tonks's Surgical Portraits', *Art History*, 32 (2009), 578–607; Julian Freeman, 'Professor Tonks: War Artist', *Burlington Magazine*, 127 (1985), 285–93; Marguerite Helmers, 'Iconic Images of Wounded Soldiers by Henry Tonks', *Journal of War and Culture Studies*, 3, 2 (2010), 181–99; Tom Lubbock, 'Doing Damage', *Modern Painters*, 12 (1999), 58–62.

28 Suzannah Biernoff, 'Flesh Poems: Henry Tonks and the Art of Surgery', *Visual Culture in Britain*, 11 (2010), 25–47, and Suzannah Biernoff, 'The Rhetoric of Disfigurement in First World War Britain', *Social History of Medicine*, 24 (2011), 666–85.

29 Of particular interest are the 2013 Goncourt Pierre Lemaître, *Au-revoir là-haut* (Paris: Albin Michel, 2013), and Marc Dugain, *La Chambre des Officiers* (Paris: Lattès, 1998); *La Chambre des Officiers*, dir. by François Dupeyron (ARP Selection, 2000). In Britain, see, for example, Pat Barker, *Toby's Room* (London: Hamish Hamilton,

Exhibitions featuring or even centred upon facially injured soldiers have also recently been organized in all three countries, in part triggered by the production of contemporary artworks inspired by First World War representations of disfigured combatants.[30] This book analyses Tonks's pastels alongside other works for the first time, not in isolation but in comparison to works by French and German artists, and discusses the relationships between images and texts that describe facial injuries.

Raising awareness and changing perceptions of facial disfigurement has also been the aim of recent campaigns by organizations such as Changing Faces and the French Facing Faces Institute. Their increasing visibility has encouraged body culture and disability studies historians to consider the role of the First World War in the evolution of perceptions and rehabilitation of disfigured ex-combatants. As Amy Lyford convincingly argues in her discussion of wounded men, the body had a collective ideological significance in the wake of the First World War; Deborah Cohen goes even further in stating that the maimed 'brought war home'.[31] Mistreated and damaged, sometimes beyond recognition, the body needed to be healed, or at least its scars needed to be concealed as much as possible.

The questions of aesthetics and disability, of appearance and function, are of particular interest when it comes to *gueules cassées*. Ana Carden-Coyne's 2009 *Reconstructing the Body: Classicism, Modernism and the First World War* underlines the rise of an obsession with physical beauty in the interwar years, as if people wanted to make up for the destructiveness of the

2012); Jody Shields, *The Crimson Portrait* (London: Back Bay Books, 2008); Louisa Young, *My Dear I Wanted to Tell You* (London: Harper and Collins, 2011) and *The Heroes' Welcome* (London: The Borough Press, 2014).

30 See, for example, 'Opération Gueule Cassée', *Musée des Hospices Civils de Lyon* (2005); 'Faces of Battle', National Army Museum, Chelsea (2007); 'Les Gueules Cassées: Scars from the Great War in Contemporary Art', Kunsthalle Mainz, Mainz (2014); 'Faces of Conflict', Royal Albert Memorial Museum, Exeter (2015).

31 Amy Lyford, *Surrealist Masculinities: Gender Anxiety and the Aesthetics of Post-World War I Reconstruction in France* (Berkeley: University of California Press, 2007). Deborah Cohen, *The War Come Home: Disabled Veterans in Britain and Germany, 1914–1939* (University of Michigan Press, 2000; repr. London: University of California Press, 2001).

conflict.[32] Facial injuries were not always associated with severe disability but they nevertheless often incurred functional impediments. Many veterans were suddenly unable to perform natural and long-acquired activities such as eating, speaking or smiling. In an essay for a writing class, a patient reports: 'It was several months after leaving hospital before I regained my speech, and not for a couple of years later could I speak plainly or eat solid food'.[33] The nickname given to the patients at the Val-de-Grâce, *les baveux* (the dribblers), is a telling reminder of one of the issues they faced, namely regaining control over, and re-appropriating, their own bodies. Injuries to the face, although they started to be recognized as representing a form of disability that was reflected in pension scales, did not always functionally impair the victim in the long-term and it took time for the aesthetic prejudice to be acknowledged. Facially disfigured soldiers were only one group amongst the millions of maimed veterans and to these visible scars should be added the invisible marks left by what was then called 'shellshock'.[34] The sacrifice entailed for the maimed soldiers who survived could not be commemorated in the same way as that of the eight million people who lost their lives.

Disability studies tend to focus on maiming and blindness, amputees often being singled out as a category that came to represent all disabled veterans.[35] It could be argued that facially disfigured veterans bore even more visible wounds, and that the threat to one's identity posed by a broken face is greater than that caused by the loss of a limb, which can be seen as mostly functional. Prostheses could also potentially compensate for this form of disability, which was easier for the general public to ignore. Blind veterans have also been a focus of attention since the Great War (various injury-specific organizations and training schools such as St Dunstan's were set

32 Ana Carden-Coyne, *Reconstructing the Body: Classicism, Modernism, and the First World War* (Oxford: Oxford University Press, 2009).

33 *My Personal Experiences and Reminiscences of the Great War*, 6, January 1922 (Liddle collection, Leeds University Library), p. 10.

34 See, for example, Bourke, *Dismembering the Male*, pp. 107–22.

35 *Disabled Veterans in History*, ed. by David A. Gerber (Ann Arbor: The University of Michigan Press, 2000), p. 2.

up to provide for them), one possible explanation being the fact that they were particularly dependent on other people.[36] This led their carers to be comforted rather than challenged in their own 'able-bodiedness'. Besides, although blindness could be accompanied by facial disfigurement, the victim remained unaware of the extent of the damage and of the potential shock his sight could provoke in others. It is therefore no surprise that blindness was sometimes called a 'blessing in disguise' by men who would have preferred to be spared the painful realization of their own disfigurement.

In his pioneering work on the history of disabled veterans, David Gerber distinguishes several trends that have impacted the perception of disability throughout the centuries: the sudden increase in the number (and therefore increased visibility) of disabled veterans, the 'greater normalization of [their] existence', alongside the growing attention paid to them by the state and a developing activism on their part, all shape the context of the interwar period.[37] Disabled veterans of the First World War are discussed in detail in two chapters in his collection of essays, which are both devoted to the rehabilitation and more specifically the vocational training offered to injured soldiers in Great Britain and Germany.[38] This approach contrasts with that of Robert Whalen, who underlines the German veterans' status as victims rather than heroes, alongside orphans and widows.[39] Antoine Prost had already touched upon the topic of French maimed soldiers; however, he only mentions disfigured ex-servicemen in terms of their relationship with injury-specific organizations, whilst Whalen uses the case of a facially disfigured combatant to illustrate his point about the

36 See Julie Anderson 'Stoics: Creating Identities at St Dunstan's, 1914–1920' in *Men After War*, ed. by Stephen McVeigh and Nicola Cooper (London: Routledge, 2013), pp. 79–91.

37 Gerber, *Disabled Veterans*, p. 2.

38 Jeffrey Reznick, 'Work-Therapy and the Disabled British Soldier in Great Britain in the First World War: The Case of Shepherd's Bush Military Hospital, London', in Gerber, *Disabled Veterans*, pp. 185–203, and Deborah Cohen, 'Will to Work: Disabled Veterans in Britain and Germany after the First World War', in Gerber, *Disabled Veterans*, pp. 294–321.

39 Robert W. Whalen, *Bitter Wounds: German Victims of the Great War, 1914–1939* (Ithaca, NY: Cornell University Press, 1984).

overwhelming presence of disabled veterans in Weimar Republic art and literature.[40]

The value of a comparative approach to the history of disabled veterans is demonstrated by Deborah Cohen in her study of German and British ex-servicemen. She notes that

> More than any other group, disabled veterans symbolized the First World War's burdens. […] Years after their demobilization, disabled veterans bore the sufferings war inflicted. […] Each disabled veteran appeared to bring the war's horrors home with him.[41]

Neither Gerber nor Cohen pay much attention to disfigured combatants, although both of them insist on the iconic quality of disabled veterans as symbols of the war. But not all veterans were treated equally, and an implicit hierarchy developed, directly influencing the amount of financial compensation that disabled ex-servicemen received. Amongst those who received little praise, Sabine Kienitz mentions facially injured soldiers; they are, however, then encompassed in a more general study of maimed veterans who, from the status of war heroes, soon came to be seen as burdens.[42] This analysis underlines the threat to the victim's manliness, Kienitz going so far as to ask the provocative question, 'Das Ende der Männlichkeit?' [The end of masculinity?].

The question of the impact of disability on gender perceptions is also raised by Bourke, who discusses a variety of 'masculinities' and argues that the Great War brought about a greater convergence of perceptions of the male body. The title of her essay *Dismembering the Male: Men's Bodies, Britain and the Great War* stands in stark contrast with Carden-Coyne's later emphasis on *Reconstructing the Body: Classicism, Modernism, and the*

40 Antoine Prost, *In the Wake of War: 'Les Anciens Combattants' and French Society*, trans. by Helen McPhail (Oxford: Berg Publishers Limited, 1992), p. 38. Whalen, *Bitter Wounds*, p. 56.

41 Cohen, *The War Come Home*, p. 2.

42 Sabine Kienitz, *Beschädigte Helden: Kriegsinvalidät und Körperbilder 1914–1923* (Paderborn: Ferdinand Schöningh, 2008), p. 104. Blinded veterans are described as the category of injured soldiers praised the most.

First World War. But if there is no denying that *gueules cassées* challenged perceptions of masculinity, the physical and psychological upheaval caused by disfigurement went beyond this gendered dimension and questioned the victims' very identity as a human being.

Towards a cultural history of facially disfigured veterans

Existing studies about facially injured men reveal disparities between countries; whilst the topic has been discussed by scholars from different disciplinary fields, the only cross-disciplinary study of facially disfigured men has been published in France by Delaporte. The fact that French disfigured men coined and claimed a name for themselves – *gueules cassées* – and set up a powerful organization, accounts for their greater visibility and the subsequent academic interest they have attracted. This book sheds a new light on the French case through a comparison with other countries and moves beyond Delaporte's work through the discussion of previously unexplored sources, especially artistic documents, from an interdisciplinary perspective. This book investigates the tensions between the visibility of *gueules cassées* and their desire to go unnoticed, its comparative approach illuminating our understanding of national variations and convergences in interwar Western societies.

The study of facially injured soldiers is of particular interest in the twenty-first-century context. The passing of the last veterans of the First World War and the commemoration of the centenary of this conflict are incentives to re-consider the history and historiography of the Great War. In recent decades, scientific and technological advances, such as the development of cloning procedures, have contributed to a questioning of the link between the face and identity, whilst the multiplication of surgical possibilities and the democratization of aesthetic surgery have made disfigurement something that can be successfully treated for the first time. Furthermore, the return of disfigured soldiers from combat in Iraq or Afghanistan, as well as the awareness-raising campaigns of modern-day charities, call for a greater understanding of the evolution of Western perceptions of, and care for, facially injured people. The rise of interest in First World War veterans since the middle of the twentieth century may also be interpreted as the result of a will to perpetuate the memory of prominent First World War figures, particularly at the time of the centenary of the War.

Acknowledging the status of *gueules cassées* as particularly potent reminders of the war, the present study uses cultural history as its main framework of analysis. Drawing upon existing research on the memorialization of the Great War, it shows the often paradoxical situation of disfigured men who, as they strove to reclaim their lives, were given a symbolic status, sometimes against their own will. The visibility of facial wounds turned the soldier into a public figure that science, popular media, the political sphere and the arts could appropriate and use. The fates and representations of *gueules cassées*, who were both ordinary men and embodiments of the destructiveness of war and patriotism, testify to the collective significance of facial wounds. Through a discussion of the place the veterans were given – or made for themselves – this study challenges traditional representations of the men as either victims or heroes, and contributes to the understanding of the role and integration of facially disfigured veterans in European societies during and after the First World War.

Cultural history, in part due to its focus both on the individual and on the collective, provides an excellent approach for investigating the interface between *gueules cassées* and society. It enables us to explore the ways in which people remember and try to understand events; it is 'a history of the intimate, the most moving experiences within a national community [...] a history of signifying practices [that] studies how men and women make sense of the world in which they live'.[43] This book examines historical accounts and artistic representations in an attempt to confront the documented 'real', perceived and mythologized destinies of First World War facially injured soldiers. It is an investigation into the experience of facial disfigurement and a discussion of how *gueules cassées* made sense of their injuries and envisaged their future. In turn, the gaze of society is explored, the onlooker's perception bringing to the fore the individual and collective

43 Jay Winter and Antoine Prost, *The Great War in History: Debates and Controversies, 1914 to the Present* (Cambridge: Cambridge University Press, 2005), p. 29.

challenges posed by the presence of disfigured men. The roles played by *gueules cassées*, the ways in which they remembered the war, how they conveyed the memory of this conflict and how they were integrated into wider memorial discourses, are analysed in depth.

Processes and products of remembrance are particularly complex in the context of the First World War, a conflict that marked people for generations. In 1975, Paul Fussell noted an 'obsession with the images and myths of the Great War among novelists and poets too young to have experienced it directly'.[44] Reflecting on the reasons accounting for the 'vividness' of combatants' memories, Fussell offers several possible answers, such as the psychological impact of the war experience, and also the emphasis put on 'alertness and a special kind of noticing [in military training]'.[45] But once the last survivors have died, this first-hand source is no longer available; other ways of accessing war memories have to be found. This observation has also been made by Peter Englund, who argues for a better validation and inclusion of individual memories within history.[46] He claims that with the disappearance of the last veterans of the Great War, we have also lost access to divergent memories, and consequently have lost some freedom in the way we approach this momentous event in world history, a phenomenon that he calls 'the multiplicity of war'.[47] This book therefore explores both individual and collective accounts of the lives of veterans, as well as of the organized structures in which they were gathered, both medical and social. Investigating individual life stories proves an indispensable step to gain insight into what facially injured soldiers experienced and how they coped with their wounds.

A comparative approach offers the advantage, in Winter's words, to 'help frame in a more informed way questions of particular national

44 Paul Fussell, *The Great War and Modern Memory* (Oxford: Oxford University Press, 1977), p. 321.

45 Ibid, p. 327.

46 Peter Englund, 'Remembering the First World War: Touched from a Distance', *History Today*, 61, 11 (2011), 3–4.

47 Ibid, p. 4.

experience'.[48] What is more, it allows for the analysis of shared experiences. As Winter points out with regard to his comparative study of capital cities at war,

> there are areas where the cases are so different, and the archival traces so uneven, that it is wise to use what we might term a 'geometrical approach', in placing one case at the centre, and using evidence of the other two cities to make a particular point about that particular case.[49]

The challenges of comparison on an international scale, especially in the context of the First World War and its aftermath, must also be kept in mind. Indeed, the nation is a construct that in those times, perhaps more than has ever subsequently been the case, did not refer to a homogeneous political or cultural ensemble. In the case of France and Germany, geographical boundaries changed as a result of the First World War – with Germany having to face the loss of war, the 'war guilt clause' and reparations as stipulated in the Treaty of Versailles, and in due course a troubled democracy.[50] The role played by France, Germany and Great Britain, all of which were major protagonists in the First World War, remains, however, a shared starting point. An important common point between the three countries is also the extent of the loss experienced, which points to the 'commonality of cultural history': even between previously hostile countries, the 'bond of bereavement was one of the most prominent and the most enduring'.[51] It can be assumed that German ex-servicemen and society at large found it harder to justify the privations and sacrifices endured, the lost war perhaps preventing an *a posteriori* vindication. The extent to which the situation of the *gueules cassées* was influenced by broader national trends is investigated, alongside the influence they sometimes had upon their countries. In this

48 Jay Winter, 'The Practices of Metropolitan Life in Wartime', in *Capital Cities at War*, ed. by Winter and Robert, pp. 1–19 (p. 9).

49 Ibid, pp. 8–9.

50 For a discussion of the Weimar Republic, see Peter Gay, *Weimar Culture: The Outsider as an Insider* (London: Penguin, 1988).

51 Winter, *Sites of Memory, Sites of Mourning*, p. 227.

context, the case of an injury-specific organization that emerged in France appears to be unique; as such, it will be studied in more depth.

The First World War was a turning point in the remembrance of conflicts. Referring to contemporaries as 'the first (though not the last) "generation of memory"', Winter contends that 'the images, languages and practices which appeared during and in the aftermath of the Great War shaped the ways in which future conflicts were imagined and remembered'.[52] The significance of the Great War as a formative moment in contemporary history was acknowledged as the events unfolded, evidenced in the state-led efforts at collecting documents related to the war and exhibiting them in dedicated spaces.[53] This agreement about the potent impact of the conflict on contemporaries did not, however, guarantee a uniform interpretation of events, as shown by the diversity of interpretations visible in the various war memorials and commemorations. Beyond these various organized processes, wounded veterans constituted yet another form of 'war memorial'.

Walking reminders of the war

Gueules cassées were powerful walking reminders of the war in the 1920s and 1930s; as such they were potentially controversial 'sites of memory'. Disfigured veterans, maybe more than any other mutilated combatants, had an iconic value, functioning as embodiments of the physical and psychological wounds caused by the First World War. This is visible in interwar artistic representations as well as through real-life stories.

52 Winter, *Remembering War: The Great War Between Memory and History in the Twentieth Century* (New Haven and London: Yale University Press, 2006), p. 1.

53 The National – now Imperial – War Museum in London and the Bibliothèque-Musée de la Guerre (now BDIC) in Paris, both of which were founded during the First World War, are cases in point.

In his work on *lieux de mémoire*, Nora underlines the necessity of the will to remember in order for sites of memory to emerge.[54] Whilst Nora does not limit his definition of *lieux de mémoire* to places but allows it to encompass other phenomena such as ceremonies, emblems and objects, the possibility of memory crystallizing in people – human beings as sites of memory – is not something he envisages. The question of *who* remembers, however, plays a crucial part in the process, as underlined by Winter in his preference for 'remembrance' over 'memory'. This lexical choice emphasizes the dynamic aspect of the process of recalling and the importance of 'answering the question who remembers, when, where and how? And on being aware of the transience of remembrance, so dependent on the frailties and commitments of the men and women who take the time and effort to engage in it'.[55] Positing that facially injured men came to embody the violence of the First World War against the human body requires a consideration of who came to regard them as reminders of the war, and especially to what extent this memorial value was self-attributed or ascribed to them by others. As people play an active part in the act of recalling the past they may resist being invested themselves with a particular memory, or with any memorial significance at all. This is particularly important to bear in mind when questioning the categorization of injured soldiers as heroes or as victims.

The functions of people as 'producers' and 'receivers' of memory is stressed by Jan Assmann, who highlights the constant reconstruction and changing use of collective memory, defined as 'a body of reusable texts, images and rituals specific to each society, each epoch'.[56] Underlining the role of memory in binding members of a community together and distinguishing them from others, Assmann's conclusions about the fundamental role of memory in shaping identity foreshadows Winter's 2007 analysis

54 Pierre Nora, 'Introduction', in *Realms of Memory: Rethinking the French Past*, ed. by Pierre Nora, trans. by Arthur Goldhammer, 3 vols (New York: Columbia University Press, 1996–1998), I, p. 37.

55 Winter, *Remembering War*, p. 3.

56 Jan Assmann, 'Collective Memory and Cultural Identity', trans. by John Czaplicka, *New German Critique*, 65 (1995), 125–33 (p. 132).

of identity in terms of inclusion and exclusion.[57] Winter approaches the case of 'men with broken faces' from the perspective of their particular socialization through the organization that they created. To him, injury-specific groups had a therapeutic role: they re-integrated men into social networks.[58] Winter uses this organization to exemplify the more widespread trend of forming support associations for veterans and their families in the interwar years: he asserts that these groups are evidence of a special 'kinship' that emerged between the combatants. However, it could be argued that whilst in one sense these organizations brought ex-soldiers together, they also further isolated them from other people.

Simultaneously, in a context in which ex-servicemen found it hard to verbalize their feelings and talk about their war experiences, their status as 'walking reminders' represented a means through which society could have access to the war – albeit not the reality of the front, but at least the imprint it had left on those who were there. This encounter, unlike the act of looking at photographs or films, was almost unmediated (except for the fact that medicine had attempted to repair bodies and faces). This 'accessibility' is thus a remarkable feature of human embodiments of war. Unlike war memorials, the men could be met anytime in the streets, during and after the conflict. Some encounters were staged – for instance, in Versailles and at military marches – but most were unplanned. This unpredictability broadened the scope of potential onlookers in an almost intrusive fashion. Contemporaries could avoid visiting memorials, but they could not as easily ignore these living memories. The latter were vehicles of meaning, but interpretations varied significantly, as this book shows.

Gueules cassées, like other maimed veterans, established a link between the battlefield and the home front. Because they were visually evocative of conflict, they constituted an intrusion of war into everyday life, especially once the war itself was over. This intrusion was not always well received by societies, who oscillated between a 'moral obligation' to remember and the

57 Winter, 'The Practices of Metropolitan Life in Wartime', p. 2.

58 Winter, 'Forms of Kinship', p. 48.

wish to forget.[59] The disappearance of the veterans in the course of time has not, however, meant the end of their use as memory tokens, in France at least. The name they coined for themselves, *gueules cassées*, is still in use today; and although it now also refers to soldiers mutilated during later wars, and those injured in non-war contexts such as firemen and policemen, it is still strongly associated with this first group of disfigured combatants. The role played by the first *gueules cassées*, and their leaders especially, is discussed here as a way of explaining their long-term memorial legacy.

An investigation of the memorial function of persons – what could be termed 'human *lieux de mémoire*' – suggests that typically there is only one distinctive feature or feat singled out in the person for its iconic value. In the case of facially injured men the focal point is their physical appearance, their disfigured face, which in turn points to the war and either to heroic values of patriotism and self-sacrifice, or conversely, to the shame and hardships associated with defeat. Being reduced to their wounds constituted a further blow to many disabled veterans, who wished to go unnoticed rather than draw attention to their injury. Thus, human embodiments of memory, if they come to be regarded as such during their lifetime, can experience a form of dissociation between their individual identity and their collective significance. Not only are individual men robbed of their faces, but their social identity is also altered. The missing faces of First World War *gueules cassées* became what defined them in the eyes of others.

The transgressive dimension of facial injuries

Wounds are visible, physical and tangible traces of the brutality of war, which remain otherwise often invisible, as noted by Eric Leed: 'It was precisely the memory of having inhabited for an unimaginable length of time a landscape saturated with invisible men and controlled by an unapproachable

59 Fussell, *The Great War and Modern Memory*, p. 327.

technology that remained the longest with many combatants'.[60] Wounds are evidence of transgression; they constitute a violation of the body and potentially of the mind. War wounds are transgressive on several accounts, war experience being in Leed's terms

> nothing if not a transgression of categories. In providing bridges across the boundaries between the visible and the invisible, the known and the unknown, the human and the inhuman, war offered numerous occasions for the shattering of distinctions that were central to orderly thought, communicable experience, and normal human relations.[61]

The present study explores this transgressive dimension of wounds, and by association that of the men who sustained them, in the long term. It investigates not only the brutality of the war, but also the violence of the interwar years. In the 1920s and 1930s, the presence of disfigured veterans, like that of other maimed soldiers, blurred spatial boundaries between the front and the home. It also distorted chronological boundaries between wartime and peacetime. The nature of the wounds made their bearers even more transgressive a figure: they bore at the same time features of the human and of the monstrous, echoing the so-called crisis of civilization triggered by the First World War in early twentieth-century Western societies. *Gueules cassées* evoked, on the one hand, the brutality and destruction that human beings were capable of, and the technological and scientific prowess they could achieve, on the other.

This link between death and life – facial surgeons were rather tellingly described as having God-like powers to create new faces – produces an unsettling effect on the onlooker, and all the more so since the face is a zone considered as 'the mirror of our individuality, our singularity'.[62] The story that war has written upon the face points to a traumatic event, which challenges the viewer. The onlooker, whether the disfigured

60 Eric J. Leed, *No Man's Land: Combat and Identity in World War I* (Cambridge: Cambridge University Press, 1979), p. 20.

61 Ibid, p. 21.

62 'le miroir de notre individualité, de notre singularité', Marie-Dominique Colas, *Le Visage des Hommes 1914–2014: Un Face-à-Face Avec le Blessé de Guerre* (Panazol: Lavauzelle, 2014), p. 51.

man – who struggles to reconcile the image reflected in the mirror with his face as he has always known it – or an external 'other', experiences conflicting impulses towards identification, on the one hand, and distance, on the other. The persistence of intact features triggers an impression of familiarity whilst the distorted, sometimes unrecognizable, traits render the disfigured face utterly alien. An almost uncanny feeling results from this paradoxical combination, adding further complexity to the remembrance process prompted by the sight of disfigured men. The presence of maimed veterans was a constant reminder of the war and as such may have contributed to what Richard Overy describes as the 'overwhelmingly morbid character of much of the culture and ideas of the inter-war years'.[63]

Because they are visible, facial wounds are particularly apt to bring memories to the surface. Although malformation and accidental disfigurement occurred during the 1920s and 1930s, facial wounds almost automatically pointed to the war. Whilst some tried to dismiss shell shock as a fantasy, the reality of wounds was undeniable. They had truth-value, functioning as tangible proof of war experience. Thus, wounds are a form of visual testimony. They evoke pain and trauma. The initial suffering caused by the injury was indeed often followed by months, even years, of operations, and even after plastic reconstruction had taken place, physical pain was something many men would have to live with for the rest of their lives. If wounds reminded victims of the physical pain they had experienced, they also triggered and recalled a psychological trauma that affected both their victims and those who encountered them. Disfigurement also shatters the subject's perception of self, of humanity and personality. As a surgeon who treated *gueules cassées* put it: 'We must [...] show that we can restore their humanity to those who have lost the outward markers of identity'.[64]

63 Richard Overy, *The Morbid Age: Britain Between the Wars* (London: Penguin, 2009), p. 364.

64 'Il faut [...] faire la preuve qu'on peut rendre l'humanité à ceux qui ont perdu les signes extérieurs de l'identité', a maxillo-facial surgeon, quoted in Colas, *Le Visage des Hommes,* p. 189.

This redefinition of the self led many a *gueule cassée* to despair of ever being able to lead a 'normal' life again. The many challenges awaiting disfigured men and the strategies developed to overcome them are explored in this volume. The question of symbolism is here of particular importance. As veterans and their societies tried to make sense of their experiences, the belief that soldiers were fighting for a noble cause such as the protection of one's country or the defence of civilization enabled the veteran to move from the status of powerless victim to that of heroic warrior. Thus, the injury was not passively suffered but became a sacrifice accepted for the good of the greatest number, at least in victorious countries.

Working from Gilman's notion of 'passing', it can be argued that *gueules cassées* had an iconic function; even though they often failed to 'pass' as normal, their scars preventing them from becoming invisible in interwar society, others invested them with a positive message not only of survival, but also of the symbolic triumph of science and progress over the destructive forces of modern war.[65] Indeed, the *gueules cassées*' motto 'Sourire quand même' ['Smile on regardless'], embodied and encouraged such a positive outlook in the face of adversity.

The place allocated to facially disfigured men correlates with each society's way of handling the memory of the War. Through the study of a wide range of documents, this book explores the perception and place in interwar societies of veterans who have been rarely analysed in depth, yet often used as symbols. The variety of primary sources discussed, from military files to personal testimonies, pastel drawings and literary accounts, provides an insight into the subjective experience and the many representations of facial disfigurement during and after the war. Different, sometimes conflicting, images of disfigured veterans are revealed, as we follow the journey of the combatant from the hospital to his potentially difficult reintegration into civilian social and economic circles, a process that was often facilitated by the mediation of a third

65 This is shown in literary representations but also in the staging of medical exhibits and photographs as narratives of successful rehabilitation (as underlined in Lyford, *Surrealist Masculinities*).

party such as medical nurses, fellow injured ex-servicemen and larger structures like veterans' charities.

The first chapter examines the confrontation with one's own reflection and with the gaze of others immediately after the wound was suffered and throughout medical treatment. It shows the key role played by the hospital as a space of transition and questions the image of 'passive victim' that is often associated with patients. Studying their interaction with medical staff also allows for a discussion of the representations of the latter in connection with the function they fulfilled for facially injured soldiers. The return of *gueules cassées* to civilian life is analysed in the second chapter, with special emphasis on the question of their reintegration into economic and social circles. Representations of the men as extra-ordinary figures are discussed. They are set against the normalizing treatment observed in some publications and claimed by soldiers via a newspaper written and circulated at the Val-de-Grâce hospital. The third chapter considers the sociability of facially injured men, from the friendships born in hospital to the 'institutionalization' of a special bond via the creation of the *Union des Blessés de la Face* in France. Its rise in importance and the subsequent changes it brought about in terms of the collective image of French *gueules cassées* are examined in an attempt to explain why such an organization emerged in this country and not in others. Chapter 4 shifts the focus to another expression of society's perception of *gueules cassées*, here by means of artistic representation. It investigates the functions and uses of depictions depending upon the visual medium used and the country of origin, showing several different ways of interpreting the presence of *gueules cassées* in European societies. It investigates the claims made by society upon the figure of the facially injured soldier and the latter's integration into discourses on war. The final chapter focuses on literary representations and the exploration of the veteran's psyche that they offer. It examines the treatment of mutilated veterans and their relationship to society in fiction, with special focus on the literary rendering of visually striking wounds and upon the process of reintegration as imagined by interwar authors. The question of what constitutues a sign of successful reintegration is considered, as well as the mediation of encounters between *gueules cassées* and society.

All five chapters demonstrate the visibility of facially injured men and explore different responses to their presence. They engage with documents by *gueules cassées* themselves and with sources reflecting other people's views in order to examine points of convergence and divergence in terms of experiences, perceptions and representations.

PART I

The Soldiers' Journey: From the Front to Civilian Life

CHAPTER 1

Hospitals as Transitional Spaces

Three decades before Archibald McIndoe's burnt airmen formed the Guinea Pig Club, First World War soldiers were the guinea pigs of fast-developing maxillofacial surgery. The medical advances that took place during the conflict have long been an object of scholarly attention, but the treatment of *gueules cassées* was a holistic process that encompassed more than the technical aspects of plastic surgery. The months, sometimes years, that patients and staff spent in hospital call for an approach that takes into account the times of rest as well as the times of surgery, the interactions between people as well as the operations.

This chapter explores life in maxillofacial units from the perspective of both the staff and the wounded. It draws upon accounts by patients and personnel that have rarely been studied before, especially not with a comparative focus. The prevalence of French and British sources can be accounted for by the fact that the context of defeat in Germany was less conducive to the publication of such narratives, and also that many archives were destroyed during the Second World War. Among the few remaining documents, the memoirs written by Henriette Rémi (aka Henriette Ith) have recently been identified as of German provenance; they are one of the most comprehensive accounts of life in a maxillofacial hospital.[1] They are here for the first time discussed in the light of this new development.

Henriette's testimony, as well as those of other staff and patients, shows the importance of hospitals as a key transitional space. They were both an extension of the battlefield and a stepping stone towards return to active

1 Henriette Rémi, *Hommes Sans Visage* (Genève: Slatkine, 2014), ed. by Stéphane Garcia. This book was first published in 1942.

service or civilian life. They were spaces in which men were being 'rebuilt'.[2] This reconstruction went beyond mere physical repair: it called for artistic insight and it involved a significant level of interaction between patients and staff. These aspects are investigated here, with special focus upon the roles that the artists and surgeons, and also the patients themselves, played in the 'rebuilding' process.

Treating facially injured soldiers: 'Rebuilding men'

The invisible face

In hospital, soldiers discovered the damage done to their faces and they started to be re-acquainted with their bodies. As such the hospital was a place of life-changing revelation. Facially injured combatants were observed and bandaged by others, their faces the object of all attention and care. But they themselves could often not see their faces for weeks, even months. The absence of mirrors, and sometimes even total ban upon them, postponed the confrontation between the disfigured man and his reflection.[3] The aim was to protect the patient from unnecessary distress whilst the reconstruction process was still incomplete. The mirror was the key to retrieving one's image and could become an obsession for patients, who sometimes regarded the unknown as harder to cope with than reality.[4]

2 *Rebuilding Men* is the title of surgeon Fred Albee's memoirs.

3 A novel by Dumas thematizes this traumatic confrontation (Pierre Dumas, *L'Homme qui Mourut Deux Fois* (Paris: Editions Delmas, 1943), which is also mentioned in the memoirs of nurses Rémi (*Hommes Sans Visage*) and Catherine Black (*King's Nurse – Beggar's Nurse: An Autobiography* (London: Hurst & Blackett, 1939)).

4 Nurses' accounts (such as Rémi's and Black's) mention how patients sought to introduce mirrors into the wards. This essential search for one's reflection is also visible in Dupeyron, *La Chambre des Officiers*.

Paradoxically, whilst the patient himself was left in a state of uncertainty and expectation concerning his appearance, the evolution of his treatment was recorded in minute details, especially through photographs and sketches. This abundance of documentation, both clinical and artistic, was made available for other specialists in published papers and in the museums sometimes attached to the hospitals. It would be a powerful visual reminder of the long way the injured had come and provide evidence of the war's 'ravages', of which patients were not always aware.[5] *Gueules cassées* first and foremost saw themselves through the eyes of their fellow patients and of the medical staff. This observation inspired twenty-first-century psychiatrists to mediate the initial mirror 'trial' by standing in front of their patient, looking at them, whilst the mirror is gradually brought into the patient's visual field sideways. This way, the practitioner's gaze is mediating the encounter, providing a safe and accepting presence.[6]

If documentation describing the damaged face and its reconstruction abounds, the soldier's initial confrontation with his reflection and the emotions it triggered have rarely been recorded. Whilst literary narratives hardly ever fail to describe this encounter, usually in a spectacular fashion, historical documents are generally silent on what is, after all, a very private topic. Indeed, the reaction could be brutal. In one of the few first-hand testimonies available, British soldier Percy Clare recalls that when he first saw his face, he 'received rather a shock' whilst French soldier Pierre-Marie Braillon, upon seeing his face for the first time, exclaimed: 'Alas! I was speechless ... Half of my face was destroyed ...'[7] Likewise, a corporal treated at Aldershot asked the nurse to put screens around his bed after he saw

5 'War ravages' is the title of a series of photographs taken by the British official photographer Horace Nicholls. Horace Nicholls, *Repairing War's Ravages: Renovating Facial Injuries*, London Imperial War Museum, Q30450, Q30452, Q 30455, Q30456, Q30457, Q30460.

6 Colas, *Le Visage des Hommes*, p. 186.

7 Clare, Private papers; 'Hélas! les bras m'en sont tombés ... moitié de la face détruite ...', Pierre-Marie Braillon, *Mémoires de Guerre d'un Poilu 14–18: Gueule Cassée le 11 Octobre 1918* (Lyon: Bellier, 2006), p. 105.

his face in a shaving-glass he had managed to get hold of.[8] This desire for isolation testifies to the officer's wish to protect himself from the view of others and to spare others the sight of his face. Realizing the nature and extent of their injuries led patients to experience what Biernoff describes as self-alienation: the subject is unable to recognize himself in the mirror. The reflected image is that of another being, human in the best of cases, monstrous in others.[9]

Once the man had seen his reflection, he entered a process of getting re-acquainted with his features, with the operations gradually changing his physical appearance. The fact that old photos of the soldiers, taken before their injury, were used in facial reconstruction, further complicated matters. In turn, the creative dimension of plastic surgery added to potential confusion, the patient sometimes being asked to choose his new features. Joseph Pickard, wounded on 31 March 1918 and treated at Sidcup hospital for two years, reports that he was asked what nose he wanted.[10] He replied: 'I don't care, as long as I get one!' These kinds of choices are nevertheless described by Rémi as an attempt to empower men by giving them some control over what their new faces would look like.[11]

The confrontation with the wounded face was thus inscribed in a wider experience of physical and psychological reconstruction. The hospital was the theatre of this process and the medical staff its first audience as well as its architects. Delaporte describes it as a 're-birth' for the wounded soldier: his face was remade and he learnt to cope with the consequences, on a psychological and practical level (eating and speaking, for instance). This view can be questioned, not least because of the implicitly positive implications of the term 're-birth', when in fact the outcome was sometimes tragic: haemorrhages and gangrenes were not uncommon, and there were cases of suicide.[12] This nevertheless highlights the radical, life-transforming

8 Catherine Black, *King's Nurse – Beggar's Nurse*, p. 88.

9 Biernoff, 'Flesh Poems', p. 39.

10 London, Imperial War Museum, Interview with Joseph Pickard (1986), Reel 18. Reference 8946.

11 Rémi, *Hommes Sans Visage*, pp. 54–57.

12 Ibid, p. 87.

dimension of facial injuries alongside the hope brought about by plastic reconstruction.

A holistic endeavour

Maxillofacial surgery had implications that went beyond physical restoration. Medical practitioners soon realized the need for a holistic approach to the treatment of facially injured combatants. Such an endeavour called for different skills and the intervention of several agents over a long period of time: surgeons, dentists and artists were the main actors in this process. In all three countries, their main goal, as indicated by military authorities, was to return men to active service. In order to do so, the restoration of function (for example, masticating and breathing) was emphasized. Gillies nevertheless complained that 'as soon as the healing had occurred the soldier was sent back to his battalion or battery, often looking like a travesty of his former self'.[13] The example of Percy Clare, who suffered wounds to his jaw and cheek, is telling. After a few weeks in hospital, he was sent back to duty despite the fact that he could hardly open his mouth. Too weak, he soon reported ill and was admitted into hospital again. A few months later he was back in Dover and he went through the same training designed to 'harden' returning soldiers. He was still too weak but the officers refused to let him report sick, and it was only because he could not open his mouth wide enough to wear a gas mask that he was allowed back into hospital.[14] Likewise in Germany, army surgeons were under orders to quickly send facial cases back into service: 'Appearance was of secondary importance'.[15] The emphasis put upon the number of soldiers sent back to the front by French surgeon Sébileau makes clear the pressure put upon French doctors to achieve this quick turnover, too.[16]

13 Pound, *Gillies*, p. 26

14 Clare, Private papers.

15 Pound, *Gillies*, p. 28. Based on surgeon August Lindemann's assessment.

16 Paris, Archives du Service de Santé aux Armées du Val-de-Grâce, *Hôpital temporaire du Collège Chaptal, 73, rue de Rome, Paris. Rapport du Centre de Chirurgie*

Whilst military authorities were more interested in the number of men who returned to the front, surgeons refused to give up on the aesthetic dimension of plastic surgery. Their main argument for this was the lasting psychological and social impact of disfigurement. Reflecting on his work during the First World War, surgeon Fred Albee notes that

> The psychological effect on a man who must go through life, an object of horror to himself as well as to others, is beyond description [...] It is a fairly common experience for the maladjusted person to feel like a stranger to his world. It must be unmitigated hell to feel like a stranger to yourself.[17]

This early analysis has been echoed in more recent works. In his study of facial injuries, Jacob Longacre underlines the risk of 'irreversible psychic trauma' due to the distinctive visual quality of wounds to the face: 'a facial deformity is not a secret. It is visible to everyone'.[18] This visibility leads Longacre to recommend early plastic reconstruction as a way to improve the condition of these patients, showing that First World War surgeons set out principles and practices still in use decades later.

The task awaiting maxillofacial surgeons was significant: pioneers of a new speciality, sometimes in opposition to the military authorities, they held their patients' physical and psychological condition in their hands. The German writer Joseph Roth resorts to the religious term of 'Erlösung' [salvation] to describe the work carried out at the Berlin Charité Hospital, whose maxillofacial section closed down in January 1922.[19] This section

---

Maxillo-Faciale. Mois de janvier 1917. Du Dr Sébileau à M. le Médecin-Inspecteur, Directeur du Service de Santé du G.M.P, Box 120. This pressure from military authorities to return soldiers, even those in a bad state, to active service is satirized in George Grosz's caricature *Die Gesundbeter* (1916–17), in which a skeleton is declared 'k.v.' [fit for duty].

17 Albee, *A Surgeon's Fight to Rebuild Men*, p. 110.

18 Jacob Longacre, *Rehabilitation of the Facially Disfigured: Prevention of Irreversible Psychic Trauma by Early Reconstruction* (Springfield: Thomas, 1973), p. ix.

19 Joseph Roth, 'Der Wiederaufbau des Menschen: Gesichtsplastik in der Charité – Kriegs- und Zivilkranke – Die Tragik der Nasen', *Neue Berliner Zeitung*, 6 June 1921, published in *Joseph Roth Werke, Das Journalistische Werk: 1915–1923*, ed. by Klaus Westermann (Köln: Kiepenheuer & Witsch, 1989), pp. 580–83 (p. 580).

was led by the specialist ear- and nose-surgeon Jacques Joseph, or 'Nasen-Joseph', whose reputation as the lead German maxillofacial surgeon grew during the war. In his article, Roth implies that denying access to medical treatment equals condemning patients to cruelty and death. And indeed, the story of one of Joseph's patients, Karl Hasbach, suggests that only the work conducted at the Charité made his life worth living again. Wounded in 1915, Hasbach underwent nineteen unsuccessful operations in Bonn before he was advised to wear a nose made of glycerine. This period he describes as 'certainly the worst time in my life', and he subsequently suffered a nervous breakdown. He was referred to Joseph in Berlin, and in 1918, after ten more operations, he finally came out of hospital with a new nose.[20] A letter he later wrote to Joseph's biographer testifies to his admiration for the surgeon:

> I could speak at length about Doctor Joseph, to whom I am infinitely grateful. He used to operate in the Passow Nose and Ear Clinic of the *Charité*, with local anaesthetics only. [...] He had personally designed his operation table and many of his surgical instruments. [...] After each of my ten operations, he waited up to a month to assure the nervous recovery. During my first important operation, which lasted five hours, he had to repeatedly anaesthetise me and a nurse had to wipe the perspiration from his back again and again.[21]

Hasbach went on to see Joseph in his private clinic, for the surgeon continued to look after his patients after the war ended. Hasbach's feeling of indebtedness to the surgeon is not uncommon, as many wounded servicemen saw surgeons as saviour-figures.

On the shoulders of maxillofacial surgeons rested thus not only the patient's physical recovery, but also his mental and social welfare, present and future. Joseph was fully aware of this and he included a section on

20 Karl Hasbach's memoirs, quoted in Hilko Weerda and Wolfgang Pirsig, 'Jacques Joseph und der Patient Dr. Karl Hasbach', Jacques Joseph: 100 Jahre moderne Nasenchirurgie <http://jacquesjoseph.de/Hasbach.html> [accessed 8 December 2014].

21 Karl Hasbach, Letter to Paul Natvig (15 November 1973) in Paul Natvig, *Jacques Joseph: Surgical Sculptor* (Philadelphia: Saunders, 1982), pp. 44–46.

'the psychological aspects of facial plastic surgery' in his 1931 masterpiece *Nasenplastik und sonstige Gesichtsplastik*. He had already made this observation during his wartime practice, and in a 1917 annual report he rejoiced at the fact that 'The discharged patients have all been cured of their psychic depression which the consciousness of bodily deformity always involves'.[22] This was however not an easy task. The title of Albee's memoirs highlights the difficulty of this endeavour: the 'fight' was not only to repair faces but to 'rebuild men'. Likewise, Roth's presentation of the work conducted at the Charité as 'Der Wiederaufbau des Menschen' ['The rebuilding of men'] indicates that it is a case of holistically 'reconstructing' human beings.[23] The human factor, although it does not come across in the words 'rebuilding', 'Wiederaufbau' or even 'gueule', was a prominent concern amongst surgeons. Indeed, despite the pressure to treat cases as quickly as possible, they insisted on treating individuals: 'all [staff] were impressed by [Gillies's] staunch insistence that the patient mattered, that he was more than a numbered warrior, a name on a bloody label'.[24] Modern warfare emphasized the collective over the individual: individual identities were erased through the wearing of uniforms, the pre-eminence of military hierarchy, and the emphasis put upon numbers – the number of combatants, of casualties, of weapons. Fighting was often anonymous, as was death, and as was healing. Disfigured men constituted an extreme embodiment of this negation of the individual. Although facially wounded soldiers were 'guinea pigs' of a developing speciality, the emphasis put by the plastic surgeon on each man thus stands out. A holistic approach to facial surgery, including pain relief, functional and aesthetic concerns, thus developed during the First World War. Gillies, Morestin, Joseph and their peers were not only surgeons, but also psychologists and artists.

22 Jacques Joseph, *Annual Report* for the Section for Facial-plasty of the Royal Ear and Nose Clinic of the *Charité* (20 June 1916–30 June 1917), 1 July 1917, Archives of the Humboldt University, Berlin, *Charité-Direktion*, No. 890/1, reprinted in Natvig, *Jacques Joseph*, p. 179.

23 Roth, 'Der Wiederaufbau des Menschen', p. 580.

24 Pound, *Gillies*, p. 49.

Artistic and medical practices at the service of the wounded

Gillies's treatise on *The Principles and Art of Plastic Surgery* and Dufourmentel's *Essai sur l'art et la chirurgie* [Essay on Art and Surgery] bring the artistic dimension of this medical speciality to the fore.[25] Albee also notes that successful plastic surgeons 'must combine mechanical dexterity with artistic feeling for the desired cosmetic result' whilst Joseph states that 'For him who wishes to practise facial surgery, it is not enough to aseptically follow the basic rule of general surgery; he must also be something of an artist, more particularly a sculptor'.[26] The aesthetic result of surgery was not the only area that called for artistic skills: surgeons also had to show creativity in their preparations. Gillies, like Albéric Pont, used sketches of the procedures they attempted. These visual representations helped them prepare for the interventions and then contributed to the dissemination of the techniques.

This artistic dimension of plastic surgery is made evident through the collaboration of doctors and artists. The surgeon was surrounded by professional artists who not only recorded the progress accomplished, but also took an active part in the surgical reconstruction. Several artists worked at Sidcup: 'Art has also been called into service, and Professor Tonks, of the Slade School, a painter of high distinction, as well as a surgeon, and Mr Edwards, an eminent sculptor, will see to it that the new creations are of types that accord with the men's features'.[27] Gillies acknowledges the contribution of the sculptor in residence at Sidcup: 'Lieutenant J. Edwards

25 Harold Gillies and Ralph Millard, *The Principles and Art of Plastic Surgery* (Boston: Little, Brown and Co., 1957). Léon Dufourmentel, *Introduction à la chirurgie constructive: Essai sur l'art et la chirurgie* (Paris: La jeune parque, 1946).

26 Albee, *A Surgeon's Fight to Rebuild Men*, p. 109; Jacques Joseph, *Rhinoplasty and Facial Plastic Surgery with a Supplement on Mammoplasty and Other Operations In the Field of Plastic Surgery of the Body—An Atlas and Textbook*, trans. by Stanley Milstein (Phoenix: Columella Press, 1987; first published in German in 1931) p. 9.

27 'Faces Rebuilt: New Hospital to Transform Ugliness into Good Looks', *Daily Sketch*, July 1917. This article is part of a collection of press cuttings on The Queen's Hospital held at the London Metropolitan Archives (hereafter referred to as LMA), reference HO2/Y01/05. This particular article can be found on p. 14.

has not only been responsible for the preparation of routine plaster-cast records, but for a very important part of our work, the reconstruction of features on the casts as a preliminary to surgical reconstruction'.[28] A 1917 newspaper article underlines the powerful impact of Edwards's casts on the onlooker: '[Edwards's casts] give vivid if grim testimony to the wonderful results attained'.[29] The benefits of the use of plaster casts are demonstrated in a short film documenting the work of Pont in Lyon: several patients are filmed holding a cast of their face before reconstruction began. The contrast between the *moulages* of the wounded faces, still and white, and the frequently smiling restored faces, is striking.[30]

Albee gives more detail about the role played by the sculptor in the reconstruction of a man's features: 'The sculptor was of great assistance to the surgeon. By making a cast of the wounded man's face from a good photograph, taken before he was wounded, the surgeon was usually able to reconstruct the badly mutilated features in such a way that his relatives would recognise the patient'.[31] Likewise, Joseph had 'Wachsköpfe' (wax heads) made after each important operation. Most of them were destroyed in the years following the war but many casts and models made in France are still held at the Musée du Service de Santé des Armées au Val-de-Grâce and have been reunited with the photographs of the cases they documented during the war (Figures 1–3).

These artefacts testify to the skilfulness of both the sculptor and the surgeon. Unlike photographs, they are three-dimensional, coloured representations. In this respect, they make the faces seem strikingly real to the onlooker. Most visual representations discussed in Chapter 4 call for the onlooker to look at the faces; casts and masks almost invite one to touch the face. At the same time, they reduce the wounded soldier to his face,

28 Gillies, *Plastic Surgery of the Face*, p. xi.

29 'The Marvels of Plastic Surgery: A New Institution For the Treatment of Wounded Heroes', January 1917, p. 3 [publication title unknown].

30 Paris, Etablissement de Communication et de Production Audiovisuelle de la Défense ECPAD, 'Service de Prothèse maxillo-faciale du Docteur Pont à Lyon', 14,18 A 910. The excerpt in question can be found at 4'17"–5'40".

31 Albee, *A Surgeon's Fight to Rebuild Men*, p. 109.

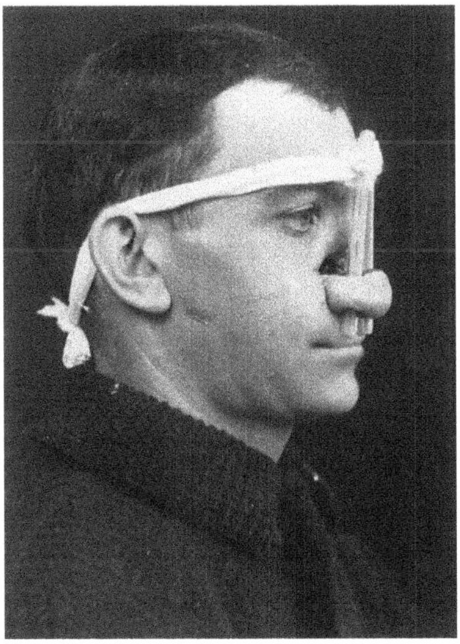

Figure 1: Patient Mascard during his treatment at the Val-de-Grâce hospital
© Musée du Service de Santé des Armées au Val-de-Grâce, Paris.

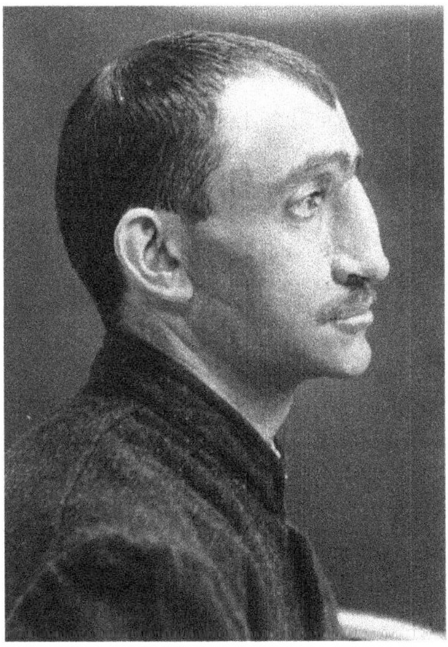

Figure 2: Patient Mascard at the end of his treatment
© Musée du Service de Santé des Armées au Val-de-Grâce, Paris.

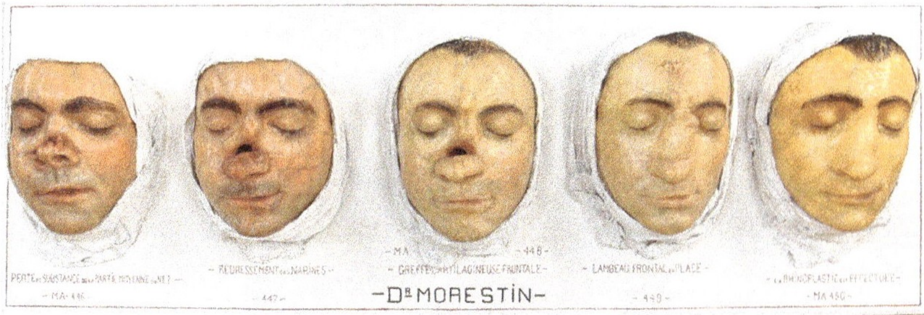

Figure 3: Series of wax models of Mascard
© Musée du Service de Santé des Armées au Val-de-Grâce, Paris.

whereas photographs usually feature hair and show the top of the chest, including clothes. Moreover, for practical reasons, *moulages* show patients with their eyes closed, thus making them appear dead. The contrast between the realistic dimension of wax (and plaster) casts and the impression of death they convey is striking. Whilst they appeal to the viewer's tactile sense, they also deny visual contact and are reminiscent of the ancient tradition of creating death masks. The disfigured man, or at least his face, becomes objectified.

Another aspect of the artists' work involved helping men whose looks had not been sufficiently improved by surgery, or who refused to undergo further treatment. A tension between surgeons and mask-makers sometimes arose. Pickerill, in charge of the New Zealand section at The Queen's Hospital, dismisses masks as a second-class solution:

> [Masks] proved to be not satisfactory from several points of view: The patients were never very happy wearing what they termed 'tin faces'. The edges of the masks were always difficult to approximate both in position and colour to the normal and mobile parts of the face on which they rested, and were, moreover, apt to become shiny. The paint on the masks, too – in towns, at least – became progressively darkened, necessitating repainting, which could only be done by a skilled artist. Patients who have been thus treated have come subsequently to have their facial losses and disfigurement remedied surgically.[32]

32 Pickerill, *Facial Surgery*, p. viii.

The surgeon recommends masks as a temporary solution only, thereby overlooking the fact that surgery could not guarantee total reconstruction in all cases. The use of masks is also documented in Germany and the help of artists in making them is mentioned by Holger Herwig and by Joseph, who deemed prostheses 'a more or less valuable makeshift measure which, at best, cannot remove the patient's feeling of being mutilated and outcast'.[33]

Most of the time, however, the work of the sculptor and the surgeon was not a competition but a collaboration, the former taking over once the latter had finished. The sculptress Kathleen Scott – wife of the Antartic explorer Robert Falcon Scott – joined Gillies's team at Sidcup, whilst Francis Derwent Wood put his art to the service of disfigured men at the 3rd London General Hospital. There, he set up the Masks for Facial Disfigurement Department, which became known as the 'Tin Noses Shop'.[34] Wood insisted that he did not seek to relieve pain or restore function and stated that he was concerned only with those cases 'in which the wounds or depredations of disease have been so severe as to remove them beyond the range of even the most advanced plastic surgical operations'.[35] In clearly distinguishing his goals from the therapeutic aims of surgery, Wood opens the door to a collaborative practice between the artist and the surgeon.

A detailed description of the work carried out by Wood is provided by Corporal Ward Muir, who followed the sculptor's progress from the time when, in 1915, they were washing dishes together. Wood is described as the 'presiding genius' in his studio, magically awakening lifeless casts in an attempt at making a mask that represents 'the man not as he is but as he was'.[36] Indeed, the masks were meant to be as close in resemblance as possible to the patient's old face: they enabled the 'passing' from 'gargoyles' to

33 Holger Herwig, *The First World War: Germany and Austria-Hungary, 1914–1918* (London: Arnold, 1997), p. 297; Joseph, *Rhinoplasty and Facial Plastic Surgery*, p. 77.

34 Ward Muir, *The Happy Hospital* (London: Simpkin, Marshall, Hamilton, Kent & Co, 1918), p. 146.

35 Francis D. Wood, 'Masks for Facial Wounds', *The Lancet*, 23 June 1917, p. 949.

36 Muir, *The Happy Hospital*, pp. 150–51.

a state of 'naturalness', a movement back in time.[37] According to Muir the only differences noticeable for a patient's friends from a short distance are the glasses and an occasional squinting.[38] Functional impediments related to masks, underlined by surgeons and acknowledged by Wood himself, are overlooked. Muir even notes an improvement in functionality brought about by the mask, which can hide a pad absorbing saliva or tears.[39] In emphasizing the aesthetic effects, he goes as far as suggesting that some patients ended up with improved looks: one 'would not be offended if told that he is now a handsomer man than he was when he joined the Army', and the eyes of another 'have become [...] straighter and more tranquil'.[40]

Muir's analysis ignores the potential pain and embarrassment men felt under their masks. Juliet Nicolson underlines that 'For most of the wearers, masks were horribly uncomfortable as the tin rubbed against the ravaged face beneath producing a nearly intolerable sensation'.[41] In her book she opposes masks, presented as visual embodiments of denial, to surgical reconstruction, described as evidence of acceptance. The issues she identifies had been noted by Joseph, who pointed out that masks had to be often repainted and French surgeon Maurice Virenque, who observed that he 'never met a man who wore a permanent facial prosthesis'.[42] Instead, the French veterans looked after by Virenque preferred to wear a piece of cloth across the wounded part of their face; this signalled the presence of the wound or scar without pretending to re-create the original features. Masking the physical marks left by war did of course not make up for the functional impediments, nor erase the trauma and disfigurement. However,

37 Ibid, p. 149.

38 Ibid, p. 152.

39 Ibid, p. 153.

40 Ibid, pp. 153–54. Rémi also reports a wounded man assuring his friend that his new nose – which is not the nose he wanted – makes him look better than he used to (*Hommes Sans Visage*, p. 57).

41 Nicolson, *The Great Silence*, pp. 66–67.

42 Maurice Virenque, quoted in Sophie Delaporte, 'Gueules Cassées de la Grande Guerre' in François Delaporte, Emmanuel Fournier and Bernard Devauchelle, eds, *La Fabrique du Visage: De la Physiognomonie Antique à la Première Greffe du Visage* (Turnhout: Brepols, 2010), p. 301.

Muir insists on the positive effects on the onlooker who, thanks to the mask, is able to look at the disfigured man without embarrassment. These devices not only protect the wearer, they also shelter the viewer from a disturbing confrontation.

Unlike 'scientific' accounts by surgeons or sculptors, which provide a factual assessment of both the damage done to the face and the result of their work, Muir's description is full of emotion. The ward orderly has a personal connection with Wood and with the other patients whom he cared for during the war. This personal link accounts for his focus on the psychological and social consequences of wearing a mask: 'Instead of being a gargoyle, ashamed to show himself on the streets, he is almost a normal human being and can go anywhere unafraid – unafraid (a happy release!) of seeing others afraid. Self-respect returns to him. His depression departs'.[43]

According to Muir, the main emotion associated with facial disfigurement is shame. Wood himself acknowledges this psychological impact: 'The patient acquires his old self-respect, self-assurance, self-reliance, and, discarding his induced despondency, takes once more to a pride in his personal appearance. His presence is no longer a source of melancholy to himself nor of sadness to his relatives and friends'.[44] The question of 'normality' is a recurring motif, not only in terms of wounded men's appearance, but also their behaviour: 'normal' looks condition 'normal' interaction with others. The benchmark against which conformity to 'normality' is assessed is not clearly specified.

Covering the damaged face would also permit an easier return to employment, yet another 'sign' of conformity to the norm. Thanks to masks, disfigured men were better able to return to their occupations and to be self-sufficient; at least, this is what the Commanding Officer hoped:

> The soldier is by nature independent, and the men who had the pluck to throw up their jobs and go to the help of the country are not the men who will wish to exist on pensions granted by the Government; they will prefer to resume their former

43 Muir, *The Happy Hospital*, p. 152.

44 Wood, 'Masks for Facial Wounds', p. 949.

> tasks when possible. The formation of this new department will, I am sure, make this possible for many.[45]

Restoring the disfigured soldier's appearance is described as key to a successful professional reintegration and to the regaining of his self-esteem.

Muir's description suggests that disfigurement is an outward sign of mental problems, the broken faces being depicted in an evocative fashion as 'macabre and sometimes brutish physiognomies metamorphosed into sane and reasonable ones', 'the "wrongness"' being 'exorcised' by the wearing of masks. These religious undertones emphasize the parallel between the sculptor and a god, fully assumed by Kathleen Scott. Thinking about the chin she was to make for a man, she comments: 'I feel terribly like God. The surgeon said without a smile, "Don't make it longer than you need or we shan't have enough flesh to cover it." God! It's a fantastic world'.[46] In a similar fashion, the result of the sculptor's work is confirmed by Muir as a blessing.

The chapter on 'Masks and Faces' – the last one in Muir's book – ends with a focus on the individual sculptor, the author allowing him a category of his own, apart from medical practitioners. The artist is depicted as a solitary figure: his area of expertise is outside the scientists' reach but he too appears as a powerful agent whose skills can make up for the destructiveness of the war. Muir's positive assessment contrasts with that of the surgeons; Gillies, for instance, writes that 'one can appreciate a sweetheart's repugnance at being expected to kiss shapely but unresponsive lips composed of enamelled phosphor-bronze'.[47] This lack of expressivity points to the theatrical dimension of masks, which is underlined by Roth in an article subtitled 'Tragik der Nasen' [Tragedy of Noses].[48] It is also particularly visible in photographs of Wood's 'Tin Noses Shop' and Ladd's 'Studio for

45 'Sculptor and Surgeon. How they Collaborate at the 3rd L.G.H. A Note by the C.O.', *The Gazette of the 3rd London General Hospital. Wandsworth*, May 1916, pp. 205–6.

46 Kathleen Scott, quoted in Louisa Young, *A Great Task of Happiness: The Life of Kathleen Scott* (London: Macmillan, 1995), p. 189.

47 Pound, *Gillies*, p. 50.

48 Roth, 'Der Wiederaufbau des Menschen', p. 580.

Portrait Masks'. Masks are to some extent theatrical props, and they were even at times used as such by injured men.[49] The alignment of before/after plaster casts in Anna Coleman Ladd's Studio evokes a kind of mass production of faces, and beyond this, of selves. Moreover, they remind the viewer of the false faces visible at a carnival. Referring to performing arts, as well as to religion, can be seen as a way of making sense of the presence of facially disfigured men, enclosing them within the sphere of the grotesque or the metaphysical.

Ladd was inspired by Wood to open her American Red Cross Studio for Portrait Masks in the Latin Quarter of Paris. She went on, according to a Red Cross report, to surpass Wood in skill.[50] Marie-Louise Brent and later Jane Poupelet, two French artists, joined the team, as well as Robert Wlérick who had already been using his sculpting skills in the service of maxillofacial surgery. The unit was incorporated into the Val-de-Grâce military hospital in 1919.[51]

Although sculptors had the skills to recreate the features of mutilated faces, the sight of disfigured men was a shock, even to them. A letter written by Brent to Poupelet testifies to her difficulties: 'this afternoon we had one who is so horrible to look at, it almost makes me sick. It is not a human face but some kind of gargoyle! Thankfully he is blind and does not suspect how terrible he looks'.[52] The adjectives 'horrible' and 'terrible' and the comparison with a gargoyle echo Muir's writings; they emphasize the inhuman dimension of facial injuries. The 'gargoyle' motif even suggests that the disfigured face itself is a sculpture, carved by war on men's

49 Pound, *Gillies*, p. 50.

50 American Red Cross archives, Washington D.C., 'The Making of Portrait Masks by Mrs Ladd', *The First Year of the American Red Cross in France: Activities for the year ended July 1, 1918*, pp. 32–33.

51 Elisabeth Lebovici, 'L'art répare les gueules cassées', *Libération*, 11 November 2005 <http://www.liberation.fr/culture/0101548040-l-art-repare-les-gueules-cassees> [accessed 18 August 2015].

52 Marie-Louise Brent, Letter to Jane Poupelet, 11 September [1918?], in *Jane Poupelet, 1874–1932: 'La beauté dans la simplicité'*, ed. by Anne Rivière (Paris: Gallimard, 2005), pp. 48–49.

bodies. This comparison also testifies to the attempt to find images to which one can relate.

Perhaps to combat this de-humanization, Ladd and her team made the Studio into a homely, warm environment. Photographs and a short film reveal that the place was nicely decorated, including flowers. The *Red Cross Magazine* underlines the pleasant settings: the sculptors welcomed the men in a 'bright studio', surrounded by an 'attractive courtyard overgrown with ivy and peopled with statues' and the workshop itself is 'a sunny room' to which 'patients have grown attached'.[53] The re-humanizing aspect of the sculptors' work is stressed in newspaper articles published during and after the war. In particular, Poupelet's work is praised in French publications: 'Miss Poupelet sacrificed her future for the benefit of humanity. She put her talent to the service of the facially disfigured, creating models, taking no rest from making casts that would help re-sculpt human faces for the miserable heroes disfigured by the stupid bullets.'[54] Here the spirit of self-sacrifice with which soldiers are generally credited transfers to the artist. This article also insists upon the heroism of mutilated veterans, although the adjective 'miserable' shows the author's pity. The sculptor's work was on occasion even put on a par with that of the medical technicians: 'The hands that moulded beauteous forms were softening paraffin, becoming the pious hands of the nurse at the same time as those of a brilliant artist'.[55]

53 Grace S. Harper, 'New Faces for Mutilated Soldiers', *American Red Cross Magazine*, November 1918, p. 44. Film: Red Cross film documenting the work of Anna Coleman Ladd at the American Red Cross 'Studio for Portrait Masks', *Red Cross Work on Mutilés at Paris, 1918*, National Museum of Health and Medicine, Armed Forces Institute of Pathology, United States of America <http://archive.org/details/RedCrossMutiles> [accessed 18 August 2015].

54 'Mademoiselle Poupelet a sacrifié son avenir à l'humanité. Pour les mutilés de la face, elle a obscurément donné son talent, créant des modèles, se fatigant à faire des moulages pour resculpter des visages humains aux misérables héros défigurés par la mitraille imbécile', André Salmon, *La Jeune Sculpture Française*, 1919, p. 74, quoted in Rivière, *Jane Poupelet*, p. 49.

55 'les mains dispensatrices de belles formes devinrent-elles des mains pieuses d'infirmière sans cesser d'être celles d'une grande artiste', Anon., *Le Petit Parisien*, 6 August 1928, p. 3, quoted in Rivière, *Jane Poupelet*, p. 49.

The masks have largely been lost and Ladd and her colleagues forgotten. In contrast, the legacy of surgeons such as Morestin, Joseph and Gillies, appears more lasting. Masks, through their association with the restoration of a previous, better state, can be seen as symbolizing a longing for a lost pre-war history. They illustrate what Nicolson describes as a form of denial.[56] Her assessment largely corresponds with the point of view of surgeons. In the light of the testimonies discussed here, it nevertheless appears that in many cases masks and attachments complemented the surgical reconstruction, even if only temporarily. As will be discussed later in this chapter, the surgeon and the artist both come across here as heroic figures; however, it is the voice of the former that has prevailed throughout the twentieth century. In turn, the facially disfigured man remains in the background, the raw material or object upon which talented professionals display their skills.

A re-creation of the family sphere

Reconstructed or masked faces thus protected the veteran, at the same time as they preserved others from a disturbing sight. To borrow Gilman's terminology, plastic reconstruction, attachments and masks favoured the 'passing' of disfigured men into society, transforming 'gargoyles' into humans. In this respect, they were part of a psychological healing process, which also relied on the soldier's relationships with fellow patients and medical staff. Delaporte notes the significant role played by the latter in the combatants' acceptance of their disfigurement and reintegration into society. Doctors and nurses were the first people with whom wounded men were in contact, making their reaction particularly important. In wards where mirrors were banned, the looks of fellow patients and the reactions of medical staff gave wounded soldiers an indication as to the damage done to their own face.

56 Nicolson, *The Great Silence*, pp. 54–68.

Moreover, the duration of the treatment meant that the contact between medical staff and patients was prolonged, making their relationship all the more significant. Studying the wounded man's interaction with others in the context of the hospital illuminates our understanding of the *gueule cassée*'s later reintegration into professional and social networks. Delaporte's model of familial relationships will be explored here with an international perspective. The implications of the familiarity implied by this parallel will be questioned and alternative approaches investigated.

Nurses and female staff: Lovers and mothers

Nurses and voluntary aids spent time with the servicemen, caring for their physical needs but also supporting them emotionally. Their written testimonies portray the men's difficulties in coping with the painful operations and the many questions and fears raised by disfigurement. Although medical staff were confronted with injuries on a daily basis, their attitude towards facially disfigured men emphasizes the distinctive quality of these wounds in the 'hierarchy' of war injuries.

Three testimonies by female staff will be examined here in order to assess the various roles played by them in the rehabilitation of facially injured combatants. One testimony is found in the memoirs of British nurse Catherine 'Blackie' Black, one is by the French Val-de-Grâce worker Hélène Baillaud and the third is by Henriette Rémi, a Swiss woman who worked in a German hospital.[57] Black worked with Gillies at Aldershot and later went on to care for King George V. Her memoirs were written several decades after the First World War but her time caring for facially wounded men appears to have made a strong impression upon her. Baillaud, like Muir, adopts a cheerful tone in her account, describing her work with facially injured soldiers as hard but enriching. She started working at the

57 Black, *King's Nurse – Beggar's Nurse*; Rémi, *Hommes Sans Visage*; Hélène Baillaud, Letter (14 pages), Paris, Archives du Service de Santé aux Armées du Val-de-Grâce (Box 148b).

Val-de-Grâce in 1914 without any qualifications or experience. Her short testimony mentions her work in different services but dwells upon her time at the specialized maxillofacial unit, under the headship of Morestin. Rémi's testimony is the longest and most comprehensive account. She focuses solely on her experience of caring for facially wounded soldiers in an unidentified hospital. Existing literature about facially injured soldiers treats this narrative as a text about a French hospital; however, Stéphane Garcia's recent findings reveal that the author was married to a German officer and lived in Germany for the duration of the war, and therefore could not have worked in a French hospital.[58] Rémi's decision to set her narrative (published in 1942) in France can be accounted for by her divorce and subsequent return to Switzerland in the 1920s, where she re-married. The tensions in Europe at the time of writing and her personal circumstances (she was involved in a pacifist movement and married to a pacifist militant who had served a prison sentence) further explain the deliberate vagueness of localization, and the pen name.[59]

The length of Rémi's narrative allows for a more detailed insight into her own emotions as well as the evolution of her relationships with her disfigured 'friends'. She describes her writing as a cathartic endeavour, also benefitting facially disfigured men whose imaginary voices plead, two decades after the events, for the world to see them and to understand: 'Give them our faces to see, that they may see us as we are, that they may hear the echo of our sufferings; since they have eyes to see may they watch and understand ... at last!'[60] Rémi's account thus gives a voice to *gueules cassées*.

58 Stéphane Garcia details his findings in his postface to the re-edition of *Hommes sans visage* (2014). Henriette Wille (La Chaux-de-Fonds, 1885 – Genève 1978) married Hans Danneil, from Hanover, in 1914. She moved to Germany and stayed with him during his time in a *Lazarett*, probably in Verden, where she lived between 1915 and 1920. Henriette moved back to Switzerland and divorced Danneil in 1928, before marrying a Swiss pacifist militant.

59 Rémi might also have hoped to find a more sympathetic audience by shifting events from Germany to France.

60 'Donne-leur nos visages en pâture, qu'ils nous voient tels que nous sommes, qu'ils aient un écho de nos souffrances; puisqu'ils ont des yeux pour voir, qu'ils regardent – et qu'ils comprennent ... enfin!', Rémi, *Hommes Sans Visage*, p. 8.

Their undetermined national origins add to the pacifist dimension of her endeavour, making them appear to be a universal indictment of war, in a way reminiscent of Ernst Friedrich's use of photographs of disfigured men in his antiwar pamphlet (1924).[61] The stories of facially injured men, like their photographs, appear to transcend national boundaries.

Baillaud, Black and Rémi's accounts underline how special the experience of caring for facially wounded soldiers is. Two key features highlighted by the authors are their attachment to patients and the difficulty of their task. Experienced nurse Black describes it as the most difficult period of her time in the military medical services:

> In all my nursing experience those months at Aldershot in the ward for facial wounds were, I think, the saddest. Sadder even than the casualty clearing stations to which I went afterwards, for there death was swifter and more merciful, and it is not so hard to see a man die as to break the news to him that he will be blind and dumb for the rest of his life. And that was something we had to do so often in that silent ward where only one in every ten patients could mumble a few words from the shattered jaws, for the facial wounds were in many respects the most serious of the War casualties.[62]

Black provides an emotional description of her own reaction, comparing it to her other war experiences. Death is perceived as more desirable than facial injuries. This account points towards the staff's identification with their suffering patients. The passage also stresses the tensions between silence and speech: the silence, understood here as the inability to communicate, surrounds injured men. The only sound is the voice of the nurse who has the responsibility to tell soldiers about the seriousness of their injuries. If death puts an end to any communication, facial injuries isolate their victims but leave them alive and conscious of their loss.

61 In *War against War!* (London: The Journeyman Press, 1987, first published in Germany in 1924), written in four different languages (German, English, French and Dutch), the Socialist militant Ernst Friedrich uses photographs to denounce the war and capitalism more generally. This pamphlet, which features a large section on facially injured soldiers, will be discussed in more detail in Chapter 4.

62 Black, *King's Nurse – Beggar's Nurse*, pp. 86–87.

Rémi's experience is similarly difficult, all the more so since she has no qualifications or training. She starts to help at the maxillofacial hospital in response to a call for help from her 'aunt Marie' (who might have been one of her husband's relatives), who works there. Rémi's 'initiation' is brutal: although she knows about the patients' disfigurement, facing them is a shock. She describes her first day as an experience of overcoming her own emotions. She has to deal with the sight of mutilated bodies, 'the most atrocious sight I have ever beheld!', as well as with the unpleasant smell of the ward.[63] Rémi's initial response is horror, her explanation of what she can see underlining the 'inhuman' nature of *gueules cassées*: 'about twenty monsters, men who have almost nothing human left, bodies featuring mutilated debris in lieu of faces'.[64] Disgust and pity overwhelm her at times and although they cannot see her, she struggles to look at them at first. The problem of visual contact is also mentioned by Muir in his account, in which he describes the onlooker's discomfort at the sight of wounded faces more than at the sight of any other mutilation.

Rémi is most preoccupied by a sense of guilt, as if the men were accusing her, holding her and the rest of society responsible for their plight: 'It was as if they were shouting "It is your fault if we are like this. No exception, no excuse. It is the weakness of every person that made this slaughter possible. You played a part too, you played a part too!"'[65] To Rémi, wounded soldiers are visual testimonies of the atrocities of war and the message they convey is one of generalized indictment of society for its participation in war, or its passivity in letting it happen. It again echoes Friedrich's antiwar pamphlet and is indicative of a use of facially injured soldiers in way of promotion of pacifist goals. In the context of the 1930s however, when Rémi was writing, this image of German veterans as antiwar symbols was no longer consistent with the growing militarism in the country. This

63 'ce que j'ai vu de plus atroce de ma vie!', Rémi, *Hommes Sans Visage*, pp. 36, 40.

64 'une vingtaine de monstres, d'hommes qui n'ont presque plus rien d'humain, de corps portant des débris mutilés de visages', Ibid, p. 36.

65 'Et il me semblait que tous me criaient: "C'est ta faute si nous sommes ainsi. Pas d'exception et pas d'excuse. C'est la faiblesse de chacun qui a permis cette boucherie. Tu as ta part, tu as ta part!"' Ibid, p. 45.

further accounts for Rémi's choice to situate her memoirs in an unidentified national context.

Caring for facially injured combatants marked staff, and Rémi and Baillaud stayed in contact with patients after the end of the conflict, Rémi still referring to hers as friends, two decades later. The physical and psychological trauma experienced by injured soldiers extended to the people who cared for them, Rémi mentioning the haunting memories that the writing of her memoirs triggered. Although they did not share a common experience of the front, they went through the long reconstruction process together. Bonds developed between female staff and patients throughout this time. Friendly, sometimes even flirtatious, relationships are mentioned by Clare, who reports that Voluntary Aid Detachment (VAD) nurses at Croydon hospital were 'quite willing to be taken out for an evening now and then: surreptitiously of course!'[66] Some nurses and female visitors even married former patients, despite efforts to prevent romances in the wards. Thus, Baillaud mentions that the French military medical authorities had a deliberate policy of choosing young women, aged between eighteen and twenty-five, to care for facially wounded men because those patients were the ones VADs were less likely to fall for.

Delaporte argues that a mother-son bond emerged, this female presence playing a significant part in the social rehabilitation of facially disfigured men.[67] Rémi's writings confirm this interpretation; from her first day, she emphasizes the importance of being useful to wounded men: 'you feel relied upon, wanted, needed and the maternal feeling that lies in every woman soon enabled you to find your true place.'[68] The parental role fulfilled by nurses and female volunteers, like Rémi, is claimed as their rightful position.

The maternal care provided by female staff is expressed in different ways. In addition to medical issues, practical help with everyday life was

66 Clare, Private papers.

67 Delaporte, *Les Gueules Cassées*, p. 148.

68 'on sent qu'ils comptent sur vous, qu'ils s'accrochent à vous, qu'ils ont besoin de vous et le sentiment maternel qui vit en toute femme vous fait bien vite trouver votre vraie place'. Rémi, *Hommes Sans Visage*, p. 38.

valued. Clare's account of the good treatment he received from nurses before he was evacuated to England emphasizes the attitude of the female staff, who are described as devoted, gentle and hard-working. Likewise, Baillaud and her colleagues cared for their patients' physical needs but they also comforted them when they woke up after an operation. Black underlines the challenges faced in everyday life:

> The problem of feeding was acute, for very few of the patients in that ward could take even a particle of anything solid, and yet their strength had to be kept up at all costs. So we had to ring the changes as best we could in two-hourly feeds … tomato soup made with milk, Benger's food, iced coffee, egg flip. Often we would use as many as three hundred eggs a day in that ward alone.[69]

In addition to providing for their practical needs, Rémi recalls reading, writing and posting letters for patients who could not do it themselves.[70]

Rémi and her colleagues also participated in the men's preparation for the future: for example, teaching them Braille (mentioned by Baillaud and Rémi) enabled the men to communicate and took them out of their isolation. Crafts exercised the patients' physical abilities and helped restore their self-esteem, whilst also keeping them busy. As Baillaud underlines, the functional consequences of injury forced the wounded to rely on other people. Like children, they had to learn basic skills; in this learning process, nurses played a significant role: 'We mainly taught them how to be self-sufficient, how to move around and to recognize us even before hearing our voices'.[71] Like parents, Baillaud and her co-workers tried to help the wounded regain some independence. This reflects a view of the injured soldier as a helpless figure needing not only to be physically re-humanized, but also to re-learn basic skills such as communication. The process of being fed and given liquid food, mentioned by Black, further emphasizes the infantilization experienced by facially wounded soldiers.

69 Black, *King's Nurse – Beggar's Nurse*, p. 87.

70 Rémi, *Hommes Sans Visage*, p. 71.

71 'Nous leur apprenions surtout à se suffire à eux-mêmes, à se diriger, à nous reconnaître sans que nous ayons à leur parler'. Baillaud, Letter, p. 9.

In addition to practical help, the emotional support provided by staff is another important aspect in the study of relationships between patients and their carers. Black highlights psychological issues that sometimes left medical staff powerless:

> Hardest of all was the task of trying to rekindle the desire to live in men condemned to lie week after week smothered in dressings and bandages, unable to talk, unable to taste, unable even to sleep without opiates because of the agony of lacerated nerves, and all that while knowing themselves to be appallingly disfigured.[72]

Black does not specify how she sought to alleviate her patients' depression; this passage nevertheless indicates her awareness of the psychological suffering men were going through. The stress is upon 'inability', both of the patients locked away in their damaged bodies, and of the staff powerless to help them.

The occasional silence between nurses and wounded men – the latter sometimes needed to come to terms with their disfigurement by themselves – did not prevent staff and patients from being close. Baillaud's fondness for her 'particularly endearing' patients shows through, echoing a poem by an anonymous Val-de-Grâce nurse.[73] In this piece, she expresses her admiration for her patients, described as valiant combatants; she also confesses her love, her thankfulness and her hope to be remembered by them.[74] The role of all women is, according to her, to be carers and confidantes of wounded soldiers. Another nurse, publishing in a later issue, writes that female staff had to keep their distance and harden themselves to be able to perform their duties. This indifference was only a façade: 'Our hearts are beating! If you could see it you would recognise the heart of a Frenchwoman, of a Mother'.[75]

72 Black, *King's Nurse – Beggar's Nurse*, p. 87.

73 'particulièrement attachants'. Baillaud, Letter, p. 7.

74 A. Nurse, 'Réponse aux Blessés de la Trogne', *La Greffe Générale*, 2 (15 January 1918), p. 3. Bibliothèque nationale de France, Paris, FRBNF32783911.

75 'Le Coeur bat! S'il pouvait se montrer à son aise, Vous reconnaîtriez celui d'une Française, celui d'une maman'. Philè, 'Aux Blessés de la Face', *La Greffe Générale*, 5 (10 March 1918), p. 3.

Female staff and volunteers shared the patients' joys and sorrows. Rémi was with Lazé, one of her patients, as he waited for his wife and son to visit, and he asked for her advice as to how to behave and whether he should kiss his son. It was also Rémi who accompanied him to his hometown to see his family later on. As they walked together from the station to his village, he opened up, sharing some of the difficulties of life at the hospital, in particular the smell in the wards and the necessity to abide by military rules.[76] Perhaps because they are outside the hospital, Lazé shares his pacifist belief and his conviction that men on both sides are being manipulated. More than the enemy soldiers, it is military authorities that Lazé holds responsible for the slaughter. This is the only passage in her book in which Rémi permits the pacifist views we know she held to be voiced – by one of the facially disfigured soldiers.

The dramatic reunion between Lazé and his son, the child failing to recognize his father and running away, terrified, underlines the perverse effect of the lengthy period of time spent by wounded soldiers, especially blind ones, in hospital. Surrounded by men like them, and by staff who have grown accustomed to their wounds, they evolve in a safe environment. This protected space is presented as necessary for their recovery but it also had adverse effects insofar as it did not prepare them for the confrontation with the world. In creating an artificial sense of 'normality', the hospital could in some cases delay moments of realization, making it all the more painful to accept reality. It was only when his son did not recognize him that Lazé understood that not only his body, but his whole life, had irremediably changed. Unable to face it, he committed suicide. Rémi's emotional reaction to this event testifies to her close relationship with her patients and her maternal feelings. The final scene of her book depicts her standing beside the surgeon, mourning together, a picture of parental grief at the loss of a son. Rémi and her colleagues thus also played the role of intermediaries. Firstly, between surgeons and patients, supporting them through their operations and sometimes transmitting messages between them: it is, for instance, Rémi who secures the major's permission for a patient's family

76 Rémi, *Hommes Sans Visage*, pp. 99–100.

to come and visit him, when the head surgeon had denied it to the man himself. Secondly, nurses and aids were mediators between the wounded men and their families. One of Rémi's colleagues, Sister Berthe, devised a procedure aimed to make the first encounter between a wounded soldier and his family less shocking: nurses made relatives walk through the main ward first, bringing them to see the most mutilated men, so that when they finally met their own relative, they were relieved. Not only did nurses comfort patients, but they also dealt with visiting relatives. Rémi recalls one of her patients asking her to stay with him as his father visits him for the first time, 'like a child wanting his mother to be there and calm down the angry father'.[77] Their medical background made them trustworthy interlocutors for patients and relatives. Rémi saw wives confide in her; they expressed their shock upon seeing their husbands for the first time, sometimes also their guilt at not being able to accept them. Her memoirs reveal the significant role played by nurses in the early encounters between men and their relatives, thus emphasizing the importance of the hospital as a space of transition.

The patients' attitude on Rémi's first day indicates that they, in turn, valued the presence of female helpers: they offered her sweets, were concerned that she would catch a cold and they wondered if she was ill when she did not eat. The men's affection for their nurses also appears in a (possibly fictional) letter from a Val-de-Grâce patient to his parents, published in *La Greffe Générale*, a newspaper written by disfigured soldiers to communicate with each other and with people outside the hospital. In his letter, the patient declares that he wants photographs of his nurses, so that he can one day show them to his children.[78] His affectionate description of his relationship with the nurses dwells on their gentle demeanour and gives a picture of a close community of patients and staff. He also expresses his initial surprise when a nurse gave him a pet name, as if he was her son.

77 'comme un enfant qui veut la présence de sa mère pour adoucir la colère du père'. Rémi, *Hommes Sans Visage*, p. 49.

78 'Lettre de Pitou à ces [*sic*] Chers Parents', Hôpital du Val-de-Grâce, 8 March 1918, copied by Francillon, *La Greffe Générale*, 5, pp. 19–20.

He later realizes that her maternal tone shows how much she cares about him. The nurses' affection created a form of 'sanctum', a safe environment in which patients were sheltered and accepted, at least for a time.

Further evidence of the patients' friendly feelings towards their nurses is found in Clare's letters, one of them describing in detail one particular Sidcup nurse: 'she is a "brick", and we all love her and vie with each other to do jobs for her, not to curry favour (which wouldn't be tolerated) but to please her'.[79] This reciprocal affection accounts for the cheerful atmosphere usually described as reigning at the hospital. Baillaud, like the British orderly Muir, emphasizes the joyful atmosphere and even the laughter which was not uncommon in the wards.[80] The nurses' mission was, she says, to fight physical pain and psychological gloominess. Contemporary accounts thus mention both moments of silence and of gaiety. Baillaud does not deny that some patients suffered from depression; however she dwells in more detail on cheerful anecdotes. The young women sought to prove to the men that their lives were not over, that there was hope for the future. In Baillaud's account, female staff members and visitors act as substitutes for mothers or lovers, re-affirming patients in their masculinity and helping them regain their independence and self-confidence. The closeness of these bonds means that some links were maintained after soldiers left hospital.

Rémi's focus on soldiers' moral qualities balances the negative description of their unsightly looks. Difficult patients are rarely mentioned. The tendency to highlight disfigured men's inner values is recurring, as if with the loss of a face there was nothing else left to praise. Besides, individual patients are often singled out, by contrast with other accounts by medical staff, especially those by doctors. To Rémi, they are not just numbers or monsters. Very little emphasis is put on them being in the army; her testimony suggests that the likelihood is that her friends will not return to active service; the focus is therefore upon their place in society, in their family in particular, not upon their military rank. To learn to identify the

79 London, Imperial War Museum, Percy Clare, Letter (manuscript), 8 January 1918. Reference 06/48/1.

80 Baillaud, Letter, p. 8.

men quickly, she uses their different and specific injuries to memorize their names. Men are thereby perhaps reduced to their wounds; yet on the other hand, Rémi's attempt also testifies to the medical staff's awareness that recognizing the men, calling them by their names, helped to affirm them as individual human beings.

Because hospital staff were the first interlocutors with the wounded soldiers after their injuries, their attitude mattered. Rémi soon realized that they observed her every reaction: 'I sense – and my feeling is later confirmed – that our 'boys' are very sensitive about the effect they have on other people and that we must avoid upsetting them or hurting them by showing disgust or simply pity'.[81] The key rule is, according to Rémi's more experienced aunt, to treat disfigured men like anybody else. Her constant battle against her emotions is described in terms of overcoming, much like the process of wounded men accepting and learning to live with their disfigurement. Furthermore, Rémi explicitly compares herself to a soldier: 'I am like a soldier who no longer lowers his head when he hears the bullets whistle'.[82] Coping with disfigurement is equated with a fight, for both the patient and the onlooker. It is a process of mutual growth, the war being prolonged or displaced from the battlefield to the medical sphere. Patients and carers are a class apart, combatting enemies such as pain and depression.

Male staff: A fraternal relationship

The symbolic function fulfilled by female staff differs from that ascribed to male helpers in contemporary accounts. The role the latter played was not one of parental authority or affection, but rather of brotherly

81 'Je pressens – et cela m'est confirmé par la suite – que nos "gars" sont très sensibles à l'effet qu'ils produisent, et qu'il faut avant tout éviter de les offenser ou de les faire souffrir, en laissant deviner du dégoût ou simplement de la compassion'. Rémi, *Hommes Sans Visage*, p. 42.

82 'je suis comme le soldat qui ne baisse plus la tête en entendant siffler les balles'. Ibid, p. 44.

fellowship, thus prolonging the comradeship often described as inherent to the experience of the front. The testimonies discussed here – one by a French and one by a British author – also make plain the tensions between the onlooker's identification with, and alienation from, disfigured veterans.

The French author Georges Duhamel enlisted in the army and worked in various capacities in the military medical force, including the role of stretcher-bearer. In *Civilisation*, he recalls scenes involving facially wounded soldiers.[83] Although the author expresses his own feeling of powerlessness when faced with the suffering and death of his comrades, these anecdotes end on a hopeful note. One of them reveals the strong impact he received from an encounter with a facially wounded combatant:

> From Louba we could not expect words: the bursting of a shell had blown away his face. Nothing remained of it but an immense, barbarous wound, one crooked, displaced eye, and the forehead, the humble forehead of a peasant. One day, however, while we were saying some friendly words to him, Louba wished to show us his pleasure, and he gave us a smile. They will always remember it, those who saw the soul of Louba smile without a face.[84]

This account shows that despite his looks, the soldier was not completely isolated from his comrades. Louba was left practically unable to communicate: his ability to speak, and seemingly his sight as well, were gone. Staff and fellow patients had become used to the state he was in and were not expecting any responses. They nevertheless continued to speak to him, their words making him smile. This very simple action is depicted as a miraculous

83 Georges Duhamel, *Civilisation: 1914–1917* (Columbia: University of South Carolina Press, 2009), first published in France (Paris: Mercure de France, 1918). This novel is based on Duhamel's own war experience and it was awarded the *Prix Goncourt* in 1918.

84 'De Louba, nous ne pouvions pas attendre des paroles: l'éclat d'obus lui avait effondré la face. Il ne restait rien de son visage qu'une immense plaie barbare, un œil dévoré, déjeté, et le front, un humble front de paysan. Un jour, pourtant, comme nous lui disions des choses fraternelles, Louba voulut nous témoigner son contentement, et il nous fit un sourire. Ils s'en souviendront, ceux qui ont vu l'âme de Louba sourire sans son visage', Duhamel, *Civilisation*, p. 37.

achievement. It is also notable that Duhamel does not distinguish between himself and other staff and patients; they are all presented as a community, his testimony emphasizing camaraderie and solidarity.

Muir's writings are more detailed and give us an insight into the daily routine of a hospital ward. A trained journalist, he is also the author of several novels and editor of *Happy – Though Wounded*, a hospital publication. Excerpts of his 1918 *The Happy Hospital* were released in newspapers and magazines before appearing in book form.[85] He points out in several places the distinctive features of the 3rd London General Hospital, emphasizing, for instance, the quality of the food served and the joyful atmosphere. Whilst pain and death were part of the daily life, they are hardly mentioned in Muir's book; by overlooking the suffering and focussing upon positive aspects, he underlines the soldiers' resilience but also presents such qualities as necessary to survive, to remain sane. Muir's frequently humorous depictions of hospital patients and staff again insist upon the comradeship amongst men.

Of the fourteen chapters in this book, only two deal with the aspects of Muir's work that he found more difficult: one is a short and rather general reflection entitled 'A Note on "Horrors"', and the other deals with the author's confrontation with facially injured soldiers. 'Masks and Faces', which presents sculptor Wood's workshop, is the very last chapter. The final position of this section, as well as its content, makes it seem more definitive and climactic than otherwise, thereby increasing the impact it has upon the reader. Muir found caring for disfigured combatants a distressing experience:

> An English war-hospital, on the whole, furnishes forth fewer horrible sights than happy ones. But there is one perturbing experience which, for the worker in such an institution, is inevitable. It is this. He finds that he must fraternise with fellow-men at whom he cannot look without the grievous risk of betraying, by his expression, how awful is their appearance. Myself, I confess that this discovery came as a surprise. I had not known before how usual and necessary a thing it is, in human

85 *The Spectator*, *The Nineteenth Century*, *Country life*, *The Daily News*, *The New Statesman*. Note, Muir, *The Happy Hospital*, p. 8.

> intercourse, to gaze straight at anybody to whom one is speaking, and to gaze with no embarrassment.[86]

Although the author acknowledges that they are still human beings, his 'fellow-men', he finds himself unable to interact with them. He is concerned about his own reaction, a phenomenon still common today and that psychologists have identified as one of the causes of difficult interaction with people presenting visible facial differences.[87] Muir later identifies the 'embarrassment' betrayed by his attitude as a form of repulsion, although this only comes, according to him, once the wounds are healed. This is due to the fact that healed wounds suggest treatment to be over, and thus the looks can no longer be improved. Muir's fears focus upon the gaze; he is sure that his eyes, the 'lamp of the soul', will 'let the poor victim perceive what I perceived: namely, that he was hideous'.[88] Although pity is not openly referred to in this passage, it is implied in the descriptions of the 'wrecked face' of the 'poor victim'.

Muir's work makes clear the challenges caused by facial disfigurement in terms of communication with the mutilated men. If even medical staff were made uncomfortable by such a sight, much more would the rest of society. The author only briefly depicts what a mangled face looks like, and this description is almost comical. The 'mournful grotesquerie' of some faces, also compared here to 'broken gargoyles', proves to be 'something of an ordeal' for anyone who wants to talk to these men.[89] However, as with the rest of the book, the author moves on from the tragic facts to the more optimistic prospect of the sculptor restoring damaged faces. The title 'Masks and Faces' betrays this emphasis on solutions to help relieve patients and, beyond that, to normalize their relationships with society.

Clare's private papers provide another insight into relationships between wounded men and staff. The cheerful attitude of stretcher-bearers carrying men onto the ship which was to take them back to England

86 Muir, *The Happy Hospital*, p. 143.

87 Stock et al.,'Young People's Perceptions of Visible Difference', pp. 46–47.

88 Muir, *The Happy Hospital*, p. 143.

89 Ibid, p. 144.

made a lasting impression on him: 'they invariably went out of their way to say cheery and encouraging words to the wounded and showed that fellowship with suffering which only men in the fighting forces felt and understood'.[90] Most of the staff he was in contact with during his time in hospitals were female, which makes this anecdote particularly significant. It further evidences comradeship between men, whether patients or staff.

The family model illuminates important aspects of the interactions between patients and their female or male staff, interpreted respectively as maternal and fraternal bonds. The reassuring dimension of a family-like pattern provides a comforting presence to soldiers who are experiencing alienation from their own bodies and, on occasion, from their families too. In this respect, the hospital is both a re-creation of the past and a projection into the future: the wounded man finds himself in an environment bearing similarities to a home, whilst at the same time it conveys an implicit promise of reintegration into a family sphere after the conflict. However, the comparison between patient-staff relationships and family bonds can be misleading, insofar as the commonality of experiences shared by the different protagonists in the maxillofacial ward is not replicated outside the hospital, where the divide between combatants and non-combatants constitutes a significant obstacle to communication.[91] Reintegration into real-life families proved problematic in many cases. Furthermore, the implications for the patient in terms of self-image are far from negligible, especially since the family model suggests a degree of infantilization against which many men reacted.

90 Clare, Private papers.

91 This failure to relate to family is experienced by the main protagonist in Erich Maria Remarque's *All Quiet on the Western Front*, leaving the young man devastated (Erich Maria Remarque, *All Quiet on the Western Front* (trans. by Brian Murdoch (London: Vintage, 1996), first published under the title *Im Westen nichts neues* (Berlin: Ullstein, 1929), pp. 108–28). In contrast, the difference in terms of experiences between nurses, ward orderlies and patients is minimal.

The figure of the surgeon

The surgeon stands out in testimonies recording life in maxillofacial units. In narratives in which the collective prevails over the individual, he is one of the rare actors to be singled out, both by his fellow medical staff and by patients. Although his relationship to patients often resembles a paternal one, his role far exceeds it and accounts for the heroic, even mystical, aura with which he is often endowed.

A paternal figure

Biographies of the surgeons reveal little of their perceptions of and interactions with wounded soldiers. The great number of cases they treated accounts for the limited contact they had with facially injured men; however, some information can be found in the accounts of other medical staff. On some occasions they present the surgeon as a fatherly figure, in both the caring dimension and the disciplinary aspect traditionally associated with the father. In her memoirs, Black underlines Gillies's concern for patients:

> Then came the stream of wounded, men with half their faces literally blown to pieces, with the skin left hanging in shreds and the jawbones crushed to a pulp that felt like sand under your fingers. 'Don't worry, sonny, you'll be all right and have as good a face as most of us before we've finished with you,' Captain Gillies would say and the poor huddle of splints and bandages that had once been a handsome young guardsman would believe him and try to shake off his blank despair.[92]

Clare also reports that Gillies was willing to give his patients permission to stay out late to visit their families: 'Patients are required to be in at 5 o'clock but I understand that if one sees Major Gillies and gives his word

92 Pound, *Gillies*, p. 26.

of honour that he is going to his own home in London he (Major G.) will make an exception to the rule'.[93]

Gillies was ready to spend his own money to help his patients: 'Strength had to be built up in order to enable them to endure a long series of operations, sometimes twenty and more. For that purpose Gillies prescribed a supply of egg flip which he caused to be laced with brandy at his own expense'.[94] The collaboration of two patients in the preparation of his medical treatise suggests that he trusted them. In his preface, he acknowledges their help: 'The heavy secretarial work has been chiefly performed by the author's patients (for the most part E.J. Greenaway; partly also R.W.D. Seymour), who have stuck to their task with persistent, cheerful loyalty, in the intervals between their operations'.[95]

The surgeon did not only resort to patients for administrative tasks, he also trusted them to assist during operations. Clare reports helping in the operating theatre:

> For two hours yesterday I had to hang on to a man's tongue (by means of a catgut passed through it) to prevent him rolling it into his throat and choking. [...] I had to keep swabbing blood and clots away with my left hand while gently resisting the pull of his tongue with my right. I 'played' him as an angler would a fish but had to be very gentle and not let the catgut tear the hole in his tongue larger.[96]

Gillies's concern with his patients' and ex-patients' welfare did not stop once their treatment was complete. Biddy Stevens remembers the warm welcome that the surgeon gave to her father when he visited him in the 1940s, over two decades after his stay at Sidcup. Harry Burbeck was wounded during the First World War and spent three years at Sidcup (1917–1920). When he became unwell in the 1940s, Gillies examined him and reassured him, expressing his satisfaction at Burbeck's successful professional and family

93 Clare, Letter, 8 January 1918.
94 Pound, *Gillies*, p. 34.
95 Gillies, *Plastic Surgery of the Face*, p. xi.
96 Clare, Letter, 8 January 1918.

life. Moreover, the surgeon personally employed some of his ex-patients during or after their treatment, and one of them married Gillies's sister.[97]

In France, the presence of a large number of patients at Morestin's funeral in 1919, some of them in tears, indicates their attachment.[98] The emotion of soldiers and staff goes beyond the respect paid to a skilled doctor and testify to the powerful role that surgeons played in the lives of their patients. The *Union des Blessés de la Face*, founded later, also acknowledged the work of Morestin, 'a benefactor of humanity', and supported a request by ex-patients that part of the street where the hospital was located be renamed in his honour.[99] In Germany Hasbach's letter, written decades after he met Joseph, mentions that he saw the surgeon at least once after being discharged from hospital, and that he admired him greatly.[100] The continuation of surgeons' support is all the more significant as the maxillofacial centres to which they were attached closed down after the war. Many of the men still needed treatment when the Paris and Berlin specialized units stopped receiving government funding. The privately-funded Queen's Hospital, in Sidcup, continued to welcome facially injured soldiers for the longest (until 1925). The closing down of these hospitals and the surgeons' shift to beauty surgery did not, however, completely sever the doctors' links with their military patients. The surgeons' concern for ex-patients is also manifest in Rémi's account. Indeed, although it underlines on several occasions the apparent coldness and distance of doctors, it ends with a depiction of the surgeon as a human and sympathetic figure, mourning with her over the death of a patient: 'The door opens. The chief medical officer comes in. He remains silent for a moment, next to the bed, then he

97 South African Sergeant Robert Bowen was left disfigured and blind following a gunshot wound. He was treated at Sidcup and received support from the blind soldiers' organization St Dunstan's. He went on to study law and married Miss Gillies in March 1919 (St Dunstan's members' file, London: Blind Veterans UK archives).

98 Baillaud, Letter, p. 93.

99 'ce Bienfaiteur de l'Humanité', *Bulletin de l'Union des Blessés de la Face*, 6 (February 1923), p. 1. *Bulletins de l'Union des Blessés de la Face* hereafter referred to as *Bulletins*.

100 Natvig, *Jacques Joseph*, pp. 44–46.

lays his hand on the forehead of the dead man, and two tears roll down his cheeks. He is a father, too.'[101]

Surgeons were also figures of authority. They implemented discipline. As a consequence, their relationship with patients could be tense. This is made obvious in one episode recounted by Rémi, in which a wounded man, Bertrand, complains about the major's refusal to let his wife and daughter visit him. He accuses the doctor of not understanding his plight and being unable to sympathize.[102] He dismisses the major's explanation that further surgery is needed and that he should not impose the unpleasant sight and smell of his wounds upon his family. The refusal appears to be justified by medical reasons; yet the wounded man's rhetoric and the impersonation he makes of the major add to the ridicule of the scene. The latter remains silent whereas the patient comes across as a stubborn child. Permission is finally given, following Rémi's intervention to support her patient's request. The familial model mother/father/child is therewith followed through.

Delaporte notes the often distant attitude of surgeons, and interprets it as an attempt to hide the disgust they felt towards disfigured patients.[103] The patients, according to Rémi, perceived the major as a harsh man; his lack of reaction when one patient comes back distressed from a disastrous reunion with his family confirms this.[104] But if the paternal comparison provides a good basis for understanding the relationships between surgeons and facially injured men, historical archives as well as literary and artistic documents also underline another dimension of the surgeon-patient dynamic. The familiarity implied in this model does not do justice to the out-of-the-ordinary qualities attributed by staff and patients to the surgeon. Whether these perceptions were deserved or idealized, they make the relationship between the doctor – often described as a solitary

101 'La porte s'ouvre. Le médecin-chef s'approche; il reste un instant silencieux à côté du lit. Puis, doucement, il pose sa main sur le front du cadavre, et deux larmes coulent de ses yeux. Il est père, lui aussi.' Rémi, *Hommes Sans Visage*, p. 110.

102 Ibid, p. 64.

103 Delaporte, *Les Gueules Cassées*, p. 140.

104 Rémi, *Hommes Sans Visage*, p. 105.

figure – and those around him worth studying from another angle: that of surgeons as heroes.

A heroic figure

The special status given to facial surgeons is evidenced by the comparatively numerous biographies devoted to them (as opposed to accounts of patients' lives).[105] Literary fiction emphasizes the heroic work of surgeons, who are described as god-like figures.[106] Rémi recalls the work of a surgeon who specialized in noses: 'he "re-humanised" monsters […]. In the hospital, this man is considered to be a god'.[107]

Similarly, in a 1917 article in *Le Figaro*, Morestin is described as a miracle-maker.[108] This parallel between surgeons and gods is a recurring motif in all three countries. A 1917 British article, having described the consequences of facial injuries as 'hell', goes on to describe the surgeon as doing a 'Christ-like work'.[109] References to miracles and to doctors as 'wizards of surgery' can also be found, underlining their seemingly magical quality.[110] Facially injured patients were remote from normality because of their 'inhuman' appearance; equally, surgeons were often pictured as exceptional. To cope with 'monsters', 'gods' were needed.

The title of Albee's autobiography suggests that doctors were 'fighting', something that can be seen not only in terms of their attempts to defeat

105 See, for instance, Monestier; Natvig, *Jacques Joseph*; Pound, *Gillies*; and Riaud, *Première Guerre Mondiale et Stomatologie*.

106 See, for instance, Dumas, *L'Homme qui Mourut Deux Fois*, p. 49, and Roth, 'Der Wiederaufbau des Menschen', p. 581.

107 'il a "réhumanisé" des monstres […] à l'hôpital, cet homme est considéré comme un dieu', Rémi, *Hommes Sans Visage*, p. 54.

108 Louis Latzarus, 'Ils veulent rire', *Le Figaro*, 23 September 1917 [page number unknown].

109 *Kent Messenger*, July 1917, [Article title unknown], LMA HO2/Y01/05, p. 16.

110 'Opening of the Queen's Hospital', *Sidcup Times*, 27 July 1917, LMA HO2/Y01/05, p. 5; 'Faces Rebuilt: New Hospital to Transform Ugliness into Good Looks', *Daily Sketch*, July 1917, LMA H02/Y01/05, p. 14.

death and restore the soldiers' damaged bodies, but also in their conflict with the medical Establishment. A solitary figure in his status as a pioneer, Gillies's resourcefulness and determination are underlined by Black: 'There was no such word as impossible in his vocabulary. He would not admit defeat [...] [Rebuilding faces] was a task that demanded infinite time and patience, for sometimes as many as fifteen operations were necessary for one patient, but he was tireless in his determination to succeed'.[111] Extraordinary courage and perseverance characterize the plastic surgeon, alongside the expertise of his surgical skills: 'Nothing seemed to daunt them', reports a 1921 article.[112] As a consequence, patients, nurses and colleagues alike stood in awe. Baillaud stresses the medical profession's admiration for Morestin: 'surgeons often came to our unit to observe Morestin; they were, like us, in awe' and according to her, Morestin sacrificed his life, his work at the Val-de-Grâce leading to his premature death.[113]

Visits from other doctors, sometimes travelling long distances, testify to the friendly competition that existed among countries and individual surgeons. Indeed, a form of competition emerged between surgeons, adding an extra incentive to innovate and develop this emerging medical specialty: 'at [Sidcup] hospital the rapid evolution of the successful remedy of apparently hopeless facial injury has largely been the result of friendly rivalry between a number of active intelligences brought to bear upon collected material of an unusual character'.[114] The co-existence of several units at Sidcup, led by different surgeons, was conducive to collaborations and friendly competition. On an international level, the war was becoming more reliant on science and technology (with the increased use of gas, aircraft and submarines for instance), as both sides looked for new or improved means of destruction. But the battle was also fought in the field of medicine, the

111 Black, *King's Nurse – Beggar's Nurse*, pp. 85–86.

112 'The triumphs of Sidcup', *The Manchester Guardian*, 5 November 1921, LMA HO2/Y01/05, p. 8.

113 Baillaud writes that '[Morestin] est mort à la tâche (je suppose de tuberculose) quand il était encore auprès de nous' (Letter, p. 3).

114 'Intensive Medical Treatment', *The Lancet*, 8 December 1917, LMA HO2/Y01/05, p. 27.

priority being to return as many men as possible to active service. Reports by French maxillofacial and dental surgeons in Bordeaux underline the superiority of Allied techniques over German procedures.[115] In contrast, in a 1921 article, the German writer Joseph Roth presents Germany as ahead of the rest of the world when it comes to facial reconstruction, and according to him Berlin's Charité hospital is world leader in the field.[116] This description, probably ironic, matches wartime propaganda that depicted Germany as ahead of other countries.

Even between those who were fighting the same enemy, a form of rivalry, or a lack of acknowledgement, can be observed. Inter-Allied congresses brought medical practitioners together, and visits from foreign surgeons were not unusual, yet little mention is made of exchanges. There is evidence of Gillies visiting Valadier and Morestin in France and the latter's attitude shows his unwillingness to be observed. In a letter, Gillies writes: 'Morestin was very unkind to me in the way of not letting me see his war surgery, but he was a very jealous and secretive person.'[117] Gillies later acknowledged the influence of German surgeons, especially Johannes Esser, on his own practice, writing that reading a German publication had 'stimulated in [him] the desire to do this reconstructive work'.[118] This might have been one of the sixty-eight publications by Esser, who worked in the Austro-Hungarian and Prussian armies. The Dutch surgeon had first

115 Paris, Archives du Service de Santé aux Armées du Val-de-Grâce, 'Missions Etrangères', *Rapport sur le Fonctionnement du Service de Chirurgie Maxillo-Faciale et Stomatologie. Du Ier Août au 31 Août 1916 Par Monsieur le Professeur DENUCE, Médecin Principal de 2e Classe. 18e Région*, p. 7. Box 127. Another article is found in *Rapport sur le Fonctionnement du Service de Chirurgie Maxillo-Faciale et Stomatologie. Septembre 1916 Par Monsieur le Professeur DENUCE, Médecin Principal de 2e Classe. 18e Région*, pp. 1–2. Box 127.

116 Roth, 'Der Wiederaufbau des Menschen', pp. 580–83.

117 Harold Gillies, Letter to Ralph Millard, 12 September 1951 (London: Royal College of Surgeons Gillies Archives).

118 Ibid.

offered his services to the French and British, who had declined them, and he is often credited with the invention of the rotation flap.[119]

In turn, visitors to Sidcup were frequent: Varaztad Kazanjian (United States), René Bloch (France) as well as at least two Japanese surgeons came.[120] A 1918 article in *The British Medical Journal* points to an Austrian monograph whose publication 'indicates that enemy dental surgeons are dealing with their war problems on much the same lines as our own', and mentions the 'opportune service' done to surgery by the translation of a French treatise on facial injuries.[121] Pickerill reports the 'healthy rivalry existing between the various sections – British, Canadian, Australian, New Zealand – into which the hospital was divided, each autonomous up to a certain point, but co-ordinated and commanded by an officer, Lieutenant-Colonel Colvin [...]'.[122] The setting up of specialized collections and exhibitions within maxillofacial hospitals or in war museums is documented in both France (Val-de-Grâce) and Great Britain:

> The Museum attached to the [Sidcup] Hospital has been formed with much care. The plaster casts together with photographic and pictorial records showing the nature of wounds and the methods of dealing with them were exhibited at the Inter-Allied Medical Congress at Rome and at the Imperial War Exhibition (Medical Section), Crystal Palace, where they attracted considerable attention.[123]

This initiative was first described as 'weird', especially the masks, which were also said to 'almost take one's breath away with amazement as to what has been achieved'.[124] Journalists stressed its necessary but shocking

119 Jan Hilbert and Johannes Hoenig, 'The Plastic Surgeon Johannes Fredericus Samuel Esser (1877 to 1946) and His Unknown Period During 1917 and 1925 in Berlin, Germany', *European Journal of Plastic Surgery*, 32 (2009), 127–30 (p. 128).

120 London, Wellcome Library archives, *The Queens Hospital, Sidcup: Visitors' Book, from 15 August 1919*. Reference Hist. pam/QUE.

121 'Injuries of the Face and Jaw', *British Medical Journal*, 13 April 1918, p. 429.

122 Pickerill, *Facial Surgery*, p. vii.

123 Wellcome Library Archives, London, *The Queen's Hospital, Sidcup, Kent, for Sailors and Soldiers Suffering from Facial and Jaw Injuries; Report on Work: 1917–1921*, p. 4. Reference RAMC/1296, Box 284.

124 'Opening of The Queen's Hospital', LMA HO2/Y01/05.

nature, describing it as an 'interesting, but ghastly, museum' and a 'place of marvels'.[125] In France, items from various maxillofacial services in the country were sent to the military medical services headquarters at the Val-de-Grâce. Although Sidcup centralized most 'facial cases' in Great Britain, smaller units independently carried out similar work, and documented it. Thus, exhibits from the Facial and Jaw Centre at the 2nd Western General Hospital, a three hundred-bed medical unit, were displayed at the Disabled Service Men's Exhibition in Manchester.[126] The general public were given access to them and could see for themselves the extent of the progress made.

The architect of bodily reconstruction, the surgeon, is brought to the fore in most accounts. Maxillofacial specialists, like their disfigured patients, are described in terms that exceed the limits of a human status. In literature, the doctor is portrayed as the *gueules cassées*' saviour, capable of 'resuscitating [...], building, really creating, bringing to life living flesh on the dead half of a face'.[127] The power of the 'surgeon creator' to shape new facial features or to restore human traits is reminiscent of God's work, although there is also a dark side that is sometimes hinted at, as in Duhamel's recollection of memories *A Muster of Ghosts*.[128] Thinking about Morestin, with whom he worked before the war when he was operating on patients suffering from tongue cancers, the French author writes: 'The artist was transformed into a wild beast'.[129] This description of a surgeon turned into an uncontrollable and somewhat frightening figure is however an isolated instance and it contrasts with the vast majority of depictions,

125 'The Queen's Hospital: An Institution for the Treatment of Facial Wounds', *Westminster Gazette*, July 1917, LMA HO2/Y01/05, p. 9; 'Facial Surgery for Sailors and Soldiers: Some Great Achievements', *Morning Post*, July 1917, LMA HO2/Y01/05, p. 11.

126 'Facial Wounds: Merciful Work of Modern Surgery', *The Manchester Guardian*, p. 3.

127 'ressusciter [...] bâtir, créer véritablement, faire naître de la chair vivante sur une moitié de visage mort', Dumas, *L'Homme qui Mourut Deux Fois*, pp. 35 and 41.

128 'New Faces for Old: Surgeon creator tells the story of his triumphs', *Daily Express*, September 1920, LMA HO2/Y01/05, p. 64.

129 'A Muster of Ghosts' in Georges Duhamel, *Light On My Days: An Autobiography*, trans. by Basil Collier (London: J.M. Dent & Sons Ltd, 1948), p. 275.

which indeed underline the 'civilized' nature of the doctors who restored the wounded men's faces back to a human state. Depictions of surgeons as benevolent geniuses, remote from ordinary mortals, and as god-like figures are a more frequent motif in all three countries. These religious undertones are also present in Roth's article *Lebende Kriegsdenkmäler* [Living War Monuments], in which he writes that 'Soldiers with facial wounds are people created by God in his image and whom the war remade in *its* image. Here we see the face of these heroic times. This is what the war looks like'.[130] The war deprived soldiers of their likeness with God and left its own evil imprint on their faces. According to Roth, there is nothing heroic about the war, which robs men of their resemblance with God. Roth's visit to the Charité in Berlin, where he witnessed both the horror of injuries and the miracles of surgery, left him with mixed feelings, especially when witnessing what he describes as the supernatural powers of the surgeon, which enable him to take over the Maker's work.[131] The credit for restoring the disfigured man's body and spirits is unreservedly given to the surgeon; he is presented as the soldier's saviour. The doctor gave his patients reason to hope, and Black too reports that Gillies 'made life worth living again for thousands of despairing war-disfigured men'.[132] Likewise, a former patient in a Manchester hospital confesses:

> When I left the battlefield I did not recognise myself. I was stricken with horror when I happened one day to catch a glimpse of my injuries. I said to myself, 'I am done for. No surgeon living can put me right again'. I was a pessimist then; I am an optimist now.[133]

130 '[Kieferbeschädigte] sind Menschen, die Gott nach seinem Ebenbilde schuf und die dann der Krieg nach *seinem* Ebenbild umarbeitete. Hier siehst du die Fratze der Großen Zeit. So sah der Krieg aus'. Roth, 'Lebende Kriegsdenkmäler', *Neue Berliner Zeitung*, 31 August 1920, in *Joseph Roth, Werke: 1915–1923*, ed. by Klaus Westermann, 6 vols (Köln: Kiepenheuer & Witsch, 1989), I, pp. 347–52 (p. 351).

131 Roth, 'Der Wiederaufbau des Menschen', p. 580.

132 Black, *King's Nurse – Beggar's Nurse*, p. 85.

133 'Disfigured Faces Restored', *The Manchester Guardian*, 26 September 1916, p. 4.

Hasbach's gratitude and Rémi's description of a nose specialist adored by his patients are other examples.[134] The mythical and religious dimensions attributed to surgeons accounts for the distance between them and their patients, as well as for the fact that their destinies and their work are better known to us than the fates of the men they treated.

Summary

The hospital was the place where facially injured soldiers were first confronted with their disfigurement and with the gaze of others. Accounts of the experiences of patients and staff underline the nature of the hospital as a transitional, albeit enclosed space, in which men were 'works in progress'. Relationships that developed were of key importance in the physical and psychological recovery of the wounded. In particular, the reassuring aspect of family-like relationships with nurses and surgeons helped mutilated men cope with the pain and depression caused by their conditions. At the same time, the hospital was an extension of the battlefield: staff and patients were fighting a common battle against death, disfigurement and despair. In the ward as well as on the front, the collective prevailed over the individual. However, amongst the masses of anonymous men, the surgeon stands out. Alternately a pioneer, a paternal figure, a genius and a god, he is the one true heroic figure. The embodiment of the beneficial impact of war on science and mankind more generally, his achievements helped make sense of a conflict that was otherwise characterized by its destructiveness.

This chapter has shown the implications of the parental model and heroic depictions of surgeons and sculptors, especially the way such images emphasize the infantilization and powerlessness of the soldiers. As this discussion showed, however, the wounded were not always as helpless as this model suggests. The combined skills of the surgeon and sculptor,

134 Rémi, *Hommes Sans Visage*, p. 54.

whose work is less known, aimed to make the wounded fit and presentable again. The hospital prepared men for their return to active service or to civilian life; it was there that they re-learned to relate to other people. An early description makes this future-oriented dimension clear: Sidcup hospital '[endeavoured] to secure the welfare and future of the men whilst brightening their lives during convalescence'.[135] The maxillofacial ward was a protected environment, a safe place where disfigurement was the norm. Upon the soldiers' discharge however, the confrontation with the outside world in which their injured faces were not the norm but the exception, and an extremely noticeable one, could be brutal. Medical treatments did not in all cases enable soldiers to go unnoticed, or in Gilman's terms to 'pass' into society. Those who remained severely disfigured constituted a transgressive presence in civilian and peacetime societies. This chapter has highlighted a communal point of departure between France, Germany and Great Britain. However, interwar societies responded to the presence of *gueules cassées* in different ways, which will be explored in the following chapters.

135 'The Queen's New Hospital for Treatment of Severe Facial and Jaw Injuries', *Rotherham Advertiser*, January 1917, LMA H02/Y01/05, p. 1.

CHAPTER 2

Facing the World: Economic and Social Reintegration

In 1918 Grace Harper, Chief of the Bureau for the Rehabilitation of *Mutilés* of the American Red Cross in France, began an article on Anna Coleman Ladd's Studio with the following words:

> Of all the results of war horrors, facial disfigurement seems the most cruel. What answer is there to the appeal: 'How can I work with such a face? How can I live with my family or they with me?' Many can help the cripple, but few can administer to the need of such as these.[1]

Harper's responsibilities within the organization give credibility to her description of the difficulties facing the disfigured veteran trying to find a place in a profession or within his family. The loss of his status as breadwinner and father is emphasized even more than the aesthetic prejudice. Harper was in regular contact with veterans and her depiction of the doctor's efforts to make patients 'less repulsive' implies that complete recovery was impossible.[2]

The social impact of facial wounds upon the victim and the onlooker was also underlined by professionals. Maxillofacial specialist Varaztad Kazanjian, who visited The Queen's Hospital, wrote:

> There is no person more severely handicapped than the patient with severe facial disfigurement. Since the face is the centre of attention wherever social interaction occurs, the region where the sense of self is generally located, the dominant part of

1 Harper, 'New Faces for Mutilated Soldiers', p. 44.
2 Ibid.

> the body image and the most revealing area of personality traits, those who have gross facial deformity undergo countless indignities and social deprivations.[3]

This assessment, if it is very pessimistic in tone, foreshadows the findings of later research in psychology. An article from 2003 demonstrates that 'Facial deformities have a significant negative effect on perceptions of social functionality, including employability, honesty, and trustworthiness'.[4] The number of disfigured veterans and the widespread understanding of the cause of their injuries may have mitigated this negative prejudice in the post-war years, yet the concerns expressed by Kazanjian suggest that disfigured combatants have long faced obstacles to their professional and social reintegration. In particular, the popularity of physiognomy and phrenology in nineteenth-century Europe contributed to the belief that facial features were a direct reflection of personality traits. More recent scientific research confirms the persistence of a 'hierarchy' between injuries: disfigurement is more negatively perceived than any other mutilation or disability, for:

> The face is the focus of social interaction and is an important source of social information, and hence a facial disfigurement would be particularly obtrusive, as well as being hard to conceal. Although a wheelchair is generally a negative stimulus and is also very visibly noticeable, it lacks the negative aesthetic impact of a facial disfigurement.[5]

Starting from the observation that from the outset, specialists were concerned about the return of disfigured veterans to civilian life, this chapter examines the challenges posed by the presence of ex-soldiers within society, and the efforts made to facilitate their economic and social reintegration. It questions the assessment made by the German surgeon Walkhoff who,

3 Varaztad Kazanjian and John M. Converse, *Surgical Treatment of Facial Injuries* (Baltimore: Williams and Wilkins Company, 1959), p. vii. The first edition was published in 1949.

4 Marlene Rankin and Gregory Borah, 'Perceived Functional Impact of Abnormal Facial Appearance', *Plastic and Reconstructive Surgery*, 11 (2003), 2140–46 (p. 2140).

5 Anna Stone and Toby Wright, 'When Your Face Doesn't Fit: Employment Discrimination Against People with Facial Disfigurements', *Journal of Applied Social Psychology*, 43 (2013), 515–26 (p. 516).

drawing upon his experience in the 1870 Franco-Prussian war, said that 'those suffering from injuries of the face and jaws are heroes today; but later, if untreated, are objects of dread and loathing to their fellow-countrymen'.[6]

With the exception of a short chapter in Delaporte's essay, the reintegration of First World War facially wounded soldiers has only been touched upon as a peripheral question in existing literature. Even less attention has been paid to their place in the world of employment. This chapter aims to show that efforts were made to prepare veterans to settle back into the civilian world, but society was sometimes at a loss to know how to relate to them. It draws upon primary sources, some of which have never been discussed before, including newspaper articles, official reports and individual testimonies, in order to investigate strategies designed to promote the reintegration of *gueules cassées*. The last section confronts the different journalistic treatment of facially wounded soldiers and proposes an alternative frame of interpretation to the more common depictions of disfigured men as extraordinary figures.

Professional reintegration

Training in hospitals

In wartime, patient-soldiers were expected to continue their active service, especially between operations and during convalescence. Alongside the expectation that men, even wounded, would contribute to the war effort, was the suspicion that some hospital patients were taking advantage of their situation to stay away from the front. A report by the French surgeon Temoin in 1916 specifically warns against malingerers amongst facially injured combatants, arguing that they can easily use their impressive jaw

6 W.H. Dolamure (translated and shortened), 'The Treatment in Germany of Gunshot Injuries of the Face and Jaws', *British Dental Journal*, 37 (1916), 105–84 (p. 105).

wounds to their advantage, convincing unsuspecting doctors that they are unfit for service.[7]

As well as being of immediate use, starting the process of professional reintegration when wounded soldiers were still in hospital presented advantages in terms of their future rehabilitation. The development of occupational therapy during the First World War stems from the realization that keeping men busy had a positive impact on their recovery. Boredom and depression weighed on patients' self-perception and their apparent inactivity influenced what other people thought of them. Having an occupation proved that they could still contribute to the war effort and post-war reconstruction. An article published in January 1917 in a British newspaper explains:

> No effort must be spared to give these men – many of them mere lads – a fresh interest and a new start in life – preferably in the country, and make them realise that they are not useless wrecks. If this is not done, many will drift to the towns on their discharge from the services, only to become mere objects of pity and frequently the recipients of misdirected charity.[8]

This fear of disfigured veterans becoming burdens echoes Walkhoff's warning. The article discusses professional training with an emphasis upon its beneficial results in practical and emotional terms. A 1919 newspaper article further underlines this positive impact: 'In some cases, where sufferers had become depressed to the point of contemplating, and even attempting, suicide, the work had brought a powerful counteracting interest'.[9] In psychological terms, professional activities opened up prospects for the future and reassured soldiers about their abilities and status. Some occupations put men in a position to earn money or provide for their fellow

7 Paris, Archives du Service de Santé aux Armées du Val-de-Grâce, Temoin, Report on the *Centre de Prothèse Restauratrice Maxillo-dento-faciale, 8e Région, Place de Bourges*, May 1916, p. 2. Box 122.

8 'The Queen's New Hospital for Treatment of Severe Facial and Jaw Injuries', January 1917, LMA H02/Y01/05, p. 1.

9 'Soldier Craftsmen: Display of Work by Hospital Patients', *The Times*, 9 December 1919, p. 11.

patients; for example, patients helped with the production of eggs, fruit and vegetables at Sidcup hospital.

The functional consequences of facial disfigurement prevented some patients from returning to their previous occupations once discharged: a lawyer had to abandon his career due to a fractured jaw, a horologist's only remaining eye was not enough to carry out precise work upon clocks and watches, and many a labourer had to give up his physically demanding activity because of the weakness induced by his changed diet.[10] In order to tackle these problems, nurses and hospital visitors trained soldiers in new professional and social skills, such as reading Braille, stenography, or simply the means of recognizing people. Baillaud recalls the successful case of one blind patient she took under her wing, who went on to pass his BA in sciences.[11] He then secured a teaching job and married the woman he was engaged to before his injury. A similar commitment to help blind patients regain their dexterity and to prepare them for life outside hospital was observed in Sidcup. Clare expresses his surprise at a blind patient's embroidery skills; a cushion he made was even presented to Princess Victoria when she visited the hospital.[12] The beauty of the item is here underlined, in contrast to its maker's disfigurement.

In addition to practical issues, the aesthetic consequences of facial wounds meant that many *gueules cassées* had to change jobs. Vocational training in occupations suitable for disfigured veterans was offered in many hospitals. Patients themselves often looked for people to teach them new trades and skills.[13] The official report on the work carried out at The Queen's Hospital between 1917 and 1921 details the various workshops set up, amongst which the most popular were toymaking (322 attendees), woodwork (253), business (120) and beadwork (67).[14] Overall, customer-facing trades were rare. Some activities were directly related to the workings

10 *Bulletin*, 11b (June 1925), p. 7.

11 Baillaud, Letter, p. 9.

12 Clare, Letter, 8 January 1918.

13 Baillaud, Letter, p. 9.

14 *The Queen's Hospital, Sidcup, Kent, for Sailors and Soldiers Suffering from Facial and Jaw Injuries: Report on Work, 1917–1921.*

of a maxillofacial hospital; for example, farming provided food for patients and staff, and dentistry students made prostheses. Only a few months after the opening of the hospital, an article reported that 'at least two Frognal patients are already engaged at work in the dental laboratory whilst undergoing treatment for their own wounds'.[15]

The speedy establishment of the dental workshop suggests that the idea had been considered beforehand, maybe modelled upon similar French initiatives and those in other British hospitals, such as Roehampton. Delagenière and Lebedinsky had already suggested the setting up of a similar workshop in Le Mans, France, in March 1917; they argued that it would be doubly beneficial, as the men would make prostheses useful to their comrades at the same time as learning a new trade themselves.[16] In Bordeaux, the author of a report on an *Ecole des Mutilés* [School for the Mutilated] gives a positive description of the work carried out there, and provides an example of successful professional reintegration: 'one of these mutilated men, D ... has just left our workshop to take up a position paid 300 Francs a month and guaranteed for two years. He was with us four and a half months'.[17] It is also suggested that apprentices, being trained in the work of rubber and metals, could reuse these skills in other trades. Beyond the financial gain, through their participation in their own treatment, patients moved from a passive to an active role, contributing to the reconstruction of their faces and of their lives.

Cinema-operating classes were also run at Sidcup. They are particularly interesting, not least because of the support that the Cinema Trade

15 'A Christmas Wonder Tale: How They Spend Yule in the Military Hospitals', *Pall Mall*, December 1917, LMA HO2/Y01/05, p. 26.

16 Paris, Archives du Service de Santé aux Armées du Val-de-Grâce, Delagenière and Lebedinsky, *Rapport sur l'organisation et le fonctionnement du Centre de Stomatologie et de Prothèse MF. 4e région. Place du Mans.* Section on 'Centre de Prothèse Elementaire pour Edentés', 1–31 March 1917, p. 10, Box 121.

17 'un de ces mutilés, D ... vient de sortir de nos ateliers, avec des appointements de 300 Fr. par mois et un engagement de deux ans. Il y était resté 4 mois ½'. Paris, Archives du Service de Santé aux Armées du Val-de-Grâce, *Rapport sur le Fonctionnement du Service de Chirurgie Maxillo-Faciale et Stomatologie. Octobre 1916, Par Monsieur le Professeur DENUCE, Médecin Principal de 2e Classe. 18e Région*, p. 2. Box 127.

Benevolent Fund gave to maxillofacial hospitals.[18] The development of cinema in the first decades of the twentieth century created new jobs, some of them particularly suitable for men who did not wish to be seen by other people. However, the low number of trainee projectionists (four) is surprising, especially when compared to the number of men training as hairdressers, a customer-facing job featuring an aesthetic dimension.[19] Toy-making, woodwork (also referred to as carpentry) and commercial classes were attended by larger cohorts. The items made by toy-making and carpentry students were displayed and sold to the general public, their quality underlined in newspapers: 'It is a tribute to their quality that more than one well-known firm has offered to take any surplus [toys] remaining'.[20] Their exhibition at Chelsea House and the royal endorsement through the visit of the Queen, Princess Mary and Princess Helena Victoria also drew attention to the items.[21] The primary purpose of such instructional workshops – which were similar to those offered in other institutions, for example, at St Dunstan's – was to provide an occupation for patients and to train them in a trade that they could pursue later (not unlike the recreational and therapeutic activities that have been employed in hospitals ever since). They empowered the wounded and showed society that facially injured men were able and willing to work.

The challenges of returning to civilian employment

This preparation, however, was no guarantee of an easy professional reintegration into civilian society. The wartime and post-war economic context

18 This support is acknowledged for the Brook Street Red Cross Hospital for Facial Injuries in 'Hospitals for Facial Injuries', *The Official Journal of the British Red Cross Society*, 5 (15 October 1918).

19 The novelty of the venues may account for this reluctance to get training in cinema-related occupations, as well as the association with the celebrity cult.

20 'Queen's Hospital Industries', *Morning Post*, December 1919, LMA HO2/Y01/05, p. 59. This reflected well on the companies too.

21 'Soldiers Craftsmen', p. 11.

created problems for all workers and the situation of disabled veterans was particularly precarious. In *The War Come Home*, Cohen underlines national divergences in terms of the state's treatment of disabled veterans: 'In contrast to Britain, where civil servants sought to divest the state of responsibility to the disabled, the Weimar Republic – a pioneer in the field of social welfare – regarded rehabilitation as its highest obligation'.[22] She contrasts the 1918 King's Roll – the only measure taken in Britain to support the employment of ex-servicemen – with the numerous laws passed in Germany, which had the perverse effect of leading 'most Germans [to think] that the disabled were the favoured wards of the welfare state'.[23] In France, Prost notes that early in the war, 'the inadequacy of pensions and the difficulty of finding work sometimes meant heartbreaking destitution for the disabled'.[24] The pensions to which facially disfigured soldiers were entitled were regarded as insufficient, especially because the aesthetic consequences of their condition were not always taken into account in the calculation of the pension rate. However, there was a growing awareness that something had to be done to keep discharged soldiers off the streets.

Pensions were expensive for the state and did not cover the needs of disabled veterans. In all three countries, there is evidence of authorities or private organizations trying to improve the situation of disabled veterans through employment schemes. A 1917 article urged the British government to copy a tax scheme set up in France, under which the state subsidized employers so that recruiting disabled employees would not be financially disadvantageous.[25] Existing research has shown that the degree of state involvement varied depending upon the national context. Germany is an example of strong state intervention, and Great Britain one of significant private support networks. Instead of drawing upon official documents, this section will focus upon individual stories in order to investigate the challenges faced by *gueules cassées* in terms of professional reintegration.

22 Cohen, *The War Come Home*, p. 5.

23 Ibid., p. 9.

24 Winter and Prost, *The Great War in History*, p. 29.

25 'Treatment of Disabled Soldiers: British and French Methods', *The Manchester Guardian*, 7 August 1917, p. 6.

The veteran's confrontation with the labour market provides an insight into society's perception of disfigured ex-servicemen and into the place they were given in civilian society.

In contemporary accounts, work is a key source of concern for disfigured men. Rémi recalls a farmer's son questioning his prospects, having suffered injuries to the face and hand. Likewise, she reports a father's assessment of his son's future in the family hairdressing business: 'Do you really believe that posh men and elegant ladies will want to be touched by this: [...] A *gueule cassée*, ha-ha-ha, it would remind them of too many things they would rather not think about. [...] He's screwed, screwed, he would be better-off dead!'[26] Here, disfigurement is perceived as too evocative of the war to enable the veteran's return to his previous occupation. Society, it is implied, wants to move on.

Existing literature tends to focus upon failed attempts to return to a previous job. The testimonies show, however, that the real-life destinies of facially wounded combatants were much more varied. A number of French disfigured men made a career in politics and in Britain, prominent figures such as the BBC's executive director John Reith and the commanding general of the Arab Legion John Baggott Glubb – nicknamed *Abu Hunaik* [little jaw] in Arab – enjoyed successful careers despite their injuries.[27] Many veterans in fact managed to secure a stable place in the work sphere. Karl Hasbach could hardly face standing in front of a classroom whilst wearing his prosthetic nose, but after his rhinoplasty he went on to

26 'Croyez-vous que les messieurs chics et les belles élégantes voudront se laisser toucher par ça? [...] Une gueule cassée, ha-ha-ha, ça leur rappellerait trop de choses auxquelles ils n'aiment pas penser. [...] Il est foutu, foutu, mieux vaudrait être mort!' Rémi, *Hommes Sans Visage*, pp. 85–86. This quotation is the only instance in Rémi's account in which the term *gueule cassée* is used. The author herself never employs it, which is surprising considering the popularity gained by the *Association des Gueules Cassées* by the end of the 1930s. This can be interpreted as further evidence of the fact that Rémi is not talking about French disfigured men.

27 Emily Mayhew, *Wounded: A New History of the Western Front in World War I* (Oxford: Oxford University Press, 2014), p. 215.

become a grammar school teacher.[28] Harry Burbeck secured the post of Assistant Clerk only a few months after his discharge from Sidcup; he was later promoted and he finally became Chief Financial Officer to Downham Rural District Council.[29] His disfigurement was not a major hindrance, yet it was something that he and his superiors thought worth mentioning in applications. A testimonial written for him in 1924 specifies that 'he saw five and a half years of hard War Service and bears the marks of very severe wounds'.[30] Burbeck himself gives more detail about his injury in his application letter:

> Whilst on active service in France I received severe facial wounds and after ten operations and four grafts from my leg and arms, all of which were successful, I was discharged from hospital on October 31st, 1920 with a presentable appearance, and I am perfectly fit and healthy.[31]

The emphasis upon the success of the treatment received and the absence of long-term consequences ('fit and healthy') invites the reader to picture a capable, 'normal' candidate. The very fact that he thought it necessary to specify his condition however shows that employers were believed to have concerns related to the veterans' health.

Even for those men whose faces were not improved by surgery or the wearing of a mask, and who suffered from permanent functional loss, career prospects were not necessarily bleak. Baillaud's blind patient who became a

28 Susanne Lenz, 'Hilfe vom Nasenjoseph', *Berliner Zeitung*, 4 June 2014 <http://www.berliner-zeitung.de/kultur/gesichtsplastiken-im-ersten-weltkrieg-hilfe-vom-nasenjoseph,10809150,27347646.html> [accessed 10 December 2014].

29 Notes on Harry Burbeck's professional career, from family archives. Personal archives consulted and testimony collected in 2012 during an interview with Mrs Biddy Stevens, daughter of Harry Burbeck, who was facially injured during the First World War.

30 Testimonial from Edward Clark, Castle Bytham, Grantham, 12 February 1924 (courtesy of Biddy Stevens). The time Harry Burbeck spent in treatment at Sidcup is here included in the 'five and a half years of hard War Service'.

31 Harry Burbeck, application letter (draft), 15 February 1924. Courtesy of Biddy Stevens.

teacher is a case in point.[32] The French featherweight boxer Eugène Criqui (1893–1977) suffered a severe – doctors even thought it would be fatal – jaw injury in 1915. He was taken to a hospital in Lyon and underwent several operations, followed by a long speech re-education process. He then successfully returned to his boxing career, his jaw prosthetics having earned him the nickname 'Mâchoire de fer' [Iron Jaw]. He won the world title in 1923. His injury became an integral part of his reputation.[33]

In fact, injuries could work in a man's favour, as illustrated by the story of Bélagnon. A patient at the Val-de-Grâce hospital, severely disfigured, he found a job as a postman, thanks to the help of a local senator.[34] Here, the soldier's disfigurement, interpreted as a sign of patriotism, won him the support that he needed to secure a job. Where no government scheme was successfully implemented, individual initiatives enabled many a disfigured veteran to find work. Producer Charles Chilton reports that Reith 'was anxious to give employment to ex-soldiers, especially if they had been wounded or disabled in some way.' Chilton confesses his surprise when he met them:

> I received a terrible shock when first I saw their terribly burned and disfigured faces: many of them lacked noses, ears, hair, even lips. They were so badly disfigured they stayed in their office, never going out for meals, even to the BBC canteen. I used to get their meals for them and got to know them quite well. They were very kind and friendly.[35]

32 This story can be set against the announced failure of Remarque's fictional character Paul Rademacher. More than the veteran's looks and partial blindness, his speech impediment is a source of concern to him and a reason to believe that he will not be able to become a teacher (Erich Maria Remarque, *The Road Back*, trans. by Arthur W. Wheen (London: Little, Brown & Co., 1931), pp. 76–77, first published under the title *Der Weg Zurück* (Berlin: Propylaen Verlag, 1931)).

33 Eugène Criqui and Robert Bré, 'Les Aventures de ma Vie' (2), *Match: le plus grand hebdomadaire sportif*, 23 February 1932, pp. 6–7.

34 Général O.P.Ré, *La Greffe Générale*, 7 (May 1918), p. 26.

35 Charles Chilton, *Auntie's Charlie* (Leamington Spa: Fantom Publishing, 2011), p. 104.

In France, the *Union des Blessés de la Face* tackled the issue of its members' return to work, as will be discussed in the next chapter.

Facially injured soldiers thus often faced obstacles to their professional reintegration, sometimes related to the uncomfortable memories evoked by their faces. Professionals expressed some scepticism regarding the men's employment prospects, but the case studies presented in this section show that there were many successful attempts as well as failures. Arguably, the stories recorded by contemporary observers are extreme cases of rejection or success, and many remain untold. They nevertheless give a more nuanced picture of the professional situation of *gueules cassées* than the pessimistic predictions of Harper and Walkhoff suggested.

The family sphere

In 1917, a British journalist wrote that 'many of the patients are so conscious of their affliction that they refuse to return to their homes and friends until they are convinced that everything possible has been done for them'.[36] It was presumed at the time that not only were others unprepared – sometimes unwilling – to face *gueules cassées*, but that they themselves sought to avoid contact with their families. The efforts made to prepare patients for their reunions with relatives, discussed in the previous chapter, point to the crucial significance of the family in helping men to cope with their disfigurement. The observations made by contemporaries echo the findings of a recent study of body image and facial disfigurement: 'Partners and families are likely to be the main provider of support, yet they themselves may be trying to deal with their own reactions and distress surrounding

36 'The Queen's New Hospital for Treatment of Severe Facial and Jaw Injuries', LMA H02/Y01/05, p. 1.

the disfigurement'.[37] At the time of the First World War, relatives' visits in hospital were tightly regulated, although not completely forbidden. The Sidcup hospital chaplain even made arrangements to provide accommodation for visiting relatives. Familial withdrawal on the part of the soldiers themselves was not uncommon but, more often than not, men desired to re-establish their place within their families.[38]

Parents and children

The reactions of parents to disfigurement, especially the mother, were of particular importance. Percy Clare's correspondence with his mother reveals that he had to constantly reassure her about his state.[39] In his letters, he underlines that his wound is a blessing in disguise: it means he will be safe, away from the front, for a few months at least. He expresses no fear about his appearance in the correspondence, although he does mention aesthetic and functional impediments. The fact that he encourages his mother to visit suggests that he has no doubts that she will accept him.[40] However, not all patients were looking forward to this reunion, and a French journalist reports that a patient refused to be seen by his mother, although she had travelled over four hundred kilometres to see him: 'he asked that she be told that he was not visible and despite her tears and her cries, he stayed in the prison he had locked himself in to avoid scaring his mother'.[41]

When the meeting came, parents sometimes found it difficult to cope with the sight of their disfigured child. Black reports the shock experienced

37 Nichola Rumsey and Diana Harcourt, 'Body Image and Disfigurement: Issues and Interventions', *Body Image*, 1 (2004), 83–97 (p. 88).

38 This longing for a return to 'normality' within the family sphere is prominent in literary narratives, as shown in Chapter 5.

39 See, for instance, Clare, Letter, 24 November 1917 and 13 December 1917.

40 Clare, Letter, 21 November 1917.

41 'il fit répondre qu'il n'était pas visible et, malgré les larmes, les cris, resta dans sa prison volontaire pour ne point faire peur à sa maman', Georges Finaud, 'Les Mutilés de la Face', *Après le Combat*, reprinted in *Bulletin*, 8 (September 1923), p. 1.

by an officer's mother when she first saw his face: 'On the day [Corporal X's] bandages were taken off his mother visited him. She went very white and I thought for a moment that she was going to faint, but not the slightest expression of face or voice betrayed her'.[42] A similar determination to suppress emotion is reported by Rémi, who describes a patient's father collapsing in the corridor after having managed to hide his shock in front of his son. His despair turns into anger as he blames an unidentified enemy soldier for his son's injuries.[43] Rémi suggests that blindness could make this first encounter easier. Describing the reunion of a blind *gueule cassée* with his mother and sister, she reports his enthusiasm at their meeting. He seems sure that they will take care of him, although he fears that they may not recognize him at first. The two women's initial reaction, of which he remains unaware, is one of horror: 'Her face suddenly went pale, tautened into a look of terror. Her eyes widened with dread, her hands reached forward as if to keep a vision of horror at bay, her lips formed the words "My God ... It is him!"'[44] Whether the soldier's relatives managed to overcome the initial shock is left untold. Rémi reports many cases that show the strain put on relationships between disfigured men and their families.[45]

A difficult reunion could be interpreted as a foreshadowing of future rejections. Baillaud recounts the case of Canuet, whose meeting with his mother left him dejected because his mother had not recognized him.[46] Baillaud does not specify if Canuet ever saw her again, but the fact that she goes on to mention the setting up of a mansion where men who did not want to, or could not, return home, lived together indicates that he probably chose to isolate himself and remain with his peers.[47] The attitude of hospital

42 Black, *King's Nurse – Beggar's Nurse*, p. 88.

43 Rémi, *Hommes Sans Visage*, pp. 51–52.

44 'Tout à coup, son visage pâlit, une expression de terreur le crispe; ses yeux s'agrandissent d'effroi, ses mains s'étendent en avant comme pour repousser une vision d'horreur, ses lèvres murmurent: Mon Dieu ... c'est lui!' Rémi, *Hommes Sans Visage*, p. 23.

45 See, for example, the rejection of Robert by his father (Rémi, *Hommes Sans Visage*, p. 87).

46 Baillaud, Letter, p. 10.

47 Ibid.

staff, and their assumption of the role of parental figures, therefore gave a much-needed sense of acceptance in this context. They sometimes had to step in to make up for the absence or rejection of the soldier's family. Thus, one of Baillaud's patients did not ask for his mother, but called Baillaud and his favourite hospital visitor on his deathbed; this shows his desire for a caring presence, the role of a mother now fulfilled by female staff.

The reaction of a soldier's parents was of prime importance insofar as it restored continuity of the man's familial identity: despite his injury, he was still recognized by the people who knew him best. His reinstatement as an independent adult, however, also depended upon the evolution of his relationship with his children. In this particular relationship, the veteran is himself in a position of authority and fulfils what was regarded as a traditional masculine role. A child's rejection had far-reaching implications, not only emotionally but also symbolically. Children running away from their disfigured fathers are mentioned time and again in newspaper articles, the motif being used by journalists to dramatize their stories, for example, in the *Morning Post*: 'the poor fellow's children fled in terror from him' and in the *Kent Messenger*: 'his own children ran away from him!'[48] The figure of the father is traditionally associated with safety; a man whose appearance scares off his children appears unable to fulfil this role. Then again, two stories reported by Rémi illustrate different reactions from children. The teenage daughter of a severely wounded patient, when visiting him, sits beside her father and reads to him. She does not fear physical contact with him and supports him when they go for a walk.[49] Thus, the implications of confrontation with others vary: if the response is one of acceptance, the wounded soldier is heading towards the restoration of his status of man and father. If he is rejected, it can mean that his injury has definitively robbed him of his identity and place within civilian society: 'I was a man, I did my best to live out what it meant ... And this is what is left of me ... A frightening sight for my own child, a daily burden for my

48 'Facial Surgery for Sailors and Soldiers: Some Great Achievements', p. 11 and Untitled, *Kent Messenger*, August 1917, LMA HO2/Y01/05, p. 16.

49 Rémi, *Hommes Sans Visage*, pp. 75–76.

wife, a shame for humanity …'[50] With his son's rejection, Lazé feels he has lost his status as a father, as a husband, as a man and even as a human being.

For children born to facially injured men after their injuries, the disfigurement did not come as a brutal realization. Harry Burbeck's daughter recalls that she had not noticed anything unusual about her father's face until a school friend commented that he had a 'snout', not a nose.[51] Following this comment, seven-year-old Biddy realized that her father's nose was unusual, although not 'nastily different'. According to her, 'he didn't feel less of a man because of what he looked like and what had happened'; his career and family indeed point to a successful professional and social reintegration. The main reason for this, in the opinion of Burbeck's relatives, is the pivotal part played by his wife.

Romantic relationships

When he was thirty-three, Burbeck met Isabella. She was only twenty years old and her parents at first disapproved of her intention to marry Harry. They warned her that she was 'mixing up love and pity'.[52] Their concern is indicative of the widespread assumption that disfigured men triggered compassion, but were unlikely to be loved. Isabella's parents finally gave their consent and the wedding was celebrated in 1924; this marriage is described by Biddy Stevens as 'the best thing that ever happened' to them both. Harry and Isabella Burbeck were members of many clubs and did a lot for the town that they lived in. This example shows the empowerment stemming from positive relationships. The bias in fiction and the popular press, which underlines the difficulties faced by disfigured veterans in

50 'Avoir été un homme, avoir mis toutes ses forces à réaliser en plein ce que ce mot veut dire … et n'être plus que ça … un objet de terreur pour son propre enfant, une charge quotidienne pour sa femme, une honte pour l'humanité …', Rémi, *Hommes Sans Visage*, p. 106.

51 Interview with Biddy Stevens.

52 Ibid.

terms of meeting women and getting married, should not hide the many examples of successful marriages.

In the Burbecks' case, the main obstacle to their relationship was not Isabella's fears but parental opposition. This problem is also raised in *La Greffe Générale*: engaging in an imaginary conversation with parents of women betrothed to *gueules cassées*, the author assures them that should they, or their daughters, have doubts as to whether to marry a disfigured man, the best option is to break up.[53] The author presents these broken engagements as a blessing in disguise since they protected soldiers from marriage to unworthy women. In the process, the *gueule cassée* is not a passive victim but a man in control of his destiny.

Happy marriages were not a guaranteed outcome and an article published in 1917 in *The Observer* even endeavours to help men improve their domestic situation. This article acknowledges the importance of 'wife and child' in the social rehabilitation of injured soldiers, especially for blind men. The author supports St Dunstan's founder Arthur Pearson's appeal for a marriage endowment, which would prevent the blind from '[losing] the solace and inspiration of fatherhood'.[54] This plea in favour of mutilated soldiers starts with the fictional story by the French writer Maurice Donnay, which tells of a young woman who married a *gueule cassée*:

> One of the characters is a little milliner who has married the man to whom she was engaged before the war. His face having been disfigured by a wound, he had kept away from her, had not let her know he was still living; but she had sought him out, accustomed herself with a Frenchwoman's practical instinct to his forbidding countenance, and insisted on fulfilling the pledge she had made when he was handsome and prosperous. […] We are invited to look beyond the individual and see the importance of the family.[55]

Donnay's story reverses traditional gender roles: the woman pursues the man, she does not let herself be put off by his appearance, and she honours

53 Louis Latzarus, 'Le Blessé dans la Rue', *La Greffe Générale*, 2, p. 1.

54 '"The Larger Necessity": Blinded Soldiers' Children's Fund', *The Observer*, 23 September 1917, p. 11.

55 '"The Larger Necessity"'.

her promise. The disfigured veteran, in contrast, is passive and is physically and financially unattractive. This story reflects and encourages the empowerment of women following the Great War and the related alleged demise of manhood. Its use in this context is paradoxical: if the milliner's attitude was shared by real-life veterans' fiancées and lovers, no marriage endowment would be needed. This appeal emphasizes the powerlessness of the ex-soldiers at the same time as it asserts the importance of the traditional family model, a theme that is often taken up in literature (this will be discussed in Chapter 5).

Indeed, the situation of men already engaged or married before their injuries was different from that of single men. One of Black's patients, once he had seen his face, wrote a letter to his fiancée Molly, in which:

> [he] asked her to release him, told her that he had met a girl in Paris with whom he had fallen in love. He had realized that their engagement had been a mistake. Would she forgive him and let it end there?
>
> 'It wouldn't be fair to let a girl like Molly be tied to a miserable wreck like me,' he said, 'I'm not going to let her sacrifice herself out of pity. This way she will never know'.[56]

A similar story is reported in a 1918 newspaper article: 'After [the wounded man] had coaxed a nurse to let him see his shattered face in a mirror [he] had straight away broken off his engagement and refused to see his friends. Plastic surgery had the part of the good fairy of romance and made things all right again'.[57] In turn, a reunion was not only a subject of concern for soldiers: 'I have never told anybody, but I've had those words Facial Severe going through my brain ever since my husband went out', confides a subscriber to the Queen's Hospital Recreation and Comforts Fund. 'I have done some nursing and I know what those words may mean, and I have even prayed that if he is wounded it might be in some other way'.[58]

56 Black, *King's Nurse – Beggar's Nurse*, p. 89.

57 'Happy end to war romance: broke engagement because face was shattered', *Daily Dispatch*, June 1918, LMA HO2/Y01/05, p. 54.

58 '"Facial Severe": Two Words with a Terrible Meaning', *Manchester Dispatch*, June 1918, LMA HO2/Y01/05, p. 42.

In particular, kissing appears time and again as an issue, as underlined by Roth: 'the lips are missing, the lips with which he can kiss and whisper'.[59] One of Rémi's patients despairs when his wife collapses, unable to face him, let alone to kiss him. He regarded her kiss as the ultimate sign of acceptance, a token that everything would go back to normal.[60] Her willingness to hold his hand and kiss him on the forehead appear to be only a pale compensation. For the *gueule cassée*, this kiss he is denied sums everything up:

> Then Alix understood. He would never receive this redeeming kiss. He suddenly realised the fullness of the horror of … Of what? His life? He did not have one anymore; it was flowing out of him through this weeping wound, it was leaving him through this woman who could no longer kiss him.[61]

Despite the words they exchange, there is a gap in communication. This estrangement is described in terms of silence in a British article: 'There are the tragic meetings with mothers, sisters, brothers, wives, and bairns that leave men doubly depressed when silence holds them as they clasp hands'.[62] The loving attitude of another patient's wife, Dargan, makes Alix's wife feel even more guilty, as the other woman displays a readiness to accept physical contact. Madame Dargan treats her husband as if he was not disfigured.

59 'Die Lippen fehlen, die Lippen, mit denen er küssen, flüstern konnte', Roth, 'Lebende Kriegsdenkmäler', p. 351.

60 Rémi, *Hommes Sans Visage*, p. 80.

61 'Alors Alix a compris. Ce baiser rédempteur, il ne l'aura jamais. Il a saisi soudain toute l'horreur de … de quoi? De sa vie? Il n'en a plus; elle s'écoule par cette blessure qui suinte, elle le fuit avec cette femme qui ne peut plus l'embrasser.' Rémi, *Hommes Sans Visage*, p. 80. A similar observation is made by Finaud, who writes in 1923 that gueules cassées cannot hope to be kissed again, except perhaps by their mother (Finaud, 'Les Mutilés de la Face', p. 1).

62 'Music in the Wards: Making the Lot of the War-Scarred Brighter, Public Can Help, Fund for the Queen's Hospital Mounting Up', *Evening Standard*, June 1918, LMA HO2/Y01/05, p. 38. The *Bulletin de l'Union des Blessés de la Face* also reports the case of a *gueule cassée* who had been abandoned by his first wife following his injury and whose second wife, inconvenienced by his disfigurement and inability to control his saliva, wanted to leave him too (*Bulletin*, 10 (March 1924), p. 8).

The positive impact on him is clear: he is a happy man.[63] But Rémi finds out that her attitude is only pretence: she is cheating on her husband and admits that it is her lover she thinks about when she kisses Dargan. Madame Dargan confesses that the enthusiasm and joy she displays in the presence of her husband hide her own despair.

In contrast, the reunion between Sergeant Bates and his wife at Sidcup has a positive outcome. The *Sunday Chronicle* reports that the woman, unaware of the nature of her husband's injury, is warned by the matron: 'you must be brave when you see him, because – he dreads this meeting – for your sake'. Both the patient and the nurse's concerns however prove unfounded: the wife 'took one searching glance as involuntarily he turned his "good" side to her and then, deliberately choosing the other, she went right up to the bed, and with a hand on each shoulder, kissed him – ever so lightly – on the worst scar of all'.[64]

The implications of a wife's response are also noted by Baillaud, who recalls the case of another patient: 'I think that he would have killed himself if it had not been for his fiancée waiting for him in the Ardennes, his home country then occupied. Thank Heaven she did not leave him'.[65] The man later married his fiancée, found a job and had children. The French nurse notes that this happy ending, or at least, successful return to 'normal' life, was not unusual: she recalls that all of her blind patients got married. The Val-de-Grâce hospital was in fact the starting place of many a romance, for example between mathematician Gaston Julia and a volunteer, Marianne Chausson.[66] Likewise, Sidcup patients sometimes married in the vicinity.[67] Clare's testimony shows that soldiers had opportunities to meet women

63 Rémi, *Hommes Sans Visage*, p. 82.

64 'Surgical Marvels: Restoring the Men Who Went Over the Top, a National Appeal', *Sunday Chronicle*, May 1918, LMA HO2/Y01/05, p. 37.

65 'Je pense qu'il se serait suicidé s'il n'avait pas laissé une fiancée dans les Ardennes, son pays qui était alors envahi. Celle-ci, grâce au Ciel, ne l'a pas laissé tomber', Baillaud, Letter, p. 9.

66 Baillaud, Letter, p. 6.

67 HG Bingham and CE Moore, 'Farewell to Queen's Hospital, Sidcup', *British Journal of Plastic Surgery*, 29 (1976), 297–301 (p. 300).

during their treatment and his own reunion with his wife happened without any awkwardness or fear on his part.[68] Clare's fate, as well as the destinies of the other men discussed in this chapter, confirms that families had mixed responses when confronted with their disfigured relatives. The consequences of rejection, especially by a spouse or child, could be fatal. Efforts were made to facilitate this process, although no general reflection was conducted on this matter, and no official instructions given. It was down to each unit, and even to the individual surgeon, to decide on the best course of action for the patients.

Less emphasis was put upon making contact with the rest of society during treatment. Testimonies and newspaper articles suggest that reintegration into the family sphere was more of a concern to soldiers than their professional careers. In contrast, society was more preoccupied with their economic usefulness. The cases discussed show that despite initial difficulties due both to the men's self-consciousness and other people's perception of them, return to civilian life was possible. An attempt to return to traditional gender roles and to move towards the re-creation of pre-war professional and familial spheres should however not hide the fact that the war, as argued by Bourke, Lyford and Carden-Coyne, also gave rise to new definitions of masculinity, transforming perceptions of the body, of a man's place in society and of the ways in which ex-servicemen related to others.

Social reintegration

Literary works and paintings often depict problematic encounters with the public, and existing research on mutilated veterans points out their difficulties in relating to others. This discussion of their interactions feeds

68 Clare, Private papers. He admits having had a shock when he first saw his own face, still covered in blood, but once it had been washed and shaved he found himself recognizable. As a result, he did not fear rejection from his wife.

into a wider reflection upon the ways in which interwar society coped with the memory of the First World War and accommodated ex-servicemen as a new conflict loomed. It draws upon testimonies as well as journalistic accounts in order to explore two major and apparently contradictory frames of interpretation. The tendency to marginalize *gueules cassées* will be analysed first. The second approach marks a departure from this traditional frame of interpretation and emphasizes efforts at 'normalizing' facially disfigured veterans.

Spaces of contact, wartime and civilian identities

Historical accounts indicate that the hospital was far from a secluded place. Visitors were common and most institutions also received the visits of officials, benefactors and others. Unlike unexpected confrontations with people in the street, encounters at the hospital were planned and organized. Many of the visitors were doctors and dentists themselves, and thus accustomed to the sight of wounded soldiers. Visits of members of the royal family to maxillofacial hospitals, Sidcup in particular, are also documented: Queen Mary came in November 1917, followed in April 1918 by Queen Alexandra, and the Duke of Connaught in June 1918.[69] The Queen, the Princess Royal and Princess Maud also visited Lady Constance Butler's Hospital for Facial Injuries in 1917.[70] The Sidcup enterprise attracted royal attention even before the centre started operating; Queen Mary took a 'personal interest' in the setting up of the hospital, supporting its creation and giving it her name.[71] A photograph documents her visit and pictures her beside the bed of a patient. She is slightly bent over him, looking at him and seemingly speaking to him. The message conveyed is one of a conversation

69 C.J. Webber, 'Queen Mary's Hospital: 1915–1971' [no publication title], 30 November 1971. Bexleyheath, Bexley Local Archives, reference P362.11SID.

70 Court Circular, *The Times*, 5 January 1917, p. 11.

71 Webber, 'Queen Mary's Hospital'.

between the Queen and a soldier.[72] The bandages on his head spare both his royal visitor and the viewer the sight of his wound. This visual association of injured soldiers and royals emphasizes the heroic character of the men and suggests that they are not repulsive. The Queen sets an example of interaction with them. In France, military officials and political leaders also visited maxillofacial units, whilst in Germany the emperor took great interest in Joseph's work and personally offered him the Chair for Plastic Surgery at the Charité Hospital in 1915.[73]

Baillaud mentions several other categories of anonymous visitors: families, instructors, and people who came to take patients out on walks and to provide entertainment for them. A local woman recalls visiting Sidcup patients with her father to bring them cigarettes: 'We felt we were doing something to repay them for the sacrifices they had made on behalf of the cause of freedom for our nation, Great Britain'.[74] Gifts from local residents, in response to a 1917 appeal, included an organ (to be used in the chapel), a gramophone with records, a bagatelle board and a Berbice chair.[75] The sending of presents may be interpreted as an indirect way for the population to reach out to the patients, without having to face them.

72 'The Queen's Talk at a Facial Hospital – Her Majesty Listening to the Experiences of One of the Patients at a Sidcup Hospital, Established to Treat Officers and Men Who Have Suffered Facial Disfigurement', *Daily Mail*, 13 November 1917, LMA HO2/Y01/05, p. 22.

73 The fictionalized testimony of Jean-Victor Monségur's by his great-nephew mentions the visits of Clemenceau's sister and Poincaré to facially wounded men's wards (Guy Monségur, *Etrange et Tragique Destinée d'un Poilu – En Hommage à Jean-Victor Monségur, aux Gueules Cassées et à Tous les Combattants de 14–18* (Pau: Monhélios, 2004), pp. 30–31). Wilhelm II offered Joseph a Chair but Joseph refused it because the emperor had put a condition to his offer: that Joseph convert from Judaism to Christianity.

74 Doris Marden, 'My First Memories of Queen Mary's' in *Queen Mary's Hospital 1929–2004: A Collection of Stories and Photographs to Commemorate the 75th Anniversary of Queen Mary's and the 30th Anniversary of the New Hospital*, compiled by Iris Presswell and Andrew Bamji, p. 5.

75 'Generous Gifts for Frognal Hospital', *Sidcup Times*, 26 October 1917, p. 5.

The support of the local community is also visible through the organization of fundraising events, such as a children's play in January 1918.[76]

Alongside individual initiatives, organized schemes of support developed, sometimes putting convalescent soldiers in regular contact with civilians. An active trust was run by a ladies' committee at The Queen's Hospital: the Recreation and Comforts Fund was founded in 1917 to organize entertainment, especially via the appointment and funding of a resident staff member, who was in charge of recreations and instructional workshops. Some benefactresses even got involved themselves. Essays written as part of a writing class run by one lady are still in existence; the theme was the men's war reminiscences and their writings are in fact characterized by an overwhelmingly positive assessment of experience of the front.[77] Similar initiatives developed in France, here without the overarching supervision of a committee. Baillaud reports that people came to the Val-de-Grâce hospital to teach men crafts such as basket weaving, in order to entertain them and help them regain their dexterity. Others took blind men out for walks in the Val-de-Grâce gardens.[78]

Clare writes to his mother about various events, such as cinema and concerts, organized to entertain the patients at Sidcup.[79] These events, similar to those offered to soldiers on active duty, were sometimes for patients only; yet they could also serve to bring soldiers and civilians together. Thus, the musical play 'Jig-saw' was not only shown in Sidcup town to raise funds for the hospital, but the children also gave a performance for patients and staff at the hospital. *The Sidcup Times* describes it as a success:

76 '"Jig-saw", Children's Musical Play at Sidcup in Aid of The Queen's Hospital', *Sidcup Times*, 11 January 1918, p. 5. *The Times* reports other performances in London in support of the maxillofacial hospital and attended by members of the royal family (Court Circular, *The Times*, 1 December 1917, p. 11 and Court Circular, *The Times*, 26 June 1918, p. 9).

77 'War Reminiscences', essays written by patients and now held in the Liddle Collection, Leeds University Library. The positive tone of these writings can be regarded as further proof of the difficulty to express the problems associated with the experience of war, or as suggesting that a particular discourse on war was expected from the soldiers.

78 Baillaud, Letter, pp. 8–9.

79 Clare, Letter, 3 January 1918.

patients '[followed] the play with the greatest pleasure and [were] able for the time being to forget their suffering'.[80] Clare also reports being invited to the house of a family friend who lived near Sidcup for tea, and that he was encouraged to bring another patient along.[81] At the Red Cross Kennington Hospital, the support of benefactors was acknowledged too: 'The men are happy, and are fortunate in having generous friends in the vicinity, who arrange various entertainments, as well as an outing now and then, such as a motor char-a-banc drive to Bexhill for the day – a trip which has just been arranged'.[82] Similar recreational activities were offered in other hospitals: 'The men at Norfolk Street, two weeks ago, went to Chislehurst for a picnic, being driven out there in a motor char-a-banc, provided generously by a lady'.[83] These examples testify to the support of local people, as well as to the presence of facially injured men outside the walls of military hospitals – a conscious effort, then, on behalf of the home front.

Baillaud emphasizes the support of visitors, and it seems that both military authorities and patients welcomed the help of outsiders. This apparently contradicts Rémi's account, in which she mentions that visits, especially from relatives, were strictly regulated. Considering the different national origins of the two testimonies, it could be that access to French hospitals, especially those located in the centre of cities such as Paris and Lyon, was easier than to German institutions. It is also possible that contact with families was more carefully checked due to the fact that the reactions of close relatives were very significant in the patients' recovery. Although Baillaud mentions helpers coming from outside to entertain and instruct patients, she makes no reference in her short testimony to patients venturing outside the Val-de-Grâce. Unlike passers-by, visitors and families who came to the hospital did so deliberately, usually knowing what to expect. They had a reason to go, whether it was visiting relatives or entertaining the men. The boundaries between military and civilian worlds were far from

80 '"The Jig-Saw" play at Sidcup', p. 4.

81 Clare, Letter, 3 January 1918.

82 'Hospitals for Facial Injuries', *The Official Journal of the British Red Cross Society*, p. 118.

83 Ibid, p. 118.

rigid, and documents only rarely mention instances in which men were kept inside hospitals, hidden from the rest of the population.[84]

Encounters with other people could be tense, but the relationships evolved as they grew used to the sight of injured soldiers. A film documenting the work of Albéric Pont at the *Service de Prothèse Maxillo-Faciale* in Lyon, starts with a view of the hospital, set up in a primary school, from the outside: patients stand at the windows whilst civilians pass by outside on the street, some of them staring, some of them quickly walking past. Although there is no direct contact, wounded soldiers are a visible presence.[85] Similarly, it took some time for Sidcup locals to grow used to the presence of disfigured men: 'Although not initially well accepted in Sidcup High Street the ubiquitous soldiers, with their tube pedicles hanging like sausages, were soon made welcome'.[86] Even when no direct interaction took place, the locals grew accustomed to the sight of patients: 'The servicemen were often to be seen sitting along the roadside "seeing" the outside world'.[87] In turn, patients were not systematically avoiding other people, although they did not deliberately seek contact.

A distinction should be made between encounters happening whilst patients were still in treatment, and confrontation between discharged men and society. Patients were encouraged to go out and mix with the population. The assistance of nurses, also noted by a patient at the Val-de-Grâce, gave men the practical help and confidence needed to venture outside the hospital. During short leaves, such as for Christmas, Sidcup patients who had family nearby could go and visit them. This gave them their first contact with the rest of the world whilst their identity was still

84 George Gelly, in his *Appel*, seems to support this idea without giving any specific detail about these hiding places. Paris, Bibliothèque Interuniversitaire de Médecine (BIUM) archives, Georges Gelly, *Appel en faveur du 'Foyer des Gueules Cassées'* (Etampes: Imprimerie Maurice et Cerf, 1926). Reference BIUM 156766/306–16.

85 'Service de Prothèse Maxillo-Faciale du Docteur Pont à Lyon' (film). Etablissement de Communication et de Production Audiovisuelle de la Défense ECPAD, Paris, 14,18 A 910.

86 Bingham and Moore, 'Farewell to Queen's Hospital', p. 300.

87 Marden, 'My First Memories of Queen Mary's', p. 5.

associated with that of a wounded soldier; this status entitled them to some privileges, from train and bus conductors, for instance.[88] But differences can be observed between society's attitudes to injured soldiers in wartime and in peacetime. Clare remarks: 'What kind friends the Tommy ever found in those War days. When peace came it was another story!'[89] In an essay on 'The practices of metropolitan life in wartime', Winter draws attention to changes in terms of the soldier's identity: 'When a soldier was discharged, he left his wartime uniform and gear behind, and became a civilian again. Some were not so fortunate; they never escaped from their wartime identity'.[90] This can be extended to most wounded servicemen who, as long as they were in treatment, remained combatants. Upon their return 'home', their status became more ambivalent. As long as they were patients, there remained hope for improvement. Some injured combatants wished they were not wearing 'the blues', but once they had taken them off they were no longer facially wounded servicemen in convalescence, but civilians with disfigured faces.

Marginal figures

The study of how people tried to make sense of events is a key question in cultural history.[91] In the case of First World War facial injuries, one recurring pattern that developed during and after the conflict pictures *gueules cassées* as excessive figures, whether in a positive or negative light. Newspapers emphasized the out-of-the-ordinary character of facial wounds. Most articles deal with institutional aspects of injury, such as hospitals, medical treatment, soldiers' and veterans' newspapers, support organizations or fundraisers. What the articles say is almost as significant as what they leave out, especially with regard to their portrayal of the physical

88 Clare reports being allowed on a crowded bus, and to travel without paying (Clare, Private papers).

89 Ibid.

90 Winter, 'Hospitals', p. 2.

91 Winter and Prost, *The Great War in History*, p. 29.

and psychological impact of facial wounds. These articles, alongside other publications by or about *gueules cassées*, shaped society's perceptions. They created links and influenced relationships between facially injured soldiers and those around them. In press accounts, disfigured soldiers are often described as inhuman monsters, pitiable victims or superhuman heroes.

The strong emphasis put on this 'inhuman' dimension is one key feature of depictions of facially wounded men. Sensationalism and pathos characterize most journalistic descriptions, despite the acknowledgement of an 'unspeakable' quality to facial wounds. One writer admits that 'many of the cases are beyond description'; another one highlights their haunting nature; yet another expresses the difficulty he has in writing about what he saw at Sidcup: 'I shall not talk about the operating theatres, nor the instruments, nor the gifted and untiring doctors, nor the wounds. One can imagine it all with awe and sympathy'.[92] The visual images conjured up by the mere evocation of facial injury appears to be telling enough. The only reason given to justify an attempt to put into words what the onlooker sees is said to be the hope that these images inspire:

> Any word of description of that little room, indeed, its very existence would be an unpardonable offence if it were not that the portraits and casts are made to serve a scientific and beneficient [sic] purpose, if it were not for the heartening inspiring fact that these horrors always, or nearly always, come right in the end.[93]

To the author, the positive outcome makes it acceptable to talk about facially injured soldiers. This optimistic view overlooks the disfigurement that many men were left with. In dwelling upon the state in which soldiers start their treatment, the journalist operates along the same principle as Sister Berthe, who worked with Rémi: he introduces his readers to the 'horrors' first, before talking about the men's improved looks following the treatment. The silence presented as a mark of respect has to be set against the

92 'The Queen's Hospital: Appeal for Equipment', *The Times*, July 1917, LMA HO2/Y01/05, p. 12; Robert Blatchford, 'A Holstery of Healing: I Visit a Place of Noble Men', *Sunday Chronicle*, June 1918, LMA HO2/Y01/05, p. 46.

93 'The Loneliest of All Tommies: The Man Whose Face is Shot Away and Hides From His Friends', *Sunday Herald*, June 1918, LMA HO2/Y01/05, p. 41.

profusion of descriptions of the marvels achieved by maxillofacial surgeons and, paradoxically, against the detailed and often emotional descriptions of facial injuries, sometimes in the very same articles. Journalists, while they insist upon the limitations of language, still employ many adjectives pointing to the shocking nature of facial injuries and by extension, of disfigured people themselves. The alien nature of disfigured faces is emphasized, and the mere thought of facial injury is said to trigger a mental block, as if facing *gueules cassées* was too unsettling for people, even in their imagination:

> What kind of vision does your mind conjure up when you hear or see the word 'wounded'? Probably, if you are an average stay-at-home civilian, a limping man in a blue hospital suit or, at worst, an indefinite huddled figure on a stretcher.
>
> But there are other wounded that the mind instinctively avoids contemplating. There are men who come from battle still walking firmly, still with capable hands, unscarred bodies, but who are the most tragic of all war's victims, whose endurance is to be tried in the hardest days, who are now half-strangers among their own people, and reluctant even to tread the long-wished-for paths of home.
>
> In medical language they are classed as 'Facial and Jaw Cases'. Think that phrase over for a minute and realise what it may mean.[94]

Over and above the victimization of facially injured soldiers, this article highlights the gap between them and the rest of the world. Injuries affected many *gueules cassées*' speech and sight, and their own voices and views are seldom to be heard in the press. This article points to the deliberate silence and blindness on the part of society, which tried to obliterate the existence of 'facial and jaw cases' from popular consciousness. This situation weighed on some of the men still in treatment after the war, as underlined in a 1921 article: 'what makes them heart-sick is the realisation forced on them that they are being forgotten. One of them said on Monday: "The war ended such a long time ago. We are forgotten now"'.[95]

94 'Miracles They Work at Frognal', *Daily Sketch*, March 1918, LMA HO2/Y01/05, p. 36.

95 'The Men Behind the Veil', *The African World*, 16 July 1921, p. 428.

Similarly, the French writer Georges Finaud observes in 1923 that 'no one wants to remember; now people only want wild joy'.[96] In this respect the post-war experience of disfigured veterans is shared with that of other wounded men. In wartime however, people were already trying to avoid their presence. A train journey with a patient that Rémi describes is revealing: in the crowded carriage, people prefer to stand than sit opposite her and her disfigured companion.[97] When a child enquires out loud about the reason for Lazé's disfigured face, the wounded man declares, in the silent carriage:

> Look at me, little man, take a good look at me. And don't ever forget what you have seen. This is what war is like – war is this and nothing but this. [...] Remember me always, always![98]

This scene increases the uncomfortable atmosphere created in the train by Lazé's presence. He confronts the child, and beyond him the other passengers present, forcing them to face what he describes as the true face of war. This association is also to be found in the section on facially injured soldiers, titled 'The Face of War', in Ernst Friedrich's 1924 anti-war pamphlet *War against War!*[99] The silence that follows Lazé's remark highlights the uneasiness of everyone present. Rémi notes that, although there must be people who disagree with the wounded man, no one dares to challenge him. The soldier's face is apparently too powerful evidence to be contradicted.[100]

96 'On ne veut plus se souvenir, aujourd'hui, on ne veut plus que de la joie bestiale'. Finaud, 'Les Mutilés de la Face', p. 1.

97 Rémi, *Hommes Sans Visage*, p. 96.

98 'Regarde-moi bien, mon petiot, regarde-moi bien. Et ne m'oublie jamais. Ca, c'est la guerre – la guerre, c'est ça, et rien que ça! [...] Souviens-t'en toujours, toujours!', Ibid, p. 97.

99 Friedrich, pp. 204–27.

100 This is further evidenced in a man's comments, reported by Mrs Wray in a 1920 article: 'when he saw the men he exclaimed: "My God! I've not known what the war was before!"' ('Disfigured Soldiers who are Being Well-Treated at Sidcup: 300 Shy Heroes', *Dundee Evening Telegraph*, May 1921, LMA HO2/Y01/05, p. 66).

Another facet of the marginalization of disfigured men is their frequent comparison with inhuman, monster-like creatures. It can be observed in journalistic accounts as well as in contemporary literary documents. Gelly, a medically trained professional himself, portrays the men he looks after as 'monsters, whose fates are worse than death'.[101] Terms such as the 'frightful nature of the injuries' and 'terrible cases of facial smash-up' are indicative of the fact that facial injuries trigger the need for such a description.[102] When observers do not remain silent, they provide emotionally loaded depictions of 'faces shattered beyond human semblance'.[103] The very term *gueules cassées*, widely used in France, coined and claimed by veterans themselves, suggests this de-humanizing aspect: 'gueules' do not belong to humans but to animals.

The parallel between wild beasts or monsters and *gueules cassées* is not limited to the appearance of disfigured men. Comparisons are also made in terms of attitude:

> To the victims of such grievous injury, the mental suffering is acute. They suffer frequently from terrible depression, hiding themselves in corners of hospital wards, refusing to return to home or friends in dread of the pity, or even worse, the repulsion, that they know their awful disfigurement would evoke.[104]

Hiding is presented as a dominant feature of the lives of *gueules cassées*, and the author presumes that no normal interaction can take place between them and society. A similar assumption is made in another article, which describes disgust as the instinctive reaction to injuries of a 'most revolting

101 'Monstres, dont le sort est pire que la mort', Gelly, 'Appel', section published in *Revue Odontologique de France*, 7 (July 1926).

102 'The Marvels of Plastic Surgery: a New Institution for the Treatment of Wounded Heroes', LMA HO2/Y01/05, p. 3; 'New Features for Old: Wonders of Plastic Surgery', *Morning Advertiser*, July 1917, LMA HO2/Y01/05, p. 14.

103 'Face Restoring: Wonders of War Surgery', *Morning Post* (special correspondent), January 1920, LMA HO2/Y01/05, p. 61.

104 'New Features for Old: Wonders of Plastic Surgery', LMA HO2/Y01/05, p. 14.

nature', 'rendering [the men's] appearance positively repulsive'.[105] The relatively isolated location of the Sidcup hospital is one of the reasons why it was established there, so as to spare soldiers and civilians distressing encounters: '[facially injured men] did not make good progress in the ordinary hospitals, where to be out of doors meant to be braving the streets and the pitying stares or shocked, averted looks of the passers-by'.[106]

This overview of the rhetoric of monstrosity reveals a blurring of boundaries between the wounds, the man and beyond, society as a whole. All of them appear time and again as inhuman. Joseph Roth's choice to refer to disfigured veterans as *Fratze* echoes the French *gueule* and indicates that these men have lost their humanity – the German alluding to a sight of grotesque horror.[107] The use of this term in connection with the appearance of the devil further emphasizes the degrading of men with broken faces. The 'Große Zeit' refers to a popular propagandistic depiction of wartime, and the fate of the disfigured stands in stark contrast.

Lazé's pacifist speech on the train also invests *gueules cassées* with a universal message of peace whilst the state appears to be the disfigured – morally disfigured – entity. The monstrous and inhuman quality of facial wounds extends to the pro-war people themselves. A displacement takes place, from the physical disfigurement of individuals to the moral disfigurement of warmongers.

The experience of the future president of the *Union des Blessés de la Face* Yves Picot during his first outing is indicative of people's tendency to take physical disfigurement for a sign of moral degeneration. His mangled face and his glass eye led people to accuse him of being a pervert, suggesting that society was quick to associate mutilation, especially facial wounds, with questionable ethics.[108] Evidence of the fact that disfigurement may

105 'Faces Rebuilt: New Hospital to Transform Ugliness Into Good Looks', *Daily Sketch*, July 1917, LMA HO2/Y01/05, p. 14; 'Queen's Hospital, Frognal: Marvels of Plastic Surgery', *Sportsman*, July 1917, LMA HO2/Y01/05, p. 10.

106 'Miracles They Work at Frognal', LMA HO2/Y01/05, p. 36.

107 Roth, 'Lebende Kriegsdenkmäler', pp. 347–52.

108 Yves Picot, '"Un Regard Compromettant": Histoire Véridique', *La Greffe Générale*, 7, p. 27.

still be associated today with dubious moral or intellectual ability can be observed, for example in the almost systematic portrayal of disfigured people as evil characters in contemporary film.

The popular image of the veteran as either an embodiment of evil or as a superhuman sacrifice thus needs to be questioned. Literary works and historical documents are more nuanced; it is not unusual to find accounts that combine negative personal traits with victimization or pity of ex-soldiers. Even in extreme cases in which they committed criminal actions, there is a reluctance to condemn them, either morally or legally. The trial of Léon Gardeblé, a French *gueule cassée* accused of the murder of his wife's lover, is a case in point.[109] Although the ex-serviceman admitted that he committed a crime, the portrayal made in the press of Gardeblé is positive and leads the reader to sympathize with him. His wound is described as enough to justify his acquittal: 'the mere sight of his poor face eloquently pleads in his favour'.[110] In contrast, the state as the war leader is regarded as responsible for the ex-serviceman turning into a criminal and consequently must support his acquittal: the police inspector in charge of the enquiry openly praised Gardeblé and the prosecutor's closing speech was very moderate.

The idea or motif of 'a nation indebted to soldiers' appears frequently in press articles; an example is found in one report of a visit of Albert Lebrun to the *Maison des Gueules Cassées*, the house bought by French disfigured veterans. During his visit, the French president expressed 'the nation's eternal thankfulness towards its glorious wounded'.[111] British newspapers also imply the existence of a national debt:

> Around in the cool shades of the wards lie hundreds of heroes, who have never gained a decoration, pain-racked, maimed, disfigured.

109 This case is analysed in more detail in Gehrhardt, 'World War One *Gueules Cassées* and the Ambiguity of Violence'.

110 'Le seul aspect de son pauvre visage plaide éloquemment pour lui'. Georges Martin, '"Une gueule cassée" Léon Gardeblé meurtrier de l'ami de sa femme est acquitté', *Le Petit Journal*, 7 January 1930, p. 3.

111 'L'éternelle reconnaissance du pays pour les glorieux mutilés', 'M. Albert Lebrun visite le domaine des "Gueules Cassées"', *Le Petit Journal*, 28 July 1933, p. 1.

> How can we attempt to pay an unredeemable debt? One looks about in a tumult of emotion. These men have paid their debt. They have fulfilled their part.[112]

The acquittal of Gardeblé appears as one way in which the French state repays its debt; British newspapers on the other hand appeal to British society to provide for their veterans. Readers have the power to 'lighten [the soldiers'] grey lives' through gifts of money, for example, to the Recreation Fund.[113] Most of the press articles published in Great Britain were issued between 1917 and 1918, and appeal for donations. The rhetoric they use reveals a tendency to victimize facially wounded men: 'In some respects facial injury cases are the saddest'; 'Our worst broken men'; 'So intimate and sacred, somehow, and so precious a man's face to his being that the loss of a limb – grave as it is – seems to many a trifle to it'; 'Among the many sad results of wounds, facial injuries have a particularly pathetic place' and 'The most distressing of all injuries …'[114] These examples of expressions used to describe *gueules cassées* often appear in a context that depicts their situation as hopeless, and even people close to the French *gueules cassées*' organization state that 'Their fate is worse than death!'[115] Here again the boundary between death, especially war-induced, and life, becomes blurred, underlining the transgressive dimension of facial injury.

112 'Victims of War: What You Must Do to Help our Maimed Men. Wounds of the Face: a Fund to Fight Depression and Fill Monotonous Days', *Evening Standard*, June 1918, LMA H02/Y01/05, p. 39.

113 Ibid.

114 'The Queen's Auxiliary Hospital', *Ladies Field*, January 1917, LMA H02/Y01/05, p. 7; 'The Queen's New Hospital for Treatment of Severe Facial and Jaw Injuries', LMA H02/Y01/05, p. 1; 'Worst Loss of All: Public Deeply Moved by War-Time Revelation', *Manchester Evening Chronicle*, May 1918, LMA H02/Y01/05, p. 37; 'The Queen's Auxiliary Hospital for Sailors and Soldiers Suffering from Facial Injuries' [Publication title unknown], February 1917, LMA H02/Y01/05 p. 8; 'A Home of Beneficient Surgery', *Lady*, August 1917, LMA H02/Y01/05, p. 19.

115 'Leur sort est pire que la mort!', poster entitled *Les Gueules Cassées?*, by the Comité de Propagande Lyonnais [1926?]. Péronne, Historial de la Grande Guerre, 14 AFF 54.1. A similar statement is made by Finaud, who writes that 'les mutilés de la face sont des enterrés vivants' [the facially wounded are buried alive] (Finaud, 'Les Mutilés de la Face', p. 1).

In the hierarchy of wounds facial injuries are deemed the worst of all, not only in terms of physical disfigurement, but also regarding their psychological and social impact. A similar classification is visible in all three countries. Roth writes in 1921 that in Germany, facial injuries constitute the 'most awful of all wounds'.[116] In France, Gelly notes that 'There is no worse legacy of the Great War than maxillo-facial injuries'.[117] Likewise a 1918 article claims that facial injuries are 'the rudest blow that war can deal and yet let its victim live'. As a consequence, the soldier suffers from the 'torturing knowledge of that loss' and experiences 'the ravages of loneliness'.[118] Isolation is a recurring motif, facially injured men being described as 'the loneliest of all Tommies', whilst their estrangement from family and friends is emphasized.[119]

Thus, newspapers project an image of the facially injured soldier as a victim on several counts. He is a victim of the war and its physical destructiveness upon the human body, and he embodies his country's 'wounds still bleeding'.[120] But even in peacetime, he continues to sustain daily blows: he is the victim of a society unable, or unwilling, to welcome him back. In terms of impact upon the wounded soldier, the difference between wartime and peacetime is not as significant as the difference between before and after his injury. The blurring of the border between wartime and peacetime, discussed by Stéphane Audoin-Rouzeau and Christophe Prochasson in *Sortir de la Grande Guerre*, is particularly visible in the continuity of descriptions of facially injured men as victims even after the Armistice and the Treaty of Versailles.[121]

Presenting *gueules cassées* as victims suggests a specific impact upon readers. Such descriptions aim to shape society's perception of, and

116 'Entsetzlichsten aller Gebrechen', Roth, 'Der Wiederaufbau des Menschen', p. 580.

117 'Il n'est pas de plus atroce héritage de la Grande Guerre que celui des blessures maxillo-faciales', Gelly, *Appel*, p. 8.

118 'Worst Loss of All', *Manchester Evening Chronicle*, LMA H02/Y01/05, p. 37.

119 'The Loneliest of All Tommies', LMA HO2/Y01/05, p. 41.

120 'Meurtrissures encore toutes saignantes', Gelly, *Appel*, p. 5.

121 *Sortir de la Grande Guerre: Le Monde et l'Après-1918*, ed. by Stéphane Audoin-Rouzeau and Christophe Prochasson (Paris: Tallandier, 2008).

responses to, the injured men. To construct them as victims is to imply that they represent no threat to society, but that instead they need help. If the support of their families is sometimes denied to them, society is called in to the rescue. This type of representation appeals, openly or not, to the reader's pity and compassion: 'Among our wounded sailors and soldiers none, perhaps, deserve our sympathy and compassion more than those who have suffered grievous facial injuries, in many cases of such a nature as to render them at first almost unrecognisable'.[122] Ultimately, it is the public who here comes across as heroic, helping to save the disfigured. Press publications in France and Great Britain are usually accompanied by a call for action, especially for donations to relief funds: the readers' support will 'lead [disfigured men] to realise that they are not useless wrecks'.[123] More than an expression of sympathy, supporting the injured is described as a moral obligation: it is 'the duty of the nation'.[124] Unlike in Germany, where Cohen establishes that authorities took charge and yet subsequently isolated veterans from their fellow countrymen, the British, and to some extent the French, are urged to take responsibility for the welfare of their wounded, and thus society is empowered.

Alongside their representations as victims, and sometimes in the very same articles, *gueules cassées* are also given a heroic dimension. Although a hero is a more positive image than a victim, it remains a stereotypical figure remote from reality: 'these glories who can no longer speak, these faces whose appearance transcends the human to reach a superhuman Ideal'.[125] The disfigured heroes are described in flattering terms in the press, as: 'The gallants who have suffered so cruelly on our behalf', 'Noble Men', 'Shy heroes' and 'Martyrs'.[126]

122 'The Queen's New Hospital for Treatment of Severe Facial and Jaw Injuries', LMA H02/Y01/05, p. 1.

123 'Queen and our Wounded: New Special Hospital', LMA H02/Y01/05, p. 1.

124 'Facial Injuries', LMA HO2/Y01/05, p. 3.

125 'Ces gloires qui ne peuvent plus parler, ces visages qui ont quitté l'aspect terrestre pour se métamorphoser en Idéal surhumain'.Gelly, *Appel*, pp. 8–9.

126 'A Home of Beneficient Surgery', LMA H02/Y01/05, p. 19; Blatchford, 'A Holstery of Healing', p. 46; 'Disfigured Soldiers who are Being Well-Treated at Sidcup: 300 Shy Heroes', LMA HO2/Y01/05, p. 66; Gelly, *Appel*, p. 22.

The experience of coming face-to-face with *gueules cassées* led some to express their admiration for them. The socialist journalist Robert Blatchford writes: 'One does not pity these men. One feels more like standing to attention and saluting. [...] We often say of our brave dead that they have "made the supreme sacrifice" but these mutilated heroes at Frognal have paid a higher price than life for their unselfish valour'.[127] This heroic status, bordering on that of a martyr, further isolates them from others. This rhetoric triggers, or at least aims to produce, certain emotions in society, such as pity or a feeling of indebtedness. In this respect, the authors' intentions are similar, whether playing the 'victim' or the 'hero' card. Supporting veterans appears to be the duty of a society indebted to them. It is a moral necessity.

The long-term difficulties awaiting *gueules cassées*, in medical and social terms, are also emphasized in newspapers and propaganda documents. In the mid-1920s, Gelly reminds his readers of the physical and economic struggles that veterans faced, and suggests that the gratitude French society should feel is to be channelled through financial donations to the *Union des Blessés de la Face*. Similar views were already expressed before the end of the war, for instance, in a poem written by historian Arthur Chuquet, in which he praises the *gueules cassées*' courage and holds them up as examples.[128] In this poem, the war that facially injured men are fighting against depression and isolation is described as never-ending. By supporting them, readers are given the opportunity to contribute to this new war effort. Nevertheless it remains that, like the monstrous or 'inhuman' quality of their wounds, their 'superhuman' dimension marginalizes facially wounded veterans. They constitute their own category, a group that remains isolated from the rest of society, even from other veterans. It is partly in response to this that an organization was set up in France in 1921, as will be discussed in the next chapter.

127 Blatchford, 'A Holstery of Healing', p. 46.

128 Arthur Chuquet, 'A la 5e Division de Blessés du Val-de-Grâce', *La Greffe Générale*, 6 (1 April 1918), p. 22.

Normalizing depictions

Not all newspapers sought to make veterans fit into one of these stereotypical categories. Indeed, some articles fulfil a 'normalizing' function, presenting the facially disfigured soldier or veteran as a man like any other, self-sufficient and independent, of whom society need not be afraid. This last trend shows the traditional hero/victim dichotomy to be more nuanced and reflects the less spectacular destinies experienced by most veterans. It tells of a reality more diverse than the romanticized vision of the First World War veteran that has developed throughout the twentieth century. Many contemporary accounts reveal a tendency to present *gueules cassées* as ordinary people with an extraordinary physique.

Whilst acknowledging the soldiers' desire to remain hidden, newspapers still tracked them down, entering the country hospital in Sidcup and lifting the veil on the curtained cabs in which the men travelled, as shown in a 1921 article.[129] The article takes the point of view of one of the hospital's benefactresses, who takes patients on outings. In underlining the disfigured men's humanity, this article departs from other stereotypical representations of excessive figures. Its date of publication, several years after the end of the conflict, accounts for this 'normalizing' treatment, but earlier journalistic descriptions of *gueules cassées* as ordinary men can also be found. Both their physical appearance and their mental condition are time and again presented as ordinary: 'The new surgery has not only made them able to speak and eat again. It has made them look like normal men'.[130]

Likewise, a Canadian visitor observes: 'Many are being made almost normal in appearance again'.[131] Against the unknown, and potentially frightening, dimension of the stories of men who underwent plastic surgery, the

129 'Disfigured Soldiers Who Are Being Well-Treated at Sidcup: 300 Shy Heroes', LMA HO2/Y01/0, pp. 5, 66.

130 'Miracles They Work at Frognal', LMA HO2/Y01/05, p. 36.

131 Iola Plaxton, 'A Wonderful Hospital for Injuries to Face: Mrs William Carruthers of Toronto Describes Another Feature of War Work in which Britain is Leading the World – Soldiers from Every British Dominion and Colony Benefit', *Toronto Star Weekly*, November 1917, LMA HO2/Y01/05, p. 25.

press stresses ideas of familiarity and return to a safer past. One journalist notes that 'their features are being restored to something exceedingly near their original appearance'.[132] After their treatment, many 'have returned to civil life sufficiently improved in appearance to permit of their taking their place besides their fellows'.[133] At the hospital the patient is being 'made into himself again'.[134] Not only is he physically repaired, but his identity is also presented as restored. The possibility of return to a pre-war 'normality' and of erasing the traces of the war is emphasized, as if the conflict itself could be forgotten if the scars it left were hidden.

The 'normal' physical and psychological condition of facially wounded men anticipates a successful social reintegration:

> Patients acquire their old self-respect, self-assurance, self-reliance, and discarding despondency, take more pride in their personal appearance. Their presence is no longer a source of melancholy to themselves nor of sadness to their relatives or friends.[135]

> For [Sidcup patients] have gone out into the world again with faces that stirred no atom of pitying aversion among strangers, and which their children fondled as of old.[136]

Reports about visits by well-known figures gave journalists the opportunity to present Sidcup Hospital as a peaceful and homely environment. Thus, an article about the visit of General Sir Francis Lloyd is accompanied by a photograph not of wounded patients, but of the matron Miss Barber having tea with Mrs Marsham-Townshend.[137] The *Maison des Gueules Cassées*, where some French veterans withdrew from 1927 onwards, is depicted in similar terms; one journalist underlines the pleasant surroundings comprising

132 'Hospital for Facial Surgery', *Globe*, July 1917, LMA HO2/Y01/05, p. 9.

133 'The Marvels of Plastic Surgery: a New Institution for the Treatment of Wounded Heroes', LMA HO2/Y01/05, p. 3.

134 'Miracles Worked at Frognal', LMA HO2/Y01/05, p. 36.

135 'Men Shattered in War', *Evening Standard*, June 1918, LMA HO2/Y01/05, p. 40.

136 'The Loneliest of All Tommies', LMA HO2/Y01/05, p. 41.

137 'Gen. Sir Francis Lloyd Inspects New Hospital for Tommy and Jack', *Daily Sketch*, July 1917, LMA HO2/Y01/05, p. 15.

rose gardens, playgrounds and a park.[138] Moreover, newspapers present patients enjoying ordinary activities, such as the Sidcup men who work and who play indoor and outdoor games (such as tennis and billiards).[139] Photographs published in newspapers give a sense of cheerfulness; they show 'the patients [finding] pleasure in feeding the poultry' and 'enjoying a game of bowls, in which they display considerable skill', 'the men [taking] much interest in the rabbits' and 'playing with boyish zest the good old game of leap-frog while waiting for their wounds to heal'.[140] Rather patronizing descriptions of the disfigured men contributed to lessen the impact of their potentially threatening appearance.

The sense of humour displayed by *gueules cassées* and reported in the press also contributes to their 'normalization'. The pun on the words *greffe* [graft] and *grève* [strike] included in the title of the Val-de-Grâce patients' journal *La Greffe Générale* [The General Graft] testifies to this cheerfulness, as well as comments such as those by an Irish patient reported by Gillies: 'When he saw his disfigured face [he] grinned with a peculiar pleasure. When asked what had pleased him, he replied: "Sure, I was just thinking what an easy time the barber would have in future, only half a face to shave"'.[141] This cheerfulness is interpreted by Cohen as 'not only [gratifying] donors but also [demonstrating] that victory, however terrible the price, had been worth it. No matter how badly injured, the war casualties did not regret their sacrifices'.[142]

These depictions of facially injured veterans as ordinary men implicitly suggest an easy future, and to some extent prepare for it. In presenting *gueules cassées* as normal people, newspapers demystify them. Some articles go as far as to underline the benefits of their presence within society. For example, the French *Association des Gueules Cassées* organized popular fêtes

138 'M. Albert Lebrun Visite le Domaine des "Gueules Cassées"', *Le Petit Journal*, p. 1.

139 'Miracles They Work at Frognal', LMA HO2/Y01/05, p. 36.

140 'New Faces for Old: Wonderful Work for Disfigured Soldiers', *Daily Sketch*, June 1918, LMA HO2/Y01/05, p. 40.

141 Harold J. Shepstone, 'Surgical Miracles', *Worlds Work*, 618–30 (p. 625), LMA HO2/Y01/05, p. 62.

142 Cohen, *The War Come Home*, p. 130.

and contributed to the local and national economic recovery in the 1920s and 1930s (as will be discussed in Chapter 3). It is also argued in a British newspaper that 'the establishment of this hospital at Sidcup is bound to bring much additional life to that favourite Kentish suburb, and incidentally it should increase the value of neighbouring property, and especially that of the adjoining charming estate, Sidcup Place, now called Sidcup Hall'.[143]

Journalistic descriptions of facially injured men as ordinary people echo the image that the men themselves wanted to project. This appears in *La Greffe Générale*, which aimed not only to entertain patients, but also to establish contact between them and the rest of society. This soldiers' journal targeted a wide audience: facially disfigured men, other wounded soldiers, combatants on the front and civilians. Its aim was to represent wounded men and to give society a glimpse of the cheerful spirits behind damaged faces. The self-ascribed goal of *La Greffe Générale* is to 'become the moral liaison officer between the frontlines, the rear front and the home front'.[144] This role as an intermediary is telling of the potentially difficult relationships between these three groups with different war experiences. The journal, a unique endeavour since no evidence of a similar periodical exists in other countries, testifies to the desire of French facially wounded men to take control of their public image. The authors confer a positive value on their disfigurement and by contrast denounce shirkers. According to Val-de-Grâce patients, their wounds testify to their service and their sacrifice for France, physical evidence that other men cannot boast of. The journal reveals their perception of being invested, due to their visible wounds, with a greater mission of representing soldiers and establishing a link between them and the rest of society. Paul Bäumer, in Remarque's *All Quiet on the Western Front*, notes the gap in experience between the front and the home front; but the existence of a 'huge gulf in understanding and experience' between the fighting front and the home front has since been

143 'New Military Queen's Hospital at Frognal, Sidcup, Kent', *Citizen*, August 1917, LMA HO2/Y01/05, p. 16.

144 'Devenir l'agent de liaison morale entre le Front, l'Arrière-Front et l'Arrière', *La Greffe Générale*, 1 (15 December 1917), p. 4.

questioned, for example by Matthew Stibbe.[145] The presence of mutilated men, whose bodies showed the destructive power of war, contributed to the bridging of this gap.

The soldiers' journal *La Greffe Générale* explicitly aimed to help readers understand the experience of disfigured combatants, and to prepare society to face the veterans. In 'Le Blessé dans la Rue', the author suggests that the soldiers' unsightly looks are of a temporary nature and of minor importance.[146] However, the written medium, by its very nature, misses an essential feature of the relations between society and facially disfigured men: namely the visual impact of such wounds.

Summary

For those men who withdrew from society, out of choice or otherwise, making sense of their injuries was particularly important. Failure to reintegrate into professional and social networks could mean that the war had robbed them not only of their body, but also of their place in the civilian world. This made them appear as victims of the conflict and of an indifferent, even hostile, interwar society. This latter 'enemy', as shown in this chapter, was perhaps even more difficult to fight, for it was not an unidentified weapon doing harm but a familiar face: a wife unable to kiss her husband, a father refusing to take his son back in the family business, a shopkeeper hiding his employee from the sight of customers or a passer-by looking at the veteran with repulsion.

People's perceptions of facially injured men, whether they knew them or not, covered a range of reactions from pity and disgust to admiration. What soldiers had been promised was respect and gratefulness for what

145 Remarque, *All Quiet on the Western Front*, pp. 109–28; Stibbe, *Germany, 1914–1933*, p. 38.

146 Latzarus, 'Le Blessé dans la Rue', p. 1.

was presented as patriotic sacrifice. What they apparently wanted was to be allowed to forget, claiming a right to indifference from authorities and society. Journalistic accounts, mainly with the view to fundraising on their behalf, depict them as powerless but deserving, or as heroes to whom society is indebted. National differences in terms of the journalistic treatment reveal that Cohen's assessment of the public/private veteran support divide between Germany and Great Britain can be observed in the case of facially disfigured men too.[147] Appeals for funding for maxillofacial hospitals and reports on the charitable activities run by private bodies appeared in British newspapers, urging the population to help its veterans. Whereas the politicization of German veterans is evidenced in the national press, British 'men without faces' are discussed in a more emotive tone and the support of society that they need or deserve is frequently highlighted. These sensational descriptions from the press, that of course also aims to 'sell', demonstrate a certain national attitude and often jar against the normalizing depictions of *gueules cassées* who want to 'tell' their stories, or simply to express their desire for silence. Instead, *gueules cassées* were a familiar newspaper topic for some time as journalists conveyed images that sought to inform and prepare the wider public regarding their condition. In contrast, as the next chapter will show, the *Union des Blessés de la Face* aimed for something more lasting: as a body, it fostered a sense of identity among the veterans.

147 Cohen, *The War Come Home.*

CHAPTER 3

Shaping a Collective Identity

Against the many, and sometimes conflicting, perceptions and depictions of facially injured men, an apparently unified discourse concerning *gueules cassées* gradually emerged in France. This is largely due, I argue, to the creation and rise in power of the *Union des Blessés de la Face* (UBF), an organization run by and for disfigured veterans. The existence of this support group throughout the interwar years also testifies to the emergence of new social networks. The present chapter therefore investigates the interaction amongst facially injured combatants themselves and demonstrates that these links played a significant part in their reintegration into wider society. It studies the relationship dynamics between the disfigured and explores the influence of individual leaders in the formation of the UBF, which also came to be known as *Association des Gueules Cassées*.

The relationships formed in hospital were key to the later creation of the *Union des Blessés de la Face* and the comradeship between the wounded in all three countries is the starting point of this enquiry. The UBF is, however, a unique example of disfigured men collectively shaping their public profile and claiming a place within post-war society. It has been briefly discussed by Jay Winter, who uses it as a case study in his discussion of veterans' groups as an extension of 'family' networks.[1] Sophie Delaporte, in her essay, traces the development of the UBF from its inception in 1921 to the end of the twentieth century, thus offering a useful but general overview of the history of the organization. In contrast, this chapter examines the aims and achievements of the UBF in depth, looking closely at the impact it had upon the image of *gueules cassées*, and their links with wider society in the 1920s and 1930s. The *Bulletins de*

1 Winter, 'Forms of kinship', pp. 48–51.

l'Union des Blessés de la Face, a publication that has rarely been explored, constitutes the main primary source.[2] Written and published by members of the organization, these texts present the voices of French *gueules cassées* themselves. Their agenda – publicizing the organization and uniting its members – means that they offer a positive view of the UBF and rarely mention the disagreements that occurred. Taking this bias into account, this chapter seeks to examine the image that the *gueules cassées* projected of themselves. Through their *Association*, French veterans appeared much stronger than their German and British counterparts; they became symbols of resilience and models of successful national reconstruction that society was urged to imitate.

Individual and collective dimensions of identity

Facial injuries often induce a feeling of isolation from other people. At the same time, these wounds create a special bond between fellow sufferers, described by Winter as a form of 'kinship'.[3] The visibility of their disfigurement made *gueules cassées* easy to identify, and the length of their treatment brought patients into contact with one another for significant periods of time. The personal nature of wounds affecting 'the region where the sense of self is generally located, the dominant part of the body image and the most revealing area of personality traits', makes facial disfigurement an intimate and unique experience regardless of a person's national origin.[4] The wartime military context challenged the relationship between a soldier's collective and individual experiences, and helps to explain the motivation behind the creation of the *Association des Gueules Cassées* in France.

2 These bulletins were consulted at the UBF headquarters in Paris.

3 Winter, 'Forms of kinship'.

4 Kazanjian and Converse, *Surgical Treatment of Facial Injuries*, p. vii.

'Esprit de corps' *amongst* gueules cassées

The *Bulletins de l'Union des Blessés de la Face*, published from 1921 onwards, posit the existence of a special link between facially wounded men. Friendship and comradeship are also highlighted in Rémi's account and Clare's testimony. The latter describes his first impression of Sidcup as a 'wonderful place', not least because of the 'bright congenial company', which he notes on his arrival: 'Men came round the bed to enquire about me. They all seemed just one happy family, each thinking of the other fellow's welfare'.[5]

Clare's wounds are minor but he is nevertheless recognized as part of the 'family'. This contrasts with his depiction of another hospital, Summerdown, where he does not really mix with other patients.[6] His testimony consistently describes a strong bond between 'jaw cases', however, no matter where they are. For example, when he is reunited with some of his fellow patients from Sidcup at Croydon hospital, he notes 'To my great surprise and joy I was loudly greeted on entering the ward, by familiar friends who had been at Sidcup with me. They crowded round my cot to hear my story'.[7] The very presence of disfigured men is comforting to the wounded soldier as he is amongst his peers: he belongs.

Relationships extended to men who were treated elsewhere and a friendly rivalry sometimes emerged between patients from different hospitals, for instance, in the context of games. A Red Cross report on the Brook Street Hospital, London, mentions that the patients 'have recently been given a full-size billiard table, which is appreciated immensely. From time to time they put on billiard matches with Norfolk Street, and also the Maxillo Hospital at Kennington, and prizes are usually given by a generous donor to the winning side'.[8]

5 Clare, Private papers.

6 Clare, Letter, 'Summerdown'.

7 Clare, Private papers.

8 'Hospitals for Facial Injuries', p. 118. The Brook Street Hospital for Facial Injuries was opened in 1916.

The bond between disfigured men was one that transcended hierarchical differences. Although officers and soldiers were usually accommodated in separate facilities, friendships developed between them, their wounds bridging the gap between military ranks.[9] Tensions between patients are rarely mentioned; rather, Rémi notes the help offered by seeing patients to their blind comrades.[10] Clare also emphasizes solidarity: 'All the bed 'boys' are waited on hand and foot by those of us who are "up cases"'.[11] The cheerful atmosphere at the hospital is presented by Clare as part of the men's effort to face difficult situations together, and is further evidenced by their coining of expressions for hospital life: 'The boys call going under operation in the theatre "going to the pictures" because of the effects of the anaesthetic I suppose, but they make a jest about anything!'[12] The Val-de-Grâce patients' newspaper *La Greffe Générale* [The General Graft] fulfilled a similar function of strengthening the links between facially injured men and encouraging humour. The use of humour as a weapon against depression is underlined in its first article:

> We gave you [the journal] a happy name. Show yourself worthy of your calling, but do not forget the seriousness of your mission. Out of your cheeky beak will come astonishing ideas, great jokes and monstrous puns, and all the ammunition necessary to fight our old friend the blues.[13]

9 Evidence of this spatial segregation can be found for Sidcup in 'The Queen's Hospital, Frognal, Sidcup', *The Lancet*, 3 November 1917, p. 687. Delaporte underlines the friendship across military ranks, which persisted in the UBF later and contrasts with large veterans' unions such as the UNMR or the AGMG (Delaporte, *Les Gueules* Cassées, p. 174).

10 Rémi, *Hommes Sans Visage*, p. 71.

11 Clare, Letter, 28 December 1917.

12 Clare, Letter, 3 January 1918.

13 'Nous vous avons baptisé le plus joyeusement possible. Portez donc dignement votre nom, mais n'oubliez pas pour cela la gravité de la mission qui vous est confiée. De votre bec, un tantinet gavroche, tomberont les fantaisies étourdissantes, les blagues énormes, les calembours monstrueux, toutes munitions indispensables dans la lutte contre ce vieux frère de Cafard', 'Derniers Conseils à notre Enfant', *La Greffe Générale*, 1, p. 1.

The article acknowledges the risk of depression and advocates humour and solidarity in order to fight it. A similarly good-humoured and self-derisive spirit was observed at Sidcup, as shown in Percy Clare's memoirs and in a Souvenir Programme issued by The Queen's Hospital Thespian Society on 19 December 1919.[14] The puns based upon hospital life and war injuries that it contains are indicative of a desire to laugh even about very difficult topics. A darker dimension is still present, though itself gently mocked, with the advertised play being set in 'A facial hospital in Nightmareland'. The entertainment and activities provided by outsiders and organized by patients and staff also contributed to cheer up the men and encourage friendships. Team sports in particular were available, such as football, and competitions with other hospitals were organized, strengthening the *esprit de corps* amongst facially disfigured men.

The bond between *gueules cassées* often went beyond friendship: their relationships resembled family ties. In a letter, Clare, who went home for the holiday, describes the Christmas celebrations at The Queen's Hospital:

> The people here apparently had a ripping time and the Sisters, Nurses and Officers of the Hospital spared no effort or expense to make the poor boys who cannot go home, or who have no home, perfectly happy. [...] There was a ton of good things. Turkey, Christmas puddings, jellies, custards and all good Christmas fare. Entertainments, games, and a concert each night (with Officers and Sisters as Artists), Charades, Cinema and Sketches.[15]

Likewise, during his treatment at the Charité, Karl Hasbach became close friends with a fellow patient, the Turk Sadik Seki Menduch. In 1922, he asked Seki to be godfather to his eldest daughter, thereby officially making him part of his family.[16] Their friendship had started in hospital in 1916, when the two men would go out to the theatre and on excursions together between operations. This unusual couple of wounded combatants – a Turk

14 Souvenir Programme, The Queen's Hospital Thespian Society (1919), London: Royal College of Surgeons, Gillies archives.

15 Clare, Letter, 28 December 1917.

16 Hasbach's memoirs, quoted in Weerda and Pirsig, 'Jacques Joseph und der Patient Dr. Karl Hasbach'.

wearing a white bandage across his face and a German officer wearing a black bandage – drew much attention during their outings, according to Hasbach.

The soldiers' apparent freedom of speech and readiness to share, especially regarding their wounds and the war experience, had limits however. Rémi writes that the men were always in groups and did not show their true selves.[17] Prost goes further in questioning the very existence of the comradeship that so many contemporaries insisted upon, suggesting that it was mostly a façade: 'In the veterans' world, once the war was over, there was an insistence on brotherhood, promoted as a constant element of trench life, whereas callousness and insensitivity were passed over in silence'.[18] Whether real or imagined, this 'special bond' between soldiers appears in most of the literature as a compensating feature for their traumatic experiences. In the case of disfigured men, medical staff and the patients themselves describe this 'brotherhood' as genuine and lasting.[19] The strong links between patients proved particularly important for those who experienced rejection by their families in all three countries; these bonds, however, found a unique expression in France.

The creation of the Union des Blessés de la Face

The desire of veterans to gather together is made clear in the creation of a variety of organizations during and after the war in all three countries. The reasons motivating them were sometimes political and economic, sometimes social, as an implicit understanding between ex-servicemen could arise from a shared war experience. The works of Cohen, Prost and Winter on veterans in the interwar years point to national variations in this trend. German ex-servicemen appear to have been isolated from their fellow-countrymen and highly politicized, whereas British combatants enjoyed

17 Rémi, *Hommes Sans Visage*, p. 74.

18 Prost, *In the Wake of War*, p. 22.

19 Bréhamet, *Le Colonel Picot*, p. 20.

easier relationships with the rest of society. Their support is described respectively as having come either exclusively from the state, or exclusively from private charitable sources. French veterans were between these two 'extremes'; many of them joined organizations but still maintained good relationships with the wider population. Their position, especially towards society and authorities, was perhaps less clear-cut than in the two other countries, leaving room for a flourishing of self-support organizations. It is in this context that the *Union des Blessés de la Face* was born on 2 July 1921, one of the first injury-specific organizations in France.[20]

The *Bulletins de l'Union des Blessés de la Face* provide an insight into the purpose and workings of this organization. They record the challenges faced by *gueules cassées* and their attempts to solve them collectively. Between 1921 and 1939, issues of the bulletin increased in length and frequency, from a short newsletter format to a twenty-page long document. Unlike official reports and accounts by contemporary observers, they reflect the point of view of the veterans. Written by the executive committee of the UBF, with the occasional input and contribution from other members, they follow the evolution of the disfigured men's circumstances and reveal the image that they wished to project.

The organization's official name, as of July 1921, was *Union des Blessés de la Face*, immediately followed in the first bulletin by *Les Gueules Cassées*, the name under which it became better known.[21] The strong value placed upon mutual support was stressed from the first issue. Veterans did not gather primarily to express their dissatisfaction or further any claims; rather, the UBF was set up to maintain the spirit of solidarity and one of its primary aims was to 'strengthen the friendly links born between members during their hospital treatment, maintain the spirit of solidarity that united them and establish relationships beneficial to the greater number'.[22] The members'

20 *Bulletin*, 1 (Summer 1921).

21 Bulletin, 1, p. 1.

22 'resserrer entre ses membres les liens de bonne camaraderie et d'amitié contractés au cours de leur traitement dans les hôpitaux, de maintenir entre eux l'esprit de solidarité qui les unissait et d'établir des relations profitables aux intérêts de tous', *Bulletin*, 1, p. 2 and *Bulletin*, 4 (May 1922), p. 1.

moral qualities are often highlighted, as if their facial wounds enabled soldiers to bond in a more meaningful way than in relationships based upon outward appearance. Descriptions of facial disfigurement are scarce in this first issue: 'the face hidden behind bandages and cloths', 'bruised and deformed faces but hearts intact'.[23]

The association's slogan, 'Sourire quand même' [Smile on regardless], is indicative of the founding members' will not to let their disfigurement be an obstacle to happiness. Many were in fact unable to smile due to their injury. No distinction was made between officers and normal soldiers; indeed, in the first bulletin, the organization's president Picot urges readers to reach out to disfigured men regardless of their military rank. As an incentive to expand the membership, this first bulletin states that the contribution of men who manage to recruit ten new members will be officially acknowledged. This 'propaganda' strategy, as it was referred to in the bulletin, was to remain an important feature of the *Union*, which also benefitted from the support of prominent figures such as Pétain – the organization's honorary president – and many popular artists.[24]

The *Union des Blessés de la Face* aimed to support *gueules cassées* in several areas: it endeavoured to offer political, legal, economic, social and emotional help. Although the UBF shared similar goals with other veterans' organizations, such as pension reforms, it remained distinct in its recruitment and aims, as will be demonstrated later in this chapter.

The role of individual leaders

The UBF was a self-help organization, run by and for *gueules cassées*. Despite its emphasis upon the collective, individuals often stood out and some of its members held iconic status, most notably Colonel Yves Picot. He is known as the founding father of the *Union*, and the investigation of his role in the

23 'la face masquée par les bandes et les pansements', 'visages meurtris et déformés, mais, cœurs intacts', *Bulletin*, 1, p. 2.

24 Ibid, p. 4.

setting up and running of this organization provides an understanding of its development. He is said to have coined the term 'gueule cassée', under which French facially disfigured veterans came to be known, when he was refused entrance to a patriotic fête at the Sorbonne.[25] Although Picot, still in treatment at the Val-de-Grâce, was wearing his officer's uniform and bandages, the security guard did not let him in because he did not have an official invitation. Noticing how a *Député* [Member of Parliament] was allowed in after merely stating his function and quickly showing a card, Picot waited until the guard had left, came back to the door and showed his card, muttered the words 'Gueule cassée' and went in without being stopped.

More than its meaning, it is the rhyme and similarity of 'gueule cassée' with 'député' which inspired Picot to use the term. This anecdote provides a useful symbolic narrative to describe the origins of the organization. Having been denied entrance to a patriotic celebration, the soldier's resourcefulness and boldness enabled him to take a place now acknowledged to be rightfully his. This story also creates a seminal link between Picot and the *Union des Blessés de la Face*: even if setting up an organization was not his idea, he is still accredited with a pivotal role in its genesis. The widespread use of the term *gueule cassée* by facially injured veterans also contributed to a change in the expression's connotations, as shown in the headline of an article in *The Times*, which announced '"La gueule" is now polite'.[26]

The comparative significance of Picot as an individual figure is further evidenced by the wealth of information about his life, as opposed to those of other members. The UBF commissioned his biography to be written, a mark of distinction that no other member was given. This narrative presents the French colonel as a heroic figure, yet also human and humble. It describes Picot's paternal attitude towards his fellow patients, despite the difficulties he went through during his treatment. Following his injury on 15 January 1917, he was sent to the Val-de-Grâce, where he befriended

25 This narrative is based on Picot's speech at the 1927 AGM (*Bulletin*, 17 (May 1927), pp. 12–13.

26 '"La gueule" is now polite', *The Times*, London, 12 October 1920, p. 9.

another patient, infantryman Albert Jugon. Jugon later met another veteran, Bienaimé Jourdain, and it is from this initial trio that the *Union des Blessés de la Face*, which grew to number thousands of members during the interwar years, was born.[27]

The idea of founding an association emerged at the Val-de-Grâce in 1918, as the ever-helpful Jugon was trying to cheer up his comrades.[28] He implemented his idea of an *amicale* with help from his brother (who had some legal knowledge) and from Bienaimé Jourdain, who was to become the *Association*'s general secretary.[29] It is under the former's influence that Picot came to be the organization's ambassador. Indeed Picot, although he is usually regarded as the founder of the UBF, only became involved at a later stage, when Jugon, Jourdain and a few other disfigured ex-servicemen were looking for a respected president to lead and represent the organization.[30] The involvement of Picot with the *Union* appears to be a natural extension of his wartime service: when his request to return to active service was rejected, he found other ways to serve his country and the men for whom he felt responsible.

Picot's role within the otherwise rather anonymous group, is striking. His age – he was 54 when he was wounded – meant that he appeared as a more mature figure than most soldiers. His rank and the military honours he was awarded during and after the war gave him an authority based upon experience.[31] Moreover, he took on political responsibilities, serving in the French parliament from 1919 to 1932 as representative for the *Gironde*. His position in the French government was a further asset to the UBF, opening the door for it to foster ties with the state. Picot's involvement in the debate over war pensions in Parliament from 1919 onwards shows that he was committed to upholding the rights of all veterans. He also

27 In 1929, it numbered about 5,000 disfigured men (*Bulletin*, 22 (May 1929), p. 6). It reached 8,000 in the 1930s. These figures do not include *membres bienfaiteurs*.

28 Bréhamet, *Le Colonel Picot*, p. 23.

29 Jugon and Jourdain met in a waiting room; the position the latter held at the Ministry of Pensions proved useful to publicize the organization and find new members.

30 Bréhamet, *Le Colonel Picot*, p. 24.

31 In 1933 he was awarded the title of *Grand Officier de la Légion d'Honneur*.

defended several measures designed to help war victims, including maimed ex-servicemen and orphans.[32] The fact that he was asked to lead a group of disfigured members of parliament is further evidence of the respect he gained amongst veterans in general.

Picot seems to have been unanimously admired. A poem written in his honour by Edmond du Mesnil in 1925 presents him as 'a humble hero', whilst his injuries are described positively as 'a gloriously mutilated face' and 'terrible and beautiful wounds'.[33] He was also a hero in the eyes of his fellow veterans. In 1926, the organization's vice-president Roger Brunschwig, drawing a parallel between the executive committee and Greek mythology, described Picot as the *gueules cassées'* Zeus, 'the supreme God presiding over everything and everyone's destiny'.[34] This semi-divine status thereby puts Picot on an equal footing with the surgeons; but unlike doctors, who remained remote figures, Picot belongs to the group and sets an example that others are encouraged to emulate.

Picot was also a father figure: when the *Association* celebrated its first anniversary, he was officially given the title of 'Father of *Gueules cassées*'.[35] In turn, he considered *gueules cassées* as his children, explicitly addressing them as 'my children' and welcoming their support when his own son died in 1933. This substitution is made clear at the funeral when Picot watches the coffin of his son being taken away and *gueules cassées* walk towards him.[36]

Picot was credited with many a success in the early days of the *Union*. Contemporary accounts highlight his role in securing the free provision

32 The particular political context of the drafting, debating and application of the law on pensions favoured the creation of the *Union*, as underlined by members in the first AGM (*Bulletin*, 3 (January 1922), p. 2.). The fifth bulletin underlines Picot's involvement in the writing and defence of several other laws and amendments in parliament, in particular on pensions for veterans and orphans (*Bulletin*, 5 (September 1922), pp. 10–11).

33 'un modeste héros', 'visage glorieusement mutilé' and 'blessures d'une atroce beauté', *Bulletin*, 13 (March 1926), p. 15.

34 'le Dieu suprême présidant aux destinées de tout et de tous', *Bulletin*, 16 (December 1926), p. 6.

35 *Bulletin*, 5, p. 6.

36 'mes enfants', *Bulletin*, 36 (August 1933), p. 7.

of *masticateurs*, a device that helped men to chew.[37] It was also Picot, accompanied by Jourdain and the *Union*'s medical adviser Dr Sibut, who defended the claims of disfigured veterans for a pension that took into account aesthetic damage, a claim they were eventually granted in 1925.[38] In January 1927, as the UBF celebrated the acquisition of new premises, its healthy financial situation and growing membership base, the vice-president expressed the organization's debt to Picot, declaring that 'Without him, we would be nothing' (Figure 4).[39]

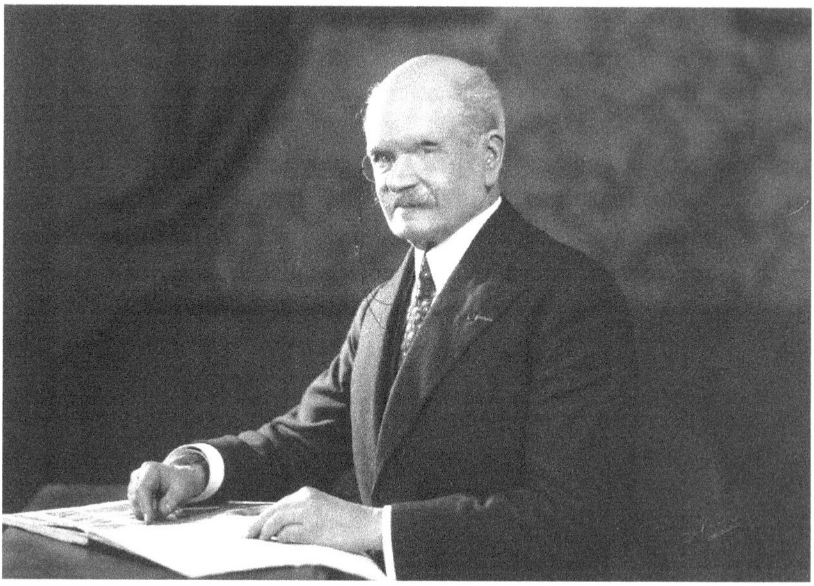

Figure 4: Portrait of Yves Picot, reproduced courtesy of Association des Gueules Cassées.

In addition to Picot's role within the *Union*, he was also a successful ambassador for the organization, for veterans more generally, and for France as

37 *Bulletin*, 6, p. 3.

38 *Bulletin*, 11 (February 1925), p. 2.

39 'Sans lui, nous ne serions rien', *Bulletin*, 17, p. 13.

a whole. Reporting on his visit to America, Brunschwig declared: 'No Frenchman has ever received such deep and unanimous admiration. [...] He is the best of ambassadors for France. [...] For us Gueules Cassées, he is the most popular representative. His mere presence makes for the best of propaganda'.[40] Picot thus conveyed the image and message of the UBF to the general public, in France and abroad. This had practical consequences, which were underlined by Jourdain in 1928: 'It is to you, my dear president, that we owe this movement of support towards the "Gueules Cassées". Your beautiful personality and your big and generous heart have galvanised magnificent energies for the benefit of our dear comrades'.[41]

When Picot was awarded the *Légion d'Honneur*, the honour was perceived as an acknowledgement of his individual achievements, but also of the organization's success.[42] Here a crucial displacement occurs: through the individual Picot, the UBF receives honour. Picot himself expressed his willingness to see his own personality merge with that of the UBF, declaring that 'it is our whole Work that is being honoured through me'.[43]

Picot's death on 19 April 1938 confirmed him as a lasting pre-eminent figure of the *Association des Gueules Cassées*. He was one of the first founding members to die, and the circumstances of his death added to his aura, as he passed away among his comrades. The special edition of the bulletin

40 'Jamais aucun Français n'a recueilli là-bas une sympathie aussi profonde et aussi unanime. [...] Il est pour la France le meilleur des ambassadeurs [...] Il est pour nous, Gueules Cassées, le plus populaire des représentants. Sa seule présence constitue la meilleure des propagandes', *Bulletin*, 17, p. 13.

41 'C'est à vous mon cher Président, que nous devons ce mouvement d'amitié vers les "Gueules Cassées", c'est à votre belle personnalité, c'est à votre cœur immense et généreux que nous devons d'avoir galvanisé d'aussi magnifiques énergies pour le plus grand bien de nos chers camarades', *Bulletin*, 21 (October 1928), p. 12.

42 *Bulletin*, 36, p. 3.

43 'C'est notre Oeuvre toute entière qu'on a voulu honorer en ma personne', *Bulletin*, 36, p. 7. A similar observation is made by Anderson on the role of Arthur Pearson and Ian Fraser in the public view of St Dunstan's in Great Britain (Anderson, 'Stoics', p. 84).

published after his death testifies to his popularity.[44] Articles retracing his life and reporting about his funeral emphasize the impact he had upon *gueules cassées* and others, and underline the necessity to keep his memory and legacy alive. His death is described as a national tragedy: many French and foreign officials paid tribute to him, as well as the anonymous crowds and the war veterans he served.[45] The presence of symbols by his coffin, such as the French flag, indicates Picot's status as a national hero.[46] Some of the objects displayed, for instance, the helmet he was wearing when he was injured, and earth and flowers picked up from the location where he was wounded, are evidence of the cult that was developing around him. Mourning for Picot extended beyond the UBF, as shown in the many services held throughout France in his memory during April and May 1938.[47] The solemn promise to continue his work that was made by *gueules cassées* reveals their determination to remain faithful to their president and follow the example that he set. Picot was buried with other *gueules cassées*, rather than in his family vault.

At first, no one was appointed to succeed Picot and all the functions of president were effectively fulfilled by the vice-president Brunschwig. This status quo was maintained for almost a year, even after the official mourning period decided by the *Union* had ended. The room where he died was kept in its original state for several months and a ceremony was held there as part of the commemoration of the first anniversary of his death.[48] Picot's role suggests that a charismatic individual was needed to represent *gueules cassées*. The development of the *Union des Blessés de la Face* in France, as opposed to other countries, thus appears to be largely due to its first president.

44 *Bulletin*, Special issue (April 1938).

45 Ibid, p. 8.

46 These elements are visible on the photographs published in *Bulletin*, Special issue (April 1938).

47 Special issue (April 938), p. 22.

48 *Bulletin*, 59 (May 1939), p. 9.

The work of the *Union des Blessés de la Face*

The role that Picot played as leader and ambassador of French facially wounded men facilitated the development of an organization that gathered over 8,000 members. Despite being limited to one category of wounded veterans, it became one of the most successful of its kind. The UBF focussed upon two areas: practical help and moral support for the veterans. In doing so, it complemented – and in some cases even took over – the economic and social functions expected from the state and from friends and family.

Meeting the veterans' practical needs

The veterans' desire to support each other remained a priority throughout the interwar years. The *Union des Blessés de la Face* set up various schemes aimed at meeting its members' practical needs, such as economic subsistence and employment.

The UBF sought to raise awareness and inform its members about their rights, through informal discussions during its regular meetings and via the bulletins. It also put forward requests, such as the freedom to choose a dentist or doctor, a right given to all other wounded. Other actions included: sending letters to the Pensions Secretary, being represented in different governmental committees and sending a delegation featuring 'a magnificent "collection of smashed-up faces", a proof of the legitimacy of their claims'.[49] On 18 July 1922, French facially injured veterans were granted the right to choose their doctor; it was however only in 1932 that they were given the free choice of their dentist and prosthetics specialist.[50] This, as well as the request for the creation of a maxillofacial centre in Paris (met

49 'une magnifique "collection d'amochés" preuve vivante de la légitimité de [leurs] revendications', *Bulletin*, 2 (January 1922), pp. 4–5; *Bulletin*, 3, p. 4.

50 *Bulletin*, 29 (June 1932), p. 4.

in December 1935), is an example of successful negotiations between the UBF and the state.

When the *Union* felt that the state was slow to meet an urgent request, it sometimes took over the responsibility for action. The provision of *masticateurs* in the early 1920s is a case in point.[51] Relationships with the state grew increasingly strained as authorities failed to respond to the UBF's request. The resolve of the *Union* was clear, however, and the executive committee eventually decided, as an exceptional and temporary measure, to help those members who urgently needed their *masticateur* to be replaced. In doing so, the UBF became a substitute for the state, although it continued campaigning until the demand was granted, in December 1922.[52]

The most significant and lasting issue, which the UBF shared with other veterans' organizations, was that of war pensions. The *Union* acted as an intermediary between *gueules cassées* and the authorities, keeping the former informed of their rights and of the administrative procedures required of them (pre-written forms were, for example, made available to facilitate individual members' applications).[53] The UBF also accompanied veterans in the legal procedures they undertook and assisted them financially, should their case be dismissed in court.

One of the initial aims of the UBF was to obtain the official acknowledgement of *la défiguration* [disfigurement] as a wound deserving a pension, regardless of any functional damage that might accompany it. In order to achieve this, the *Union* arranged to be represented at the Ministry of Pensions and to have disfigured members defending their claims in the commissions discussing such changes to the law. A decree on 5 March 1925 eventually acknowledged disfigurement as a disabling condition. This was described as a significant victory, although the application of this new piece

51 In an article (*Bulletin*, 3, p. 5), the authors stress the increase in the price of this device which, although indispensable to some *gueules cassées* who can't chew without it, is rarely paid for by the state. The UBF states its determination to see the authorities acknowledge the essential nature of this item and deliver it for free to facially injured men.

52 *Bulletin*, 6, p. 3.

53 *Bulletin*, 50 (April 1937), p. 3

of legislation was sometimes problematic. It was soon modified by another decree (20 May 1925) following the UBF's recommendations; these legal texts did not completely settle the matter, but they constituted one of the greatest successes of the UBF in the defence of its members' rights.

Throughout the 1920s and 1930s, the question of pensions remained a bone of contention in France as well as in Great Britain, as evidenced in the writings of a soldier treated at Sidcup hospital, who wrote that 'I might say I have had to fight to get my pension within anything near what it should be'.[54] A parallel can be drawn between the UBF and the British Legion, which also gave advice about pension claims to its members, and thereby contributed to maintaining less hostile relationships between veterans, the state and society, than in Germany. The role played by the UBF in channelling its members' discontent with the state was similar to the British Legion's, although its claims were more specific. The *Union*'s small membership base accounts for its success; the dissatisfaction of British veterans with their organization grew in the 1930s and led to the development of smaller and more politically active bodies such as the British Limbless Ex-Servicemen's Association.[55]

In France, parliamentary discussions around the lowering of pension rates in 1932 caused a strong response and the UBF held an emergency meeting with 800 participants on 23 October. The 'sacrifice' apparently required from ex-servicemen was perceived by *gueules cassées* as outrageous, for they considered their rights as sacred.[56] The UBF's publication from 1936 of a monthly magazine entitled *Défendons-nous* [Let us defend ourselves], devoted to legal advice, can be regarded as a response to concerns that their pensions and status were threatened. As a new war approached, the *Union* emphasized the fact that what it regarded as veterans' rights had not yet all been upheld.[57]

54 Pte Wordsworth, *My Personal Experiences and Reminiscences of the Great War*, 2, January 1922, p. 8. Liddle Collection, Leeds University Library.

55 'Our Legacy', British Limbless Ex-Servicemen's Association website <http://www.blesma.org/about-us/our-legacy/> [accessed 18 August 2015].

56 *Bulletin*, 30 (October 1932), p. 3.

57 *Bulletin*, 60 (June 1939), p. 7.

Throughout the interwar years, and maybe in reaction to shifting perceptions within French society, the UBF emphasized that veterans were not profiteers. Another facet of the organization's work was to support its members economically, so that they would not be dependent upon the state (as in Germany) or upon society's charity (a tendency observed in Great Britain). Schemes favouring the employment of *gueules cassées* were developed as part of the practical help offered, and direct financial assistance was also given. The emphasis was upon mutual support and self-help.

The UBF's aim to help its members return into employment appears clearly from its early days. *Gueules cassées* are presented as being in a worse position than other veterans, in 'a state of inferiority', and thus in need of special help.[58] The fourth issue (May 1922) denounces discrimination against them:

> If all the wounded struggle to find work, the problems faced by *gueules cassées* are without compare. The reason for this is that to the functional hindrance is added the dreadful nature of our injuries, which constitute sheer Horror … And we understand the hesitations of the employers whose forgetful customers would prefer to be served by employees with a regular smile …[59]

This article reveals no animosity between veterans and employers, for the reluctance of the latter to hire disfigured men is even presented as understandable. Against this background, the UBF sought to develop a support network for its members by means of a placement office. The organization acted as an intermediary between veterans and employers: the latter were invited to publicize offers in the *Bulletin* while jobseekers were encouraged to advertise their availability.[60] Although few offers appeared in the

58 'en état d'infériorité', *Bulletin*, 3, p. 3.

59 'S'il existe des difficultés de placement pour tous les blessés, il n'en est pas qui dépassent celles rencontrées par les "Gueules Cassées". C'est que, au degré d'incapacité fonctionnelle vient s'ajouter la nature même de nos blessures qui constitue à proprement parler l'Horreur … Et nous comprenons l'hésitation des employeurs pressés de mettre à la disposition de leur clientèle oublieuse, des employés au sourire correct …' *Bulletin*, 4, p. 6.

60 *Bulletin*, 17, p. 28; *Bulletin*, 19 (January 1928), p. 8.

1920s, more emphasis was put upon this scheme in the 1930s, and providing employment was described as equivalent to saving a comrade's life.[61] The UBF itself also employed veterans, sometimes on a temporary basis (for example on its properties at harvest-time), and gave them priority in applying for positions within the *Union*.[62]

Financial help via discounts, loans and grants was also made available. In addition to the discounts given to all mutilated veterans (for instance, by national rail services), the UBF secured offers reserved solely for its members.[63] The discount scheme enabled members to benefit from reduced prices; it also supported the businesses and professional activities of advertising members, such as the pharmacist Boesch and the mutilated artist Jeand.[64] A more organized scheme was developed in the mid-1930s, according to which members were able to buy in bulk via the *Union*.[65] From 1925, the UBF had been collecting and distributing clothes and shoes 'for our comrades in need'.[66]

Short-term interest-free loans are another facet of the financial help supplied by the *Union*. They were offered to members as an emergency measure from an early stage and in 1928, the UBF developed provisions specifically aimed to help *gueules cassées* to build or purchase a property.[67] In 1929 the group undertook preliminary actions to create a *Cité des Gueules Cassées*: a meeting with the president of the Paris city council was arranged and plans were commissioned from an architect. The financial cost put an end to this initiative. This remains as evidence, however, for the *Union*'s holistic approach, seen here in its active involvement in seeking to meet its members' practical needs. Besides this, the project testifies to the fact that

61 *Bulletin*, 50 (April 1937), p. 15.

62 See, for example, *Bulletin*, 18 (September 1927), p. 22; *Bulletin*, 21, p. 5

63 *Bulletin*, 4, p. 7 and *Bulletin*, 6, p. 10; *Bulletin*, 20 (April 1928), p. 11

64 Jeand, a singer and member of the UBF, offered to perform for veterans' organizations during their parties (*Bulletin*, 6, p. 12).

65 This concerned for example furniture, watches and perfumes. *Bulletin*, 56 (October 1938), p. 12.

66 'pour nos camarades nécessiteux', *Bulletin*, 11, p. 9; *Bulletin*, 12 (August 1925), p. 12.

67 *Bulletin*, 10, p. 3 and *Bulletin*, 21, pp. 18–20.

some *gueules cassées* wished to create a micro-community, isolated from the rest of society, and that this was in part backed by the *Union* itself.[68]

Birth, death and sickness allowances were available as a token of solidarity between members, and this system evolved throughout the years. The AGM rejected a member's suggestion to give a marriage allowance, for example, but it approved the proposal of a monetary gift to support the education of dead members' children.[69] This initiative was of both a financial and a symbolic nature. It exemplifies the inclusive policy of the organization, committed to supporting *gueules cassées* and also their families: 'Each comrade is a friend, a brother, and we propose to transfer all our caring affection onto his children after his death. This is the gesture of a man protecting his dead brother's family'.[70] No distinction is made between members in terms of military or social hierarchy. The fact that membership fees were kept low suggests that this organization intended to reach as large a membership as possible.[71]

A family structure

The UBF posited the existence of an emotional bond between disfigured men, based upon their shared suffering during and after the war. Early issues of the *Bulletin* describe a spontaneous friendship between men who have gone through similar experiences and encourage members to reach out to others.[72] This in itself was not specific to facially mutilated veterans; however, the rhetoric used in such descriptions is worth examining. The abundance of terms evoking friendship, fraternity and affection in the

68 *Bulletin*, 23 (September 1929), p. 14.

69 *Bulletin*, 21, p. 4 and p. 18.

70 'Nous vous proposons de reporter sur la tête des enfants de celui que nous considérions comme un ami, comme un frère, toute l'attention affectueuse que nous avons les uns pour les autres. C'est le geste du frère apportant sa protection aux enfants de son propre frère', *Bulletin*, 17, p. 6.

71 *Bulletin*, 15 (August 1926), p. 5.

72 *Bulletin*, 4, p. 1.

first bulletin is evidence of the founding members' desire to give a family feel to their organization. Veterans were encouraged to nurture a similar ethos of comradeship and bonding in the post-war civilian world as they were on the front.

Moral support was presented as the first mission of the UBF and regular meetings provided an opportunity for men to get together and socialize. Making it possible for *gueules cassées* to stay in contact even after the war, and to develop new friendships, was presented as the *raison d'être* of these meetings. New participants were made welcome: 'Those who attend our meetings for the first time are always struck by this spirit of excellent friendship shown by all. Here, we are "at home" ...'[73] This familiar environment contrasts with the isolation experienced by many other veterans, as shown for instance in paintings by Otto Dix and Max Beckmann (discussed in Chapter 4).

More than camaraderie, the UBF proposed to create a second family, or even substitute family, for *gueules cassées*. The fact that the origins of the organization lay in the war was openly acknowledged and this military background featured prominently, especially during its first years of existence. Members awarded medals were mentioned in the bulletin and *gueules cassées* were said to have earned their honours, like the *Légion d'Honneur*: 'your superb "gueule cassée" will be ample and admirable proof of your right to wear the *Légion d'Honneur*'.[74] Mutilated veterans are urged to be proud of their faces, presented as a visual testimony to their sacrifice on the battlefield. *Gueules cassées* campaigned to be awarded the *Légion d'Honneur* as a military award and not as civilians, thus in effect distinguishing themselves from people who had not been to the frontline. Despite this apparent hostility towards civilians, the UBF was well-anchored in civilian society. Their war experience was what united the *gueules cassées*, but unlike many other veterans' organizations, the UBF was inclusive

73 'Ceux qui, pour la première fois, viennent à nos réunions ne manquent point d'être frappés par cet esprit d'excellente amitié manifestée par tous. L'on y est "chez soi" ...', *Bulletin*, 4, p. 4.

74 'votre superbe "Gueule Cassée" témoignera hautement et fièrement de la légitimité d'arborer la Légion d'Honneur', *Bulletin*, 3, p. 5.

and sought to integrate its members' families into the *Union*. Bulletins announced weddings, births and deaths, the family news section growing bigger as the membership increased. Wives were invited to attend some of the meetings and holiday camps were organized for children.[75] Once the *Maison des Gueules Cassées*, in Moussy, had been purchased, large summer camps were run there, as the *Union* sought to entertain the children and to provide them with nourishing food.[76] In 1933, a second summer camp project started, aiming particularly to send sickly children to Le Havre near the seaside, and later to Le Coudon (a UBF property in the South of France), Wimereux, Sainte-Adresse, La Bourboule and Bielle.[77]

Annual gatherings such as Epiphany, Easter and Christmas parties also took place. On 15 January 1928, over 600 members and their families celebrated Christmas together, and children were given presents.[78] Likewise, several members are reported to have spontaneously gathered in the house belonging to the *Union* on Easter Day 1928, a 'true family gathering'.[79] Members' wives got involved, for instance, by knitting clothes for other members' children, especially orphans.[80] Two of the latter were baptised in Moussy, and godparents were chosen among *gueules cassées* and their wives, further emphasizing the familial dimension of the UBF.[81]

75 *Bulletin*, 8, p. 2. The idea was first mentioned in 1924, when ten children were sponsored to spend a few weeks in the countryside (*Bulletin*, 10, pp. 7, 10).

76 *Bulletin*, 17, p. 6. Tables including the development of the children's weight were published (*Bulletin*, 21, p. 3).

77 *Bulletin*, 34 (June 1933), p. 8. A similar interest in children's health is evidenced in the initiative, in 1935, to arrange for sickly children to stay in one of the following spa towns: St-Gervais, Vichy or La Bourboule (*Bulletin*, 41 (May 1935), p. 8). On Wimereux, see *Bulletin*, 52 (October 1937), p. 4. See also, *Bulletin*, 61 (November 1939), p. 10.

78 *Bulletin*, 19, p. 5. Similar meetings were organized on a smaller scale for members living in Marseille and Nancy (*Bulletin*, 19, p. 7).

79 'véritable réunion de famille', *Bulletin*, 20, p. 7.

80 *Bulletin*, 45 (January 1936), p. 4.

81 Ibid, p. 13.

The Maison des Gueules Cassées*: A home for facially disfigured veterans*

The UBF's vision of itself as a family, especially for those who did not have a family to go back to after the war, finds its most obvious expression in the setting up of a 'home'. From the start, the founders had envisaged the purchase of a place where *gueules cassées* could come and stay. This project is first explicitly mentioned in June 1923 by Picot.[82] A fundraising campaign started in 1925 and the purpose of the *Maison* was explained in more detail: it was to be a place of calmness and cosiness where disfigured men could spend the rest of their days.[83] The isolation of some *gueules cassées* within society was underlined, thereby emphasizing the gap between veterans and those around them; the setting up of a house that would function as a shelter was thus presented as the answer to this problem.[84] The project also had a symbolic dimension: it was to be a material symbol of the bond among *gueules cassées* and the means through which the thankful nation's gratitude could be expressed.[85] Interwar society was both blamed and praised. Its failure to accept and reintegrate mutilated men was pointed out, whilst at the same time it was described as full of noble sentiments towards veterans, which they were urged to channel into gifts of money.

Obvious benefactors were individuals, professional unions and veterans' organizations, but other donors included children and groups of students, employees and whole villages.[86] The *Maison* project seems to have been supported by all these groups, and the UBF comes across as a well-integrated association. The messages accompanying gifts of money tell touching stories of children giving up sweets to make a donation, women expressing their gratefulness to the veterans and people collecting money at a family party and a wedding. Donations from abroad are also recorded, underlining the international visibility of the UBF. Several foreign benefactors are mentioned in the *Bulletin*, from French colonies (Saigon,

82 Yves Picot, 'Anniversaire', *Bulletin*, 7, p. 1.
83 *Bulletin*, 11, p. 6.
84 *Bulletin*, 11b, p. 5.
85 *Bulletin*, 11, p. 6.
86 Ibid, pp. 6–8.

Morocco, Algeria) and other countries (Belgium, Great Britain, the United States, Australia, Canada, Argentina).[87] The largest donations came from an American woman, Mrs Strong, who gave over 500,000 Francs in 1926 and another 850,000 Francs in 1927.[88] Many gifts were the result of individual initiatives (through door-to-door collections or fundraising events). Press articles and posters were also used. Some of them gave rather dramatic portrayals of the lives of *gueules cassées*, a far cry from the otherwise largely normalizing discourse perpetuated by the UBF.

Amongst the *Maison* project's most fervent advocates was the Dental School registrar Georges Gelly. Although not a *gueule cassée* himself, Gelly took an active part in the running of the UBF from the mid-1920s onwards, in particular offering technical advice. A booklet he wrote as part of the campaign for the *Maison* testifies to his commitment. Despite Gelly's medical background, his pamphlet passes over scientific considerations to focus upon the psychological and social impact of facial wounds, thereby forming an emotional appeal to the readers' sense of duty and compassion. His descriptions oscillate between victimization, insisting upon the need to provide a shelter where veterans could withdraw, and normalization, stressing in turn the temporary dimension of convalescent stays, a stepping stone for men returning to their families and to work.[89] Gelly's use of photographic representations stands out, such visual aids being rarely used in communications emanating directly from the UBF (e.g. bulletins and posters). His medical background and the fact that he was not disfigured himself may account for his greater readiness to display wounds since 'The portraits of these unfortunate mutilated men say more than a long speech; they constitute the most impressive epic films as they faithfully reproduce the painful consequences of war'.[90]

87 See, for example, *Bulletin*, 12, p. 10; *Bulletin*, 15, p. 8; *Bulletin*, 21, p. 12.

88 Jean Bertholllin, 'La Maison des "Gueules Cassées"', *Le Gaulois*, 21 June 1927, p. 1; *Bulletin*, 16, p. 8.

89 Gelly, *Appel*, p. 3.

90 'Ces portraits de malheureux mutilés en disent bien plus que n'importe quel long discours, ils constituent les plus impressionnants films épiques, puisqu'ils reproduisent fidèlement les séquelles douloureuses de la guerre', Ibid, p. 26.

In 1926, suitable premises were found in Moussy-le-Vieux, but funding remained an issue, with an estimated cost of 700,000 Francs when the *Union* had only 400,000 Francs.[91] Fundraising efforts, which had started in 1925, intensified in 1926. Readers were encouraged to send suggestions for the workings of the house, underlining the collaborative and collective dimension of the enterprise.[92] Members were also invited to donate pieces of furniture, and gifts included books, clothes, hunting equipment, beds, ashtrays, bottles of champagne, cleaning products, and crockery and linen donated by Hotel Ritz.[93] The UBF later secured the cooperation of department stores in furnishing the house, showing the large support it gained in France.[94]

The castle of Moussy-le-Vieux was purchased on 2 August 1926 and this acquisition was announced in the December bulletin, titled 'Notre maison' [Our home], which was largely devoted to this news. The property is described as a 'smiling oasis where those who suffered most from the Great War, yet gloriously survived, can find a welcoming retreat [...]'.[95] An idyllic depiction is also given by Gelly in his *Paradis des gueules cassées* [The Gueules Cassées' Paradise], in which he forecasts the admission of fifty men into this Eden (also paradoxically described as 'the Monsters' hell').[96] Residents are promised the advantages of family life without losing their independence, but only sixteen men were living there by 1928.[97] This number did not vary much, and in 1930 the UBF expressed some disappointment, reiterating that 'We often think of those who wander aimlessly, deprived of joy and satisfactions of any kind, victims of a pathological instability, and who could come to this home where true friendships can be

91 *Bulletin*, 15, p. 3.

92 *Bulletin*, 16, p. 6.

93 Ibid, p. 8.

94 *Bulletin*, 17, p. 11.

95 'Une souriante oasis où les plus éprouvés et les plus glorieux rescapés de la grande tourmente trouveront une accueillante retraite', *Bulletin*, 16, p. 3.

96 'L'enfer des Monstres', Georges Gelly, *Le Paradis des Gueules cassées* (Etampes: Société régionale d'imprimerie et de publicité, 1926), p. 2 and p. 13.

97 *Bulletin*, 21, p. 11

found …'[98] Despite this pessimistic picture, the small number of residents suggests that most disfigured men had settled back into their families and did not wish to live in an isolated community. On the other hand, temporary residents and holiday visitors were numerous. Moussy thus appears to have been a welcome addition to the lives of most *gueules cassées*; it became a place where they enjoyed spending time, sometimes with their families. The *Maison des Gueules Cassées*, like the UBF, seems to have supplemented the social circle that most veterans already enjoyed.

The *Maison* not only helped to cement relationships between *gueules cassées*, but also to integrate them into French society more widely. The first group of *gueules cassées* visited their new home on 11 November 1926, when the UBF committee organized a trip to Moussy to celebrate the Armistice there.[99] This event is presented as a spontaneous decision to honour the local soldiers who died on the front and to meet the local population. The tribute the veterans paid to the fallen men from Moussy, alongside the local population, symbolically integrated them into the community; they to some extent 'replaced' the dead.

The *Maison des Gueules Cassées* was officially opened on 20 June 1927, the same year the UBF was granted the status of a state-approved organization (*association reconnue d'utilité publique*) The significance of this event, and indeed of the *Association* itself, was made clear by the presence of the French President Gaston Doumergue and of several high-ranking officials at the opening. In his address, Picot drew a parallel between disfigured men and the nation as a whole, portraying both of them as beacons of hope.[100] *Gueules cassées*, he argued, showed the way to their fellow countrymen, and France was to guide the world on the path of peace. In his response, Doumergue underlined the heroism of *gueules cassées*, 'the disfigured champions who shed their blood for the homeland and now will contribute to

98 'Nous pensons souvent à ceux qui errent sans but, sans joies, sans satisfactions d'aucune sorte, en proie à une instabilité maladive et qui pourraient venir là dans ce foyer où des amitiés sincères les attendent …', *Bulletin*, 26 (November 1930), p. 7.

99 *Bulletin*, 16, p. 5.

100 *Bulletin*, 18, p. 1.

making it more fertile, in the farm that adjoins their house'.[101] The veterans' past achievements are considered, but their contribution to France's post-war prosperity is also highlighted: *gueules cassées* are presented as active agents of national reconstruction. The gathering of over 2,000 people (500 of whom were members) ended with a concert featuring popular artists such as Sacha Guitry and Beatrix Dussane. The wide media coverage given to the inauguration of Moussy further increased the popularity of the UBF.

The question of the purpose of the house – whether it was to be a place of temporary or permanent stay – was discussed in several articles reporting the opening ceremony. A three-fold purpose emerged: it was to offer permanent residence to those men whose condition prohibited them from returning to work, temporary accommodation for veterans who had to undergo operations, and an affordable holiday destination to all members. The advisory group underlined the fact that inhabitants were not to be inactive and that in providing men with work suitable to their abilities, the UBF would relieve the state of their support.[102] Throughout the 1930s, visitors to the house were numerous, and included the press and officials. The French Presidents Doumergue and Lebrun went to Moussy, as did several Pensions Secretaries, usually accompanied by journalists.[103] The photographs that immortalized these events function as visual evidence of the integration – not so much of individual *gueules cassées*, but of their organization – within French society, represented by its statesmen.

In March 1934 the purchase of another property, Le Coudon, in the South of France, is mentioned.[104] The UBF justified the acquisition of this second *Maison* as a quantitative and qualitative necessity: another house was needed to accommodate all the UBF members who wished to come and visit, and the Mediterranean climate would be an added benefit for

101 'Ces défenseurs défigurés qui, après avoir arrosé le sol de la patrie de leur sang, vont contribuer à le rendre plus fertile dans une ferme attenante à leur "Maison"', speech by Gaston Doumergue, 1927, quoted in Berthollin, 'La Maison des "Gueules Cassées"', p. 1.

102 *Bulletin*, 11b, p. 7.

103 *Bulletin*, 34, p. 1.

104 Ibid, p. 7; *Bulletin*, 38 (Spring 1934), p. 4.

the wellbeing of convalescent and ageing veterans, as well as for children on holiday.[105] The inauguration ceremony of this second property, on 21 September 1936, is not described in as much detail as that of Moussy. It was less spectacular, despite the presence of politicians and military officials, including Pétain, the organization's honorary president. The economic and political climate of the mid-1930s, the fact that Le Coudon was not the first property, and its status as holiday residence, are possible reasons for this.

A change can therefore be noted between the mid-1920s and the mid-1930s, when the two properties were opened. The success of the first campaign shows the popularity of the *Union des Blessés de la Face* in French interwar society, even beyond national borders. The situation was different ten years later, when Le Coudon was purchased. Although gifts of money were still received, it appears that the UBF depended largely on its own resources to finance this new project. As in other countries, French ex-servicemen denounced society's forgetfulness of the debt they owed to the veterans, and reacted against the sometimes-scornful attitude that could be increasingly observed towards *gueules cassées*.

Publicizing the collective image of *gueules cassées*

The *Union des Blessés de la Face* participated in the definition of a collective identity for disfigured veterans and shaped society's perception of *gueules cassées* throughout the interwar years. This section explores the image promoted by the UBF, the ways in which it was publicized, and its impact upon the relationships between *gueules cassées*, interwar society and the state.

The image promoted by the UBF

The *Union des Blessés de la Face* sought to project the image of a united group. Divergent opinions were occasionally voiced as the organization

105 *Bulletin*, 38, p. 8.

grew in size but such occurrences were infrequent; this suggests that there was little disagreement, or that disputes were stifled.[106] Amongst the significant features of the collective image promoted by the *Union des Blessés de la Face*, it is worth noting the emphasis upon the organization's depiction as a distinctive but integrated group, its self-reliance, and its attempts to help other veterans.

Two paradoxical trends emerge in the self-representation of *gueules cassées*: *Bulletins* highlight both their distinctiveness from society and from other veterans, and the fact that they belonged to both these social circles. From its early days, the UBF developed links with other organizations, for example the *Fédération Nationale des Anciens Militaires* and the *Union Nationale des Combattants*.[107] *Gueules cassées* joined in shared initiatives, despite some concerns that the groups should remain completely separate. Similarly, the participation of the UBF in a committee that gathered the leaders of the main veterans' organizations was announced in 1925, as the *Union* expressed its wish to see the creation of a permanent overarching body to defend the claims of all war victims.[108] But it was only in 1937 that a larger committee defending the rights of all the wounded was born: faced with increasing difficulties, small organizations sought to join forces. These examples show the integration of the UBF into a network of veterans' organizations in France and, to some extent, on an international level. On the other hand, the distinctiveness of the *Association des Gueules Cassées* was also emphasized, and this accounts for its refusal to merge with larger groups, in which its relatively small number of members would have rendered it almost powerless. A similar distinct-but-integrated image emerges in relation to society at large. The UBF acknowledged the popular support they received: 'we had the great pleasure to see the large and generous movement of support towards our growing association'.[109] Through their organization, *gueules cassées* were collectively integrated, as

106 *Bulletin*, 18 (July 1927) for example reports the rejection of two motions, by Oddou and Labbé at a members' meeting (pp. 15–16).

107 *Bulletins* 5 and 6 mention these links, for instance, through the presence of representatives at the UBF's general meetings.

108 *Bulletin*, 11b, p. 2.

109 'Nous avons eu la joie très douce de constater un large et généreux mouvement de sympathie en faveur de notre groupe naissant', *Bulletin*, 7 (June 1923), p. 1.

shown in the success of the fundraising campaign for the house and of the UBF's participation in the national lottery.

The UBF was also keen to foster an image of self-reliance and independence, especially in economic terms. Members were encouraged to help themselves and each other. The work placement system is evidence of this attempt to enable veterans to be reintegrated into the employment market. Likewise, the way the sickness allowance was distributed illustrates this policy of encouraging self-reliance: payment only started after thirty days to encourage members to attempt to support themselves before requesting help from the *Union*.[110] On a collective level, the UBF developed a range of fundraising methods to guarantee its economic survival. Although it relied upon donated money, Picot declared: 'It is because we have proved that we are worthy that so many people have helped us. [...] Lazy people should not receive any help. The members of the *Association des Gueules Cassées* are not lazy'.[111]

In particular, the UBF presented itself as not being reliant upon the state and avoided making requests for public funding.[112] In 1935, Picot pointed out that the UBF was a 'work of solidarity that, when it can and when its members are concerned, often substitutes itself to the *Office national des Mutilés* (the state agency in charge of the war wounded). In doing so, we relieve the state of some of its burden without asking for funding in exchange'.[113] *Gueules cassées* presented themselves not as helpless victims, but as men capable of providing for their own needs. This image in turn had a positive influence on society's perception of them.

110 See, for instance, *Bulletin*, 18, in which the 30 days delay is contested by a member (pp. 8–9).

111 'C'est parce que nous avons prouvé que nous valions quelque chose que des gens de cœur nous ont aidés. [...] On ne doit pas aider des paresseux. L'Association des Gueules Cassées n'est pas une Association de paresseux', *Bulletin*, 18, p. 16.

112 Speech delivered by Colonel Picot, 27 July 1933, in *Bulletin*, 36, p. 6 (emphasis in the original text).

113 'Oeuvre de solidarité qui, dans la mesure de nos moyens et pour ce qui concerne nos membres, se substitue dans bien des cas à l'Office national des Mutilés, dont nous soulageons ainsi un peu les charges, sans solliciter de subventions en échange', *Bulletin*, 41 (May 1935), p. 4.

In order to be economically self-reliant, various fundraising methods were used throughout the 1920s and 1930s. Events such as concerts and galas were organized across France, sometimes with the participation of renowned artists. One of the most famous events was a fête at the Stade Buffalo in Paris, on 21 June 1926: the programme featured sporting competitions (cycling, fencing, athletics and boxing) and acrobatic displays. The presence of the French President bears testimony to its importance, as does the participation of other political personalities and celebrities. As the show started, one hundred and fifty veterans marched together in the stadium; this indicates that they did not fear appearing in public as a group.[114] A number of other fêtes, galas, and artistic and sporting performances were held, particularly during the fundraising campaign for the *Maison*. These events, such as the 'gala de la Reconnaissance', organized to express the nation's gratitude in 1927, are described in the bulletins as symbols of society's gratitude.[115]

In 1930, however, the UBF faced a deficit for the first time in its history.[116] Acknowledging the need to raise a large amount of money to secure its future, it launched a national lottery subscription called *La Dette* [The Debt]. Several factors account for the success of this initiative.[117] Firstly, it offered numerous prizes, ranging from bicycles to cars and small airplanes. Secondly, its endorsement by officials and celebrities contributed to publicizing the subscription, as did the active advertisement campaign led by the UBF. The campaign started in April 1931, when Picot gave the first ticket to President Doumergue as he was visiting Moussy. This launch gave credit to the enterprise and guaranteed maximum publicity. Posters were also produced, featuring striking visuals of *gueules cassées* (Figure 5).

114 *Bulletin*, 15, p. 1 and p. 9

115 *Bulletin*, 18, p. 12.

116 *Bulletin*, 27 (November 1931), p. 17. The difference between income and spending exceeded 500,000 Francs.

117 *Bulletin*, 30 (October 1932), p. 1. *Bulletin*, 31 (November 1932), p. 14.

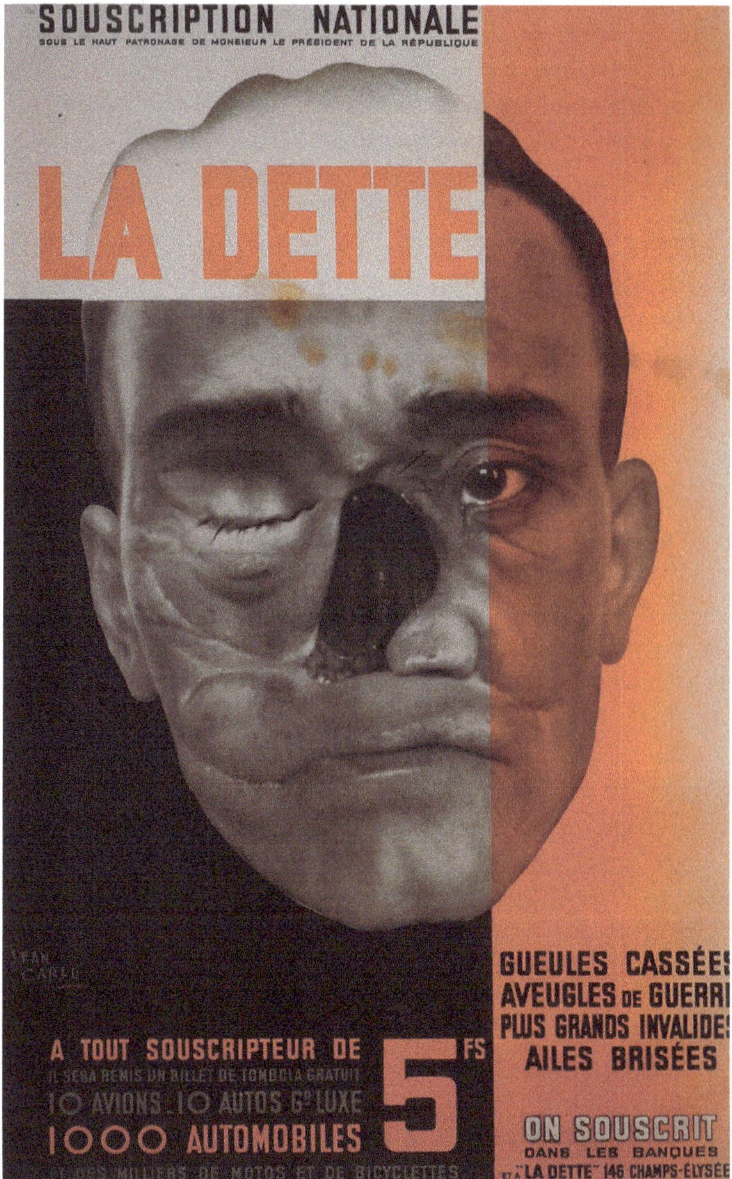

Figure 5: Jean Carlu, *La Dette* poster (1931?) © ADAGP, Paris and DACS, London 2014. Digital image, Historia de la Grande Guerre, Péronne.

In this poster, as in others publicizing *La Dette*, the focus is on the image and on the words *La Dette*. The name suggests that society is indebted to the *gueules cassées:* they suffered in defence of French people and deserve their support. The public are now given the opportunity to repay the soldiers, at least in part. The poster by Jean Carlu, then already a well-known artist, is modern in its design. The only colour, red, cannot but remind the viewer of the blood shed on the battlefield, whilst the main visual element is the face of a disfigured man, detached from its body. Part of the face is intact; the other half, which stands out against the black background, is damaged and evokes death. The overall impression is not one of pathos but of heroic sacrifice, thus further highlighting the idea that society is indebted to veterans.

This large-scale public subscription was a financial success, bringing in thirty-nine million Francs by February 1933.[118] This success encouraged the UBF to take part in other similar schemes, such as a sweepstake with the Luxembourg Red Cross in 1933 and various lotteries in 1935 and 1936.[119] However, the *Union*'s main source of income in the 1930s was the national lottery. Although this partnership only started in the mid-1930s, it secured the economic future of the group and helped to make the UBF one of the richest organizations in France, thus establishing it as a powerful veterans' association within French society.

The UBF's involvement in the French national lottery started on 22 October 1935 and it was immediately presented as a durable source of funding.[120] *Gueules cassées* began selling *Dixièmes*, worth a tenth of the value of a lottery ticket, as soon as a decree allowed the sale of fractioned tickets. Reactions to this initiative were mixed. Some veterans expressed concern that it could damage the reputation of their organization, and other groups involved in the lottery did not welcome this 'competition'.[121] The sale of *Dixièmes* was also initially criticized by other veterans' organizations.

118 *Bulletin*, 30, p. 8.

119 See *Bulletin*, 37 (December 1933), p. 14; *Bulletin*, 38, p. 8 and *Bulletin*, 39 (December 1934), p. 27.

120 *Bulletin*, 45, p. 11.

121 *Bulletin*, 48 (October 1936), p. 7.

However, by October 1936, the national lottery had become the *Union*'s main source of income.[122] Tensions eventually diminished and other groups, such as the war blind and the war amputees, joined in the venture.[123] The economic success of this operation may have helped to make the fundraising method more acceptable, whilst at the same time the popularity of the UBF gave greater credit to the lottery as a whole. The purchase of *Dixièmes* was presented to the general public as a charitable action: 'our tickets have a greater moral value in the eyes of the buyers who, whilst legitimately seeking a gain, feel that they are also supporting the group that went through the greatest suffering and represents the greatest sacrifice'.[124] By 1937, the survival of the UBF was largely dependent upon the success of this fundraising method.

In assessing the participation of the UBF in the development of the French national lottery, both the financial benefit and the impact in terms of the image of the *gueules cassées* need to be taken into account. Despite initial resistance, the sale of *Dixièmes* empowered the UBF, by increasing their income and presenting it as an entrepreneurial organization. This scheme turned men who were regarded as the worst-off of all war victims into a group that was financially independent, even prosperous. But in turn other, more personal, fundraising methods were largely abandoned, thereby again increasing the distance between *gueules cassées* and society at large.

In finding innovative ways to raise funds, the *Union* established its reputation as an independent organization and as a group that sought to help others. This is a far cry from images of helpless victims and distant heroic figures. French facially disfigured men remained the main beneficiaries of the UBF in the interwar years; however, the *Union* also supported other veterans. In doing so, it became increasingly integrated into wider

122 Ibid., p. 12.

123 *Bulletin*, 50, p. 5.

124 'Notre émission prend une valeur morale plus grande encore, près des souscripteurs qui ont le sentiment, en prenant notre billet, tout en recherchant légitimement la fortune, de soutenir le groupe qui représente la plus grande souffrance continue et le plus grand sacrifice consenti au pays', *Bulletin*, 51, p. 6.

society and it reinforced its image as a thriving organization, able and keen to benefit society as a whole.

The UBF sought to help other mutilated veterans both at home and abroad. A bulletin published in 1927 describes the difficulties faced by Belgian *gueules cassées* and considers the problems that arose due to the absence of a support organization in their country.[125] This article also mentions The Queen's Hospital and presents it as the British equivalent of Moussy, although evidence shows that in 'Sydcup' [*sic*] facially injured soldiers were no longer being treated. The UBF apparently believed that British soldiers had developed a similar structure, suggesting that little contact existed between them. The French organsiation maintained closer contacts with veterans in Belgium and, to a lesser extent, Italy. Relationships between French and Belgian ex-soldiers increased through the action of the *Comité maxillofacial de Secours Français* (a French committee set up to help people with maxillofacial injuries). This structure offered to subsidize medical consultations for Belgian patients, who had no access to such facilities in their own country.[126] The release of *Pour la Paix du Monde* [For Peace in the World] in Belgium in 1927, a film supported by the UBF, led to the organization of several fundraisers for the benefit of Belgian veterans. Although the participation of the UBF in these events enabled them to collect gifts for themselves, their main motivation is said to have been altruistic.[127] The support given by the UBF to other veterans' organizations is best seen in their inclusion of different injured men's groups in tombola and lottery schemes. *Gueules cassées* invited three other *associations* to participate in a tombola in 1931, in an early attempt to guarantee the future of their four respective organizations.[128] As a group, disfigured veterans fared better than many others, depicted in the *Bulletins* as 'Comrades who are less fortunate'.[129] The *Union* also welcomed children of other organizations' members to its summer camps, and by 1939 eighteen other associations

125 *Bulletin*, 17, p. 21.
126 Ibid, p. 22.
127 *Bulletin*, 19, p. 7.
128 *Bulletin*, 27, p. 10.
129 'Camarades moins heureux', *Bulletin*, 27, p. 18.

benefitted financially from the participation of *gueules cassées* in lottery operations.[130]

Ultimately, the *Union* came to present itself, and to be presented by others such as journalists and officials, as examples for the whole of society to follow. With the help of their organization, *gueules cassées* became the epitome of patriotism and strength in times of adversity. The image projected by the UBF shows veterans to be at the forefront of moral and national reconstruction. A journalist reporting on the successful rehabilitation of Moussy castle and arable land, commented:

> Indeed, after the example of courage and heroism they set for the whole country to follow in the war, this [the successful rehabilitation of Moussy] is the most fruitful and productive lesson the facially wounded could have given the country in peacetime.[131]

Although *gueules cassées* are often referred to as victims, in this *Bulletin* they appear to have rebuilt their lives. The author praises their entrepreneurial spirit. Their relative seclusion does not come across as isolation, but instead is depicted as a model of successful return to civilian life and of fruitful contribution to national recovery. Far from powerless, *gueules cassées* project their image as an influential group, independent and prosperous. And in the course of the 1920s and 1930s, they indeed became benefactors rather than recipients of charity.

Publicizing gueules cassées

The positive collective image of *gueules cassées* shaped by the UBF was publicized and refined in the course of the 1920s and 1930s. Both long- and

130 *Bulletin*, 56, p. 7; *Bulletin*, 60, p. 1.

131 'C'est, en effet, après la leçon de courage et l'exemple d'héroïsme qu'ils ont donné au pays pendant la Grande Tourmente, le plus fécond et le plus efficace des enseignements que les blessés de la face pouvaient lui donner pendant la paix', *Bulletin*, 27, p. 14.

short-term initiatives took place, aimed at raising the public profile of the UBF, and they often propelled the veterans into the limelight.

Long-term schemes relied mainly on two groups: *gueules cassées* themselves and the media. From the very beginning, members were urged to make the organization known, firstly to other mutilated veterans and then to potential patrons. Virtually every issue of the *Bulletin* features what is called the 'propaganda' section. At first, the emphasis was upon reaching out to all facially disfigured veterans, portrayed as desperately in need; introducing them to the UBF was the duty and responsibility of every member. The appointment of regional delegates from the mid-1920s onwards further contributed to the publicization of the *Union*. These local representatives coordinated outreach efforts in their regions, making use of the press and organizing local events. But more than the economic gain from an increasing membership, it was the symbolic power of a larger group and the legitimacy of the UBF as representing all French *gueules cassées* that were at stake. However, throughout the 1920s, a shift in the group targeted by 'propaganda' can be observed: as more *gueules cassées* joined the UBF, the focus, without ever completely moving away from veterans, was increasingly upon benefactors.

Another valuable tool in making the UBF known was the press. Early connections with publications such as the *Journal des Mutilés* are attested to by the presence of representatives at the UBF's general meetings.[132] General news publications also supported the organization, mainly through free advertisement and articles about the *Union* and its activities.[133] The support of the Parisian and regional press was frequently acknowledged and journalists were among the first to be invited to the *Maison*, even before its official opening. The good relationship between the UBF and the press is apparent in the report made by *gueules cassées* about this visit: 'We want to tell them what precious encouragement their articles full of hope for our house have been to us, and we want to express our gratitude for this

132 *Bulletin*, 5, p. 2.

133 Ibid, p. 2.

new proof of their interest'.[134] Picot went as far as declaring that 'We owe everything to journalists, who have greatly helped us. You should all know that without them, we would not have achieved what we have achieved'.[135] The relationship between veterans and the press was mutually beneficial, as articles about *gueules cassées* sold well. In turn, journalists were given privileged access to UBF events. Even at family gatherings such as Christmas parties at Moussy, representatives from the press were invited, testifying to the UBF's active publicity efforts.[136] The numerous articles published on the occasion of Picot's death further publicized the UBF and its work, as did the presence of journalists at the ceremonies commemorating the first anniversary of his death in 1939. What appear as rather intimate services and a 'pilgrimage' to Le Coudon, where Picot died, were indeed all open to reporters.[137]

In addition to the efforts of members and relationships with media professionals, the *Union des Blessés de la Face* also organized and participated in one-off events, which represented increasing contact with society as a whole. A gala series was organized as early as 1923, the first of which was held at the famous *Foire du Trône* on 27 April 1923.[138] It was described as very successful, not least thanks to the participation of the boxing world champion Battling Siki. A second gala was organized at the Neuilly fair in June, including the presence of popular singers Spinelly and Pélissier. These two instances show the support celebrities gave to the UBF early on; it was a paradoxical partnership between men usually perceived as seeking to hide, and artists defined by the limelight.

134 'Ce que nous voulons, c'est leur dire quel précieux encouragement nous avons puisé dans la lecture de leurs articles pleins de foi dans l'avenir de notre maison et quelle gratitude nous gardons pour le nouveau témoignage d'intérêt qu'ils nous ont donné', *Bulletin*, 16, p. 6.

135 'Nous devons tout aux journalistes qui nous ont puissamment aidés. Sans eux, sachez-le bien, nous ne serions pas arrivés au résultat que nous avons atteint', *Bulletin*, 18, p. 17.

136 *Bulletin*, 19, p. 5.

137 *Bulletin*, 59, p. 9.

138 *Bulletin*, 8, pp. 2–4.

During galas, the spotlight was upon the participating athletes and artists, and upon the UBF as an organization. In contrast, other publicity methods made individual members more visible. Thus, a film featuring *gueules cassées* is mentioned by Picot in July 1927, the president pointing out that the UBF not only endorsed it, but actively contributed to its production: a few members, including himself, were indeed filmed by the Gaumont studios. Their aim was to 'show to the public the sheer horror of war'.[139] Although not all *gueules cassées* were happy to be centre stage, the example given by their president Picot set the tone. Besides this, films enabled the UBF to become known internationally. Individual initiatives and collective strategies converged to publicize the cause not only in Europe but also in America and in the French overseas territories. Here, the *Association des Gueules Cassées* benefitted from the contacts of its individual members.[140] The presence of representatives from foreign veterans' organizations at general meetings is also evidence of the international profile of the UBF.[141] The interactions between ex-servicemen across the world, especially in the Americas and Great Britain, make the absence of similar groups in these countries all the more interesting. The visibility of French *gueules cassées* on the international stage started as early as 1919, when they attended the signing ceremony of the Treaty of Versailles. Although links with German veterans are seldom mentioned in UBF bulletins, relationships with England appear to have been more frequent but not very deep, as shown by the misunderstanding regarding the function of The Queen's Hospital, Sidcup.

A political body

The development and publicity of the *Union des Blessés de la Face* in France and abroad influenced and furthered its ideas. In addition to its charismatic

139 '[Montrer] au public l'horreur profonde de la guerre', *Bulletin*, 18, p. 17.

140 The work of Melchissédec in South America and Brunschwig in the United States is mentioned in several issues of the *Bulletin*.

141 *Bulletin*, 11b, p. 2.

president, its holistic approach of supporting veterans and its active propaganda, there were other factors contributing to its success. These included its integration into the political landscape of the interwar years, at a time when many veterans' organizations stood in opposition to the authorities and sometimes even to society. This integration was facilitated by the internal structure of the UBF, its contacts with the French state and its views upon war.

The stability in the *Union*'s executive committee, some members of which were actively involved in French politics, established continuity in the organization's workings and ethos. Brunschwig, the vice-president, remained in post from his election in December 1921 until the outbreak of the Second World War. The co-founders Jugon and Jourdain served as secretaries throughout the 1920s and 1930s. The uncontested leadership of Picot and his strong character are described as having secured the future of the UBF:

> Do you realise what the Union could have become, if we had experienced all the internal struggles that are so frequent in other groups [...] and that we managed to avoid? We were extraordinarily lucky in meeting a man whose high moral standards, whose age and rank, made him into an unquestionable and unquestioned leader.[142]

The continuity under Picot's seventeen-year presidency enabled the UBF to work efficiently, focussing upon the development of its social work. Long-term projects could be envisaged, such as the purchase of a house, which required careful planning and prolonged fundraising. As its membership and the scope of its activities grew, the organization also acquired premises in central Paris. Permanent headquarters were purchased in 1934 at 20 rue d'Aguesseau in Paris, where the organization is still based. This was not only a property investment, but also a sign of the *Union*'s will to leave a lasting legacy.

142 'Vous rendez-vous compte de ce qu'aurait pu être l'Union, avec ces luttes si fréquentes dans d'autres groupements, ces luttes [...] que nous avons eu le bonheur de ne jamais connaître. Mais nous avons eu cette bonne fortune extraordinaire de rencontrer un homme qui, par son élévation morale, qui par son âge, son grade, était indiscutable et indiscuté', *Bulletin*, 51 (July 1937), p. 11.

As the organization grew, its administration became increasingly professionalized. At first, members of the executive committee were not paid and volunteers carried out the administrative work. In 1926 a permanent administrative office was created and Jugon was appointed as secretary. In 1927, the internal structure evolved and several committees with different responsibilities were created.[143] But with this financial and administrative development there also came problems, and Jourdain warned his fellow members of the potential pitfalls: 'Our Union has become very important. It has always been morally significant. But now it is also materially powerful. We must be careful to protect our association and its assets, and we must lead and administer it wisely and cautiously'.[144]

The development of local branches also helped to make the workings of the UBF more efficient. The intention of the UBF to set up a network of regional delegates was announced at an early stage. There is evidence that one local correspondent had been appointed in Corsica in 1922, and in 1925 there were delegates in charge of regional propaganda in seven other cities.[145] The strengthening of these local groups is seen by the fact that they gradually started holding their own meetings, and offered weekly consultation hours, based upon the model of the Paris central office.[146] Some of them even designed their own distinct emblem and flag.[147] This structure was particularly useful in terms of the organization's social work and propaganda efforts, and despite early concerns that the *Union* would not remain united, strong links remained between regional sections and the headquarters. Bulletins from the late 1920s onwards featured a section on

143 *Bulletin*, 18, p. 13; *Bulletin*, 20 (April 1928).

144 'Notre Union est devenue très importante. Moralement elle l'a toujours été. Mais voici qu'elle est devenue considérable matériellement. Ses intérêts doivent être surveillés avec la plus grande attention et sa direction, son administration, assurées avec une sage prudence.' *Bulletin*, 21, p. 11.

145 *Bulletin*, 4, p. 2 and *Bulletin*, 13, p. 11.

146 *Bulletin*, 19, pp. 7–8.

147 *Bulletin*, 37, p. 17.

local branches and members of the executive committee regularly attended events in the different regions, including in overseas territories.[148]

The increase of the membership base of the UBF and the development of its administration brings into question whether such a big group could still be considered a 'family'. The idea of fraternity remained prevalent in the *Bulletins* and the social work conducted during this period testify to the organization's desire to remain faithful to its original aims. The stability of its leadership and the increasingly professional way in which it was run made it into a semi-professional organization, yet it remained close to its individual members. The UBF claimed to supplement – and on occasions to replace – official bodies, which were seen as too big, bureaucratic, impersonal and unstable due to frequent changes in their composition and subsequently in their policies.

At a time when tensions between veterans and the state were growing, French *gueules cassées* maintained good relationships with the authorities. In fact, the attitude of the UBF, far from being characterized by opposition, was one of active involvement in policy-making. This relatively smooth interaction reflected and facilitated the integration of the *Union des Blessés de la Face* into the French political and social landscape of the 1920s and 1930s.

The UBF was set up, in part, to defend what veterans saw as their legitimate rights before the State and Pensions commissions. This suggests that, like many veterans, they felt wronged by the authorities. The UBF nevertheless repeatedly declared its faith in them, and when tensions arose, for example regarding the provision of the *masticateur*, the *Union* did not oppose the Pensions Secretary directly, but rather it denounced the way in which the laws were applied.[149] In doing so, *gueules cassées* expressed their discontent with the state of affairs but they sided with the government, blaming not the leaders but the people in charge of applying their decisions.

In 1925, the official acknowledgement of *la défiguration* as a disabling condition led to an improvement in the relationships between the UBF

148 See *Bulletin*, 24 (May 1930), pp. 11–12 and *Bulletin*, 41, pp. 21–22.

149 *Bulletin*, 1, p. 3; *Bulletin*, 4, p. 2; *Bulletin*, 5, p. 9.

and the Pensions Secretary, whose 'encouragements' to facially disfigured veterans are highlighted.[150] The appointment of Louis Antériou to this post in 1925, and then again in 1928–1929, was welcomed by the UBF, all the more so since he was a member himself and took another *gueule cassée*, François Thomas, as his secretary. Both Thomas and Antériou were held up as examples of successful reintegration.

As the economic situation in France deteriorated, however, the UBF became increasingly critical of the ways in which its requests were being dealt with by the state. A 'Memorandum' published in August 1930, followed by a second one in November 1930, demonstrate a hardening of tone; the November 1931 bulletin marks a turning point in the relationship between the UBF and the government (Figure 6).[151]

The use of a photograph of a severely disfigured veteran on the cover page makes clear the confrontational approach adopted in the *Bulletin*. Pictures of disfigured men rarely appeared in the publication, and thus the aim here is clearly to shock the viewer and to underline what is presented as an absurd situation: a civil servant questioned the disfigured man's right to a full war pension. The French state is described as hypocritical, slow and reluctant to take responsibility. This campaign also bears testimony to the *Union*'s willingness to make use of the striking visual appearance of its members to further its claims.

The increasingly strained relationships between the state and the UBF illustrate growing tensions between authorities and veterans in general. Perhaps due to its relatively small number of members, the UBF did not resort to mass demonstrations; rather it made use of the press and other media, as well as taking advantage of the connections of some of its members. In public speeches, the UBF largely maintained a neutral or positive tone towards the state, as shown in a 1933 speech by Picot in which he claims that 'the Government has always made our task easier and ironed out any

150 *Bulletin*, 11 (February 1925), p. 1.

151 *Bulletin*, 25 (August 1930); *Bulletin*, 26 (November 1930); *Bulletin*, 27, front page (November 1931).

Fondée en 1921. — N° XXVII. (Trimestriel) Novembre 1931

BULLETIN DE L'UNION DES BLESSÉS DE LA FACE

PERMANENCE : tous les jours de 9 h. à 12 h. et de 14 h. à 18 h.

" Les Gueules Cassées "

SIÈGE SOCIAL :

46, Rue du Faubourg-Saint-Denis, PARIS (10e)

RÉUNION MENSUELLE le 1er samedi du mois, à 20 h. 30

TÉLÉPHONE : PROVENCE 62-04

Compte Chèques Postaux : PARIS 493-07

Regardez !

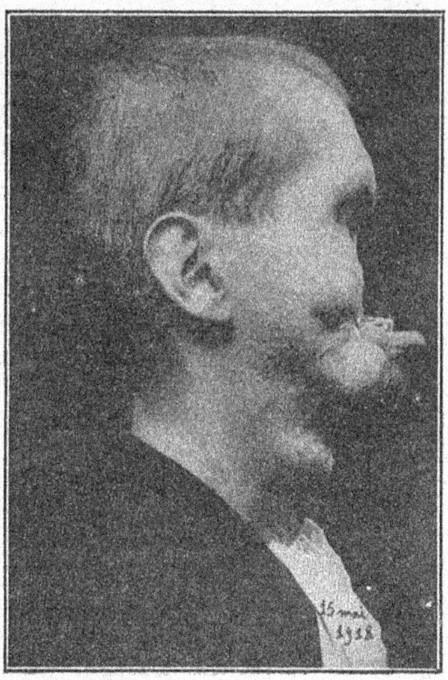

Défiguré ?

Durant dix-huit mois, et plus,
Devant cette « Gueule Cassée » en lambeaux,
L'Administration des Pensions est restée plongée en d'amères réflexions :

Est-il, ou n'est-il pas défiguré ?...

(Voir page 3)

Figure 6: Front page of *Bulletin* 27, November 1931. Reproduced courtesy of Association des Gueules Cassées.

difficulties'.[152] This, despite tensions with the French state, the methods that the UBF employed to address difficulty were always peaceful and aimed to influence authorities rather than to oppose them.

This pacifying approach was also maintained within the group; for example, discussions about politics and religion were officially banned. However, throughout the interwar years, the UBF increasingly expressed views about war, and the films it endorsed had an anti-war bias. This pacifist standpoint was presented as inscribed in the flesh of *gueules cassées*: 'in an Assembly like ours, made up of men whose flesh bears the painful traces of their longing for peace, it seems ironic to ask if we want peace!'[153]

The *Union*'s discourse on the First World War was overwhelmingly a close-up on the stories of *gueules cassées*, which ultimately merged into one narrative of patriotic sacrifice. Profiteers were denounced in the early years of the UBF, but no open criticism of France's involvement in the Great War was voiced and the *Union* presented the conflict as a trial out of which its members had emerged triumphant. This discourse enabled *gueules cassées* to make sense of their wounds, and at the same time it gave them a responsibility towards their fellow-countrymen – sometimes presented as weaker members of society – and towards the country they had saved. The *Union* sought to maintain the memory of the Great War and actively participated in events promoting its remembrance; for example, a minute of silence for the dead was observed at the beginning of each general meeting and delegations regularly visited the Tomb of the Unknown Soldier and other memorials. More than an opposition to armed conflict per se, *gueules cassées* presented the defence of peace as a duty civilians and ex-combatants alike had towards the dead of the war. Throughout the 1920s and 1930s, the UBF supported anti-war campaigns. Picot directly addressed the question of a looming war for the first time in December 1934; the UBF's concerns focussed, however, upon the socio-economic impact

152 'Le Gouvernement a toujours facilité notre tâche en aplanissant bien des difficultés', *Bulletin*, 32 (February 1933), p. 1.

153 'Dans une Assemblée comme la nôtre, composée d'hommes pour lesquels le désir de la paix est douloureusement inscrit dans leur chair, cela ressemble à une galéjade de poser la question de savoir si nous sommes pour la paix!', *Bulletin*, 30, p. 5.

of unrest and how *gueules cassées* might be helped.[154] In April 1936, Picot addressed Hitler's violation of the Treaty of Versailles and urged *gueules cassées* to set an example of unity for France to follow.[155]

The *Union*'s anti-war stance is best seen in two films with which it was involved. Their aim was to set themselves up as evidence against war, in an attempt to prevent such conflicts from breaking out in the future. *Pour la Paix du Monde*, released in 1927 in France and Belgium, reached Germany, as seen in an article by Peter Panter (one of several pseudonyms of Kurt Tucholsky).[156] The journalist points out the film's realistic dimension, achieved by the participation of *gueules cassées*:

> [...] they appear out of the darkness, in plain clothes, one following the other, like in a vision: battered, smashed-up, mangled, ghastly faces that are hardly still faces. But now the casualties are wearing their Sunday best, they are no longer soldiers but simply honest folks with nothing to distinguish them from anyone else.
>
> A heavy silence falls on the cinema theatre.[157]

Here, *gueules cassées* represent the aftermath of war. Tucholsky notes the powerful impact of disfigured men upon viewers, who fell silent at the sight of facial wounds. *Gueules cassées* thus identify with an anti-war discourse, not only by their actions, but also by their very being. Their participation in this film indicates their anti-war stance, and suggests that defending peace is a battle in itself. This is also seen in a speech given by Picot in 1931, in which he contrasts the destructiveness of war with the works of reconstruction and peace achieved by the *Association*:

154 *Bulletin*, 39, p. 1.

155 *Bulletin*, 46 (April 1936), p. 1.

156 Peter Panter (aka Kurt Tucholsky), 'Französischer Kriegsfilm', *Vossische Zeitung*, 2 November 1927. <http://www.zeno.org/Literatur/M/Tucholsky,+Kurt/Werke/1927/Franz%C3%B6sischer+Kriegsfilm> [accessed 18 August 2015].

157 'Da tauchen sie, in Zivil, aus dem Dunkel auf, einer nach dem andern, wie eine Vision: zerschossene, zerschlagene, verstümmelte, schreckliche Gesichter, die kaum noch Gesichter sind. Aber nun haben die Opfer einen Sonntagsrock an und sind keine Soldaten mehr, sondern wieder brave Leute, denen man nichts mehr ansieht. Eine schwere Stille lastete auf dem Saale', Panter, 'Französischer Kriegsfilm'.

> Thus, the mutilated veterans, the greatest victims of hatred, will again have served their country by showing what unity between men can achieve and by building a redeeming monument of fraternity upon the ruins left by the war.[158]

Picot's patriotic speech presents veterans as peacemakers. And as the risk of a new war increased, the UBF took part in another film: Abel Gance's 1938 *J'accuse*.[159] In this new version of Gance's 1919 silent production, facially disfigured soldiers feature only briefly. Their participation, and the support of the UBF, was nevertheless heavily emphasized in the publicity of the film. On posters, alongside the names of the director and main actors, 'Les Gueules Cassées' are mentioned. No individual names are singled out, but rather the group is highlighted as a whole, the veterans' participation presented as 'branding this film with a sober, moving realism'.[160] Gance made use of nine men who were among the worst mutilated, and his production notes underline his intention: 'Create lasting effect of shock and horror […]. Turn *gueules cassées* into stone statues […] whose images resist the passing of time and leave a mark in the viewers' memories'.[161] In choosing these veterans Gance guaranteed his film publicity and respect, not least thanks to the popularity of the UBF itself. But his choice was also directed by the spectacular nature of their wounds, which he utilized to make a lasting impact on viewers. Gance insists upon the memorial function fulfilled by the veterans, reminding viewers of the past and urging them to prevent such a conflict from happening again. In this respect, Gance plays upon the transgressive nature of facial injuries, and indeed of

158 'Ainsi les grands mutilés, les grandes victimes de la haine auront encore servi leur pays en montrant ce que peut l'union entre les hommes, en dressant en face de l'œuvre de ruine et de désespérance de l'abominable guerre, l'œuvre réparatrice et féconde de la fraternité.', *Bulletin*, 27 (November 1931), p. 10.

159 *J'accuse*, dir. by Abel Gance (Forrester-Parant, 1938).

160 '[Marquant] ce film d'un réalisme sobre, très émouvant', Paris, Cinémathèque française, 'Pour la presse', publicity material for *J'accuse*, B 46–134 GANCE.

161 'Créer impression d'horreur et d'épouvante inoubliable […] Faire avec les Gueules Cassées de véritable statues de pierre […] qui résistent au temps en se gravant indélébilement dans les mémoires des spectateurs', Paris, Cinémathèque française, Production notes, *J'accuse*, 616–B128 and 616–B129.

all disfigured men who exemplify an 'incomplete death'.[162] This film thus makes clear the status of *gueules cassées* as living reminders of the war and embodiments of its horror. Its inclusion of veterans in a pacifist discourse was fully accepted by the UBF.

In Picot's own words, *gueules cassées* embody the horror of war and have acted as living reminders of its reality ever since the First World War. He inscribes this participation within the trend inaugurated by Clemenceau at the signing ceremony of the Treaty of Versailles. In this context, as well as in Gance's film, *gueules cassées* were largely silent. Their bodies were deemed to be evocative enough. A similar take on war is to be found in the July 1939 issue of the *Bulletin*, which points out how the memory of the war is fading away and asks, 'how could we conceive that some men would be foolish enough to command that new massacres be perpetrated? And yet … it is now only in the hearts of those of 1914 that the infinite ideal of peace still lives'.[163]

With *J'accuse*, the UBF campaigned for peace; yet Picot, speaking on behalf of the *gueules cassées*, insisted that the French should not shy away from the war if it became necessary.[164] Indeed, when the Second World War broke out, the UBF declared its determination to support the state's decision to go to war. If few of the *gueules cassées* went back to the front, many saw their children go. The workings of the UBF as a whole were affected by this conflict, especially due to the mobilization of most of its medical advisors and the need to safeguard the organization's assets. The *Union*'s declared line of conduct was to support the war effort, especially by helping its members' sons at the front and providing for the facially wounded soldiers of the Second World War.[165]

162 'Mort inachevée', Laurent Véray, 'Abel Gance, cinéaste à l'œuvre cicatricielle', *Revue 1895*, 31 (2000), p. 42.

163 'Comment concevoir que des hommes seraient assez fous pour donne l'ordre de perpétuer de nouveaux massacres? Et cependant … ce n'est plus que dans les cœurs de ceux de 1914 que l'on peut retrouver, à l'heure actuelle, l'idéal infini de la paix', *Bulletin*, 60, p. 5.

164 *Bulletin*, 55, pp. 7–8.

165 See *Bulletin*, 60, p. 7 and *Bulletin*, 61, p. 3.

Summary

The *Union des Blessés de la Face* evolved from a small friendship network to a powerful organization. Close bonds were formed between hospital patients in France, Great Britain and Germany, as shown in the writings of Baillaud, Clare and Rémi; however, it is only in France that these relationships were given an official structure in post-war years. The development of the UBF, which became one of the richest and most respected veterans' organizations in the interwar years, was facilitated by the continuity of its leadership and the charisma of its president. Although it benefitted from the support of renowned personalities from its inception, it gained momentum in the mid-1920s, not least thanks to the success of its fund-raising campaign for the purchase of a *Maison des gueules cassées*.

This expansion was made possible by internal factors, including the absence of major controversies and the family-like atmosphere encouraged by its limited membership. At its peak, the *Union* had around eight thousand active members, and many more signed up as benefactors. Despite these limited numbers, *gueules cassées* evolved as representatives of war veterans in general. External factors also account for the success of the *Union*, the profits made from the national lottery providing an example. Continued press coverage, active propaganda efforts and the support of artists contributed to make the organization widely known.

The UBF nevertheless faced criticisms in the interwar years. During the pension campaign, *gueules cassées* were accused of trying to take advantage of the state.[166] A small membership base meant that the UBF was not always taken seriously; in 1929, for example, one journalist described it as a 'speck of dust of an association'.[167] In turn the large financial gains from the lottery caused problems, prompting the UBF to remind its detractors that the money received was used to help its members and their families,

166 *Bulletin*, 23, p. 6.

167 'Poussière d'association', *Bulletin*, 23, p. 4.

and other veterans in need.[168] With its increasing prosperity, criticisms also increased and the UBF faced hostility and competition from other organizations. Even its place in society was not without challenges. Thus, a handful of French town mayors were denounced in the *Bulletins* for being ill-disposed towards *La Dette* and for refusing to sell the tickets sent to them by the UBF.[169] This was interpreted as illustrating a lack of respect towards *gueules cassées* and a refusal to acknowledge society's debt to the veterans.

Yet despite some negative reactions, the *Union des Blessés de la Face* overwhelmingly managed to shape a positive public profile for French *gueules cassées*. The *Bulletins* were the organization's mouthpiece and consequently present it in a favourable light; they constitute a valuable source of information about the image it aimed to project. Other publications, for instance in the popular press, and the economic success experienced by the UBF during the interwar years, tend to confirm that it was well regarded by society and integrated within it. The veterans' self-reliance and attempts to help other mutilated men facilitated relationships with the state, with other veterans' organizations, and with French society as a whole. The UBF was run like a philanthropic business, extending its benefits to a wider circle. The holistic approach and traditional values upheld by the *Union* were combined with modern and original fundraising methods, enabling it to become a popular and respected veterans' organization in the interwar years. In association with their president Picot, members were seen as patriots capable of bringing a productive contribution to both wartime and peacetime society.

This positive image that was shaped by the *Association* and widely publicized helped to enhance the gueules cassées' material circumstances and self-esteem. Their organization also favoured relationships between individual members and other members of society, the strong and positive image of their organization reflecting upon them individually. A 1986 study by social psychologist Nichola Rumsey revealed that the success of an interaction between a person with a visible facial difference and another

168 *Bulletin*, 60, p. 10.
169 *Bulletin*, 32, p. 7.

person without such difference is heavily influenced by the social skills and attitude of the disfigured person.[170] These conclusions, although they apply to observations made several decades after the First World War, seem relevant to the situation of First World War *gueules cassées*, with prominent figures such as Colonel Picot rising to significant public positions despite their facial injuries. Interaction between French disfigured veterans and other members of society was facilitated by the profile of the *Association*, with which they were associated in the minds of the general public. Because this organization implemented effective communication strategies and acted as a mediator between veterans and French society, their individual 'social skills' were perceived to be enhanced.

Existing studies of German and British disabled veterans depict them as being respectively praised and ignored by the state, and regarded as either burdens or 'the objects of charity' by society.[171] In contrast, the positive image of French *gueules cassées* publicized in the media and sometimes in the arts, was claimed and reinforced by the UBF itself.

170 Nichola Rumsey, Ray Bull and Denis Gahagan, 'A Preliminary Study of the Potential of Social Skills for Improving the Quality of Social Interaction for the Facially Disfigured', *Social Behaviour*, 1 (1986), 143–46.

171 Cohen, *The War Come Home*, p. 60.

PART II

Artistic and Literary Representations

CHAPTER 4

The Faces of War: Visual Representations of Facially Injured Soldiers

Reflecting upon his visit to the leading British maxillofacial hospital and its attached museum in 1918, journalist Robert Blatchford commented:

> I shall not talk about those photographs, though I may dream of them. I shall not talk about the operating theatres, nor the instruments, nor the gifted and untiring doctors, nor the wounds. One can imagine it all with awe and sympathy.[1]

Blatchford (1851–1943) served in the army before returning to civilian life and founding the socialist newspaper *The Clarion*. He observed and wrote widely about the First World War, and it is possibly his interest in the welfare of soldiers and ex-soldiers that led him to The Queen's Hospital, the first purpose-built hospital dedicated to the treatment of face and jaw injury in Great Britain. He visited in June 1918, one year after its opening, and was left haunted by the photographs he had seen.

Photographers fixed images of war-wounded faces for posterity. Alongside them, artists captured the appearances of the men during and after their treatment, and produced works that reflect the varying responses to the return of injured soldiers. Whilst previous chapters of this book have focussed upon the experience of facially wounded combatants themselves, the visual representations studied here provide a valuable insight into the onlooker's perceptions that goes beyond the imminence of physical confrontation. These depictions help us to understand how facially injured combatants were treated and perceived by others.

1 Blatchford, 'A Holstery of Healing', p. 46.

The face has been, at least since the Renaissance, a focus of attention in visual arts. In *The Face in Western Art*, John Brophy argues that changes in the understanding of how the mind works and the development of a more acute self-consciousness brought about a renewed interest in the face, which in turn led to a stronger representation of it in the arts.[2] But if grotesque and deformed faces can be found, especially in caricatures, wounded faces have not often been depicted, not least because they challenge traditional conceptions of beauty. The canonical aesthetic notion of order and symmetry is defied, as scars disrupt the distinctive traits and common contours usually associated with the face. Not only do *gueules cassées* unsettle this 'objective' understanding of beauty, but in preventing the viewer from recognizing the men, and even more from identifying with them, the disfigured faces also threaten human relationships. They sometimes trigger a morbid fascination, as suggested by British artist Henry Tonks, but more generally they are regarded as objects of repulsion rather than sources of attraction.[3] The absence of familiar, recognizable traits in a mutilated face unsettles the onlooker, perhaps to a greater extent than a missing arm or leg.

At the time when the First World War broke out, this classical aesthetic canon of beauty that emphasized symmetry and proportion had already been challenged, in particular by the development of artistic approaches such as Realism, Naturalism and Expressionism. Artistic movements promoting life-like depictions of reality, even in its most gruesome details, grew in the century preceding the First World War and perhaps helped to encourage the production and publication of images of disfigured faces when they too became a feature of lived reality. However, wounded faces were not a common sight in visual arts before 1914, and the French art historian Louis-Paul Fischer notes that 'In painting and sculpture, facial

2 John Brophy, *The Face in Western Art* (London: George G. Harrap, 1963).

3 Henry Tonks, Letter to MacColl, reprinted in Joseph Hone, *The Life of Henry Tonks* (London: Heinemann, 1939), p. 128.

deformities caused by mutilations or by the absence of some features (lips, nose, cheekbones ...) were, we found, very rare.'[4]

First World War artists were aware of the powerful impact of *gueules cassées* upon the onlooker. Facially wounded servicemen were even used in the arts as a means of social and political criticism, to epitomize war atrocities and sometimes to promote pacifism. These depictions may all appear to be anti-militaristic, yet they present differences that are indicative of variations and similarities in the post-war situations of Great Britain, France and Germany, for example in view of the treatment and integration of the wounded. The ways in which *gueules cassées* were represented, and on occasions instrumentalized, reflect the role they played in different national backgrounds. Existing discussions of artistic depictions are often limited to individual countries or artists, whilst the comparative approach adopted here underlines the variations in societies' perceptions of disfigured combatants.[5] This chapter examines photography, medical drawings and paintings, and underlines the close relationship between medicine and the arts.

Photographic narratives of destruction and reconstruction

Amongst the many illustrated press articles reporting on soldiers wounded in recent conflicts, few feature photographs of facially injured combatants. And yet the figures tell a different story: 'At least 60 percent of the

4 'En peinture et en sculpture, les déformations du visage dues à des mutilations, à des absences d'une partie de la face (lèvres, nez, pommettes ...) avant les gueules cassées de 14–18, nous semblent rarissimes', Fischer et al., 'Les gueules cassées représentées par de grands peintres', p. 337.

5 See, for example, Maria Tatar, 'Entstellung im Vollzug: Das Gesicht des Krieges in der Malerei', in *Gesichter der Weimarer Republik*, ed. by Gilman and Schmölders, pp. 113–30; Fischer et al., 'Les Gueules Cassées Représentées Par de Grands Peintres', pp. 337–46; and Biernoff, 'Flesh Poems', in which she sets Tonks's pastels against photographic representations.

30,000-plus Americans wounded [in Iraq] endured blows to the head.'[6] Like their First World War predecessors, twenty-first-century disfigured servicemen are an uncomfortable presence. They represent 'war's dark face' and their photographs confront the onlooker with a reality that they would rather not acknowledge.

This reluctance to show the damaged face is highlighted by the essayist Susan Sontag: in *Regarding the Pain of Others*, she refers to photographs representing disfigured soldiers published in Ernst Friedrich's 1924 pamphlet as 'heartrending, stomach-turning pictures' that together form 'the most unbearable pages in [that] book'.[7] Photography was still considered a novel and exciting technique when the First World War broke out. Although photographic techniques appeared in the mid-nineteenth century, later advances in associated technologies – in printing, in communications and in literacy – made the Great War the first conflict to be widely documented, despite the interference of censorship. Jane Carmichael underlines the novelty of such coverage: 'During the First World War it was for the first time possible for people to see and read about a major conflict more or less as it happened.'[8] It was felt that photographs, unlike paintings or drawings, conveyed a greater sense of authenticity. Sontag states: 'Photographs [...] were a record of the real – incontrovertible, as no verbal account, however impartial, could be – since a machine was doing the recording. And they bore witness to the real – since a person had been there to take them'.[9] Photographs appear to give the viewer direct access to the scene pictured, with the presence of the photographer discreet or invisible. Photographs can therefore produce a very different impact upon viewers than other forms of visual representation, such as paintings or drawings, even though these forms may be more detailed or elaborate.

6 E.A. Torriero, 'Disfigured Soldiers Are War's Dark Face' *Chicago Tribune*, 26 May 2008 <http://articles.chicagotribune.com/2008-05-26/news/0805260121_1_facial-soldiers-face> [accessed 20 April 2014].

7 Sontag, *Regarding the Pain of Others*, p. 13. These images will be discusse din more detail in this chapter.

8 Jane Carmichael, *First World War Photographers* (London: Routledge, 1989), p. 4.

9 Sontag, *Regarding the Pain of Others*, p. 23.

Photographs combine artistic and documentary purposes, although attempts at rendering pictures of war more 'artistic' have long been received with suspicion: 'For the photograph of atrocity, people want the weight of witnessing without the taint of artistry, which is equated with insincerity or mere contrivance'.[10] When photographs are too obviously manipulated, be it in order to beautify or to 'uglify' their subject, they are no longer seen as reliable visual testimonies. Photographic representations of *gueules cassées* raise particular questions about the photographers' purposes, especially with regard to the way wounds are shown, highlighted or hidden. They also provide clues as to the perception and presentation of severely wounded servicemen, and beyond this, of war and its consequences.

Maimed faces have an ambiguous status: they belong to living persons but have been altered beyond recognition, even to the point of evoking the idea of death rather than life. This intermediate state – between life and death – reminds viewers of medieval visions of the apocalypse, especially at a time when apocalyptic imagery was a key artistic motif[11] The face tends to be absent from photographs of dead people, as if it was deemed too voyeuristic to show it. Likewise, to this day, soldiers often erase the face of a dead comrade on a group photograph. What then, of faces reconfigured to such an extent as to lack human resemblance? Twenty-first-century viewers often respond to these images with questions. 'How could this wounded man survive?' and 'Is life with a broken face worth living?' are typical reactions.[12]

The realistic quality of photographs raises questions not only about their impact upon the viewer, but also upon the men represented. Some of the sitters who were painted by artist Mark Gilbert as part of the *Saving Faces* project (1999) found it much easier to look at portraits of their disfigured faces, than at photographs.[13] Likewise, considering the difficulties

10 Ibid, p. 23.

11 Jay Winter, 'The Apocalyptic Imagination in Art', in Winter, *Sites of Memory, Sites of Mourning*, pp. 145–77. The casts and masks of disfigured faces are besides akin to death masks that were produced *en masse* in the 19th century.

12 This is based upon responses of university students and researchers who attended seminars in 2011–2015.

13 Paul Farrand, 'Portraiture as Therapy', *Saving Faces* art project website <http://www.savingfaces.co.uk/news-media/art-project/35-art/133-dr-paul-farrand-medical-psychologist>

some First World War soldiers experienced in coming to terms with their disfigurement, it is surprising that they would have agreed to have their picture taken at all. In a clinical context they may not have been given the choice, and thus once outside hospital, disfigured veterans were more reluctant to be photographed. For example, Karl Hasbach would only allow photographs to be taken from the left so that his right side, less well-reconstructed, would remain hidden.[14] Likewise, a 1931 French novel by Renée Girard underlines the significance of the fact that the hero, a *gueule cassée*, agrees to have his picture taken on his wedding day.[15] This act is presented as proof of his acceptance of his changed physical appearance: he is now moving on. The photograph is the visual mark of a rite of passage. This suggests that only those who had managed to come to terms with their disfigurement were represented by photographs.

The origin and nature of photographic documents explain the differences in their quality and distribution; these factors also account for the variety in the purposes of the pictures realized and in the ways the subjects are represented. The use of private cameras was not always permitted on the battlefield and regulations varied depending upon the country and the time in the war. Amateur photographers on the front – be they soldiers or nurses – were more likely to picture scenes of relaxation than the battlefield itself.[16] The quality of amateur photographs is not consistent; official photographs and those for the press were taken by professionals (when they were allowed to enter the fighting zone and hospitals) and were intended to be more widely circulated. Specific photographic departments were even set up to this end. The French War Ministry created the *Section Photographique de l'Armée* in 1915 as a response to the use of photographic documents by the Germans (within neutral countries especially). Germany was indeed one

---

[accessed 10 April 2014]. The portraits of thirty patients were realized by artist Mark Gilbert and featured in the exhibition launched in 2002.

14 Hasbach's daughter, quoted in Weerda and Pirsig, 'Jacques Joseph und der Patient Dr. Karl Hasbach'.

15 Renée Girard, *La Vie Intime d'une "Gueule Cassée"* (Paris, Les Etincelles, 1931), pp. 172–73.

16 Carmichael, *First World War Photographers*, pp. 31–35.

of the first countries to employ photographs in its large-scale propaganda efforts, especially abroad. The British authorities also appointed official photographers to record events on the Western Front and the Home Front.

Horace W. Nicholls (1867–1941) had previously covered the Second Boer War as a photojournalist and he was the first official photographer to be appointed by the Ministry of Information during the First World War. Commissioned to document the Home Front, several of his photographs represent facially injured soldiers. One set of Nicholls's before-and-after photographs (Figures 7 and 8) focuses upon an anonymous soldier and dates from 1915. Unlike the many clinical photographs taken between surgical operations, this one represents a man whose medical treatment is over. The title of the series, 'Repairing war's ravages', evokes the brutality of the conflict as well as the possibility of counteracting its effects. It highlights the fact that although scientific and technical advances increased the power of destruction, they also improved chances of survival.

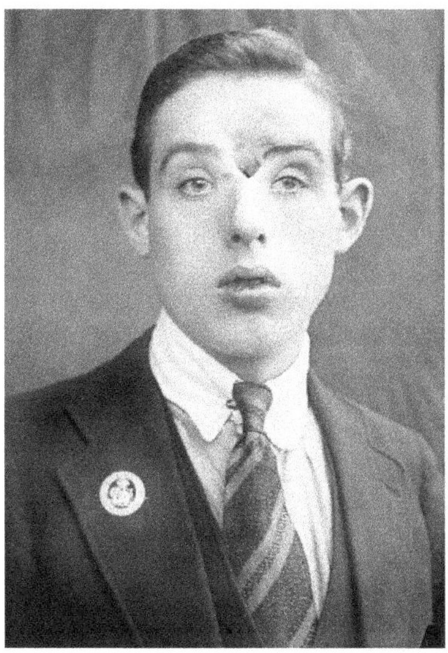

Figure 7: Horace Nicholls, 'Repairing war's ravages: renovating facial injuries. A British soldier wounded between the eyes by a piece of time-fuse, which lodged at the back of his cheek. It was extracted by massage without injury to the cheek' © Imperial War Museum (IWM), London (Q30449).

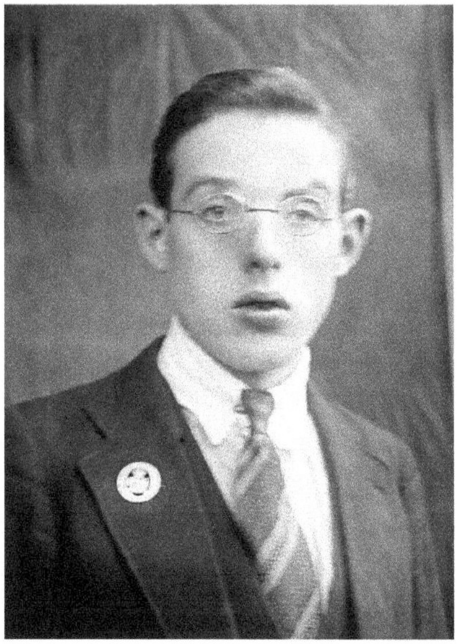

Figure 8: Horace Nicholls, 'Repairing war's ravages: renovating facial injuries. The patient after a plate was fixed for the spectacles to cover the wound. The sculptor was Captain Derwent Wood, RA, 3rd London General Hospital' © IWM (Q30450). The original photograph is blurred, probably due to the sitter moving whilst his photograph was taken.

The lack of identification – the wounded man is referred to as 'a British soldier' and 'the patient' in these official photographs, whilst medical photographs that were less likely to be disclosed do mention names – protects the sitter's identity but it also implies that he is one among many others. This emphasizes the symbolic quality of the facially injured combatant, who represents any disfigured soldier and, beyond this, the 'dark face of war' itself, as one twenty-first-century commentator puts it.[17]

In the first picture the injury is unconcealed, and the way in which the light falls upon the wound draws attention to it, with the intact side in shadow. The wound looks neat and well-healed. Unlike what the title

17 Torriero, 'Disfigured Soldiers Are War's Dark Face'.

'ravages' implies, the damage seems relatively limited and appears to be aesthetic more than functional. This photograph does not show a shocking case of disfigurement, and the framing and clothes increase the 'normal' appearance of the subject. The top of the man's chest and shoulders are visible, which enables the viewer to see that he is not wearing a hospital uniform but a suit and tie. One may assume that he is no longer a patient or a soldier, but rather has returned, or is soon to return, to civilian life. Wearing plain clothes underlines the fact that this man, despite his damaged face, leads an ordinary life, thus facilitating the viewer's identification with him, or at least providing a point of connection. This is further helped by the fact that the young man looks straight at the camera; his gaze does not avoid that of the onlooker.

In both photographs, the subject's facial expression is neutral. Although the second picture is slightly overexposed, one can see that the damaged forehead is made almost invisible by a mask attached to a pair of glasses. In spite of this improvement, the patient is neither smiling, nor showing any signs of happiness or relief. These two photographs do not diplay emotions. The emphasis is upon 'normality'; and the choice of the subject – a young, reasonably good-looking man wearing smart clothes – also points to the future and hope of smooth reintegration.[18] This reparation is, however, superficial: the man's appearance may have been put right according to a certain standard of aesthetic beauty, yet the damage is still visible. Moreover, the photographs and their captions represent physical restoration only, and do nothing to address the psychological impact of war injuries. More than the successful 'repairing' of the face, these images evidence the efficient hiding of damage.

Another series of photographs produced by Nicholls records the different stages in the making of a facial mask. This time the attention is not so much on the change it brings to the man's face but rather on the item

18 A similar take is found in Suzannah Biernoff and Jane Tynan, 'Making and Remaking the Civilian Soldier: The World War I Photographs of Horace Nicholls', *Journal of War and Culture Studies*, 5 (2012), 277–93. They underline the parallel between the physical repair of wounded men and the architectural reconstruction of damaged England.

itself, and a visual narrative emerges from these images. The setting is not a hospital ward, although the man is referred to as 'the patient'. The rooms where these photographs were taken resemble an artist's studio and were probably Wood's workshop at the 3rd London General Hospital.

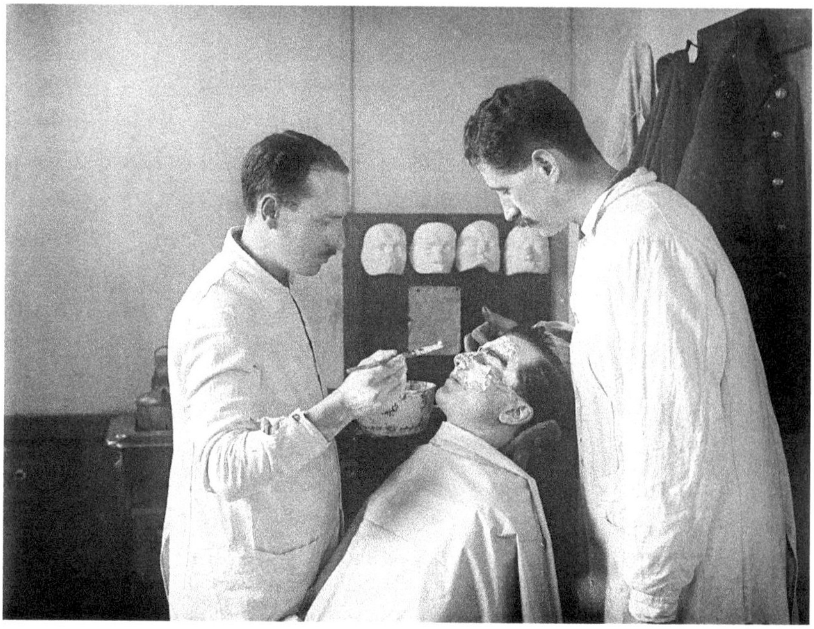

Figure 9: Horace Nicholls, 'Applying first coat of plaster for the purpose of taking the mould of the patient's face, who has been blinded in one eye. The patch is to restore that side of the face which has been disfigured' © IWM (Q30452).

The background of this first photograph in the series (Figure 9) features four masks, their light colour contrasting with the dark shelves upon which they are placed. They are positioned as if looking straight at the two men working on the disfigured soldier, and beyond, at the viewer, thus giving a slightly eerie atmosphere to this scene. A similar decor is visible in the photographs and film showing Anna Coleman Ladd's Paris studio; they testify to the artist's previous achievements and show the production process.

In this first photograph, two men are pictured bent over a disfigured soldier's face. It does not look severely damaged, thus apparently contradicting Wood's statement that 'as a general rule the cases which come to me are those in which the wounds or depredations of disease have been so severe as to remove them beyond the range of even the most advanced plastic surgical operations'.[19] The reason for this discrepancy may again lie in the targeted audience of these photographs: unlike medical photographs aimed at a limited and informed public, official photographs were likely to reach a wider audience. Too dreadful a sight would have shocked the viewers and possibly have disheartened them, at a time when keeping up the country's morale was crucial.

The two men appear focussed upon their task, as if unaware of the presence of the photographer: one is applying the plaster, the other observes. The patient himself is passive: he sits in a chair, the upper half of his body covered so as to protect his clothes, and his eyes are closed. He is the subject that the artists or technicians are working upon. This impression is even stronger in the second photograph, which pictures a patient almost completely covered in thick white plaster and Wood's assistants contemplating their work. A professional attitude also prevails in the third photograph, which shows the two men absorbed in examining the cast they have just made. In contrast, the patient is still in the same position, eyes closed, motionless, when one might expect him to look at the mask too. The first three photographs in the series thus turn the spotlight upon the sculptors and give the impression that the disfigured man is powerless or inactive, that his fate is in the hands of others. The contrast between the staff – two professionals working together – and the lonely, passive figure of the disfigured soldier, is striking.

A later photograph marks a change (Figure 10): the setting remains the same, but the focus is now upon the patient.

As the cast that will restore his looks gradually takes shape, other features are also highlighted in his appearance (for instance, his clothes) and in his posture. This photograph illustrates the confrontation between the

19 Wood, 'Masks for Facial Wounds', p. 949.

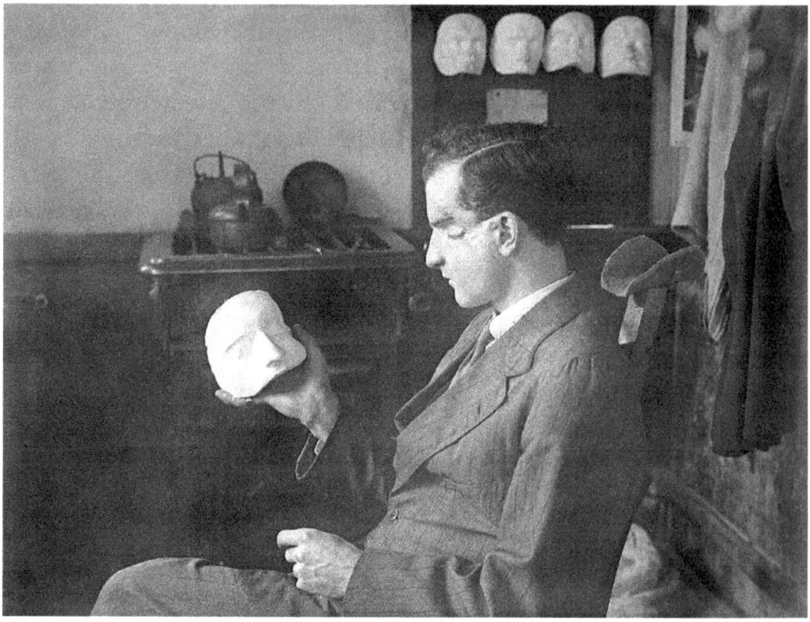

Figure 10: Horace Nicholls, 'The patient examining the mould of his own face' © IWM (Q30455).

man and the mould of his damaged face, and the viewer is the voyeur of this disturbing encounter.

Figure 11 represents the sculptor Francis Derwent Wood himself at work.

In the photograph showing the sculptor and the wounded man, the onlooker's eye is drawn to the man on the left, whose white coat stands out against the dark background and contrasts with the disfigured man's dark suit. The presence of an easel, a palette and paint brushes suggests that the scene takes place in an artist's studio. The caption confirms that the man on the left is the sculptor 'Captain Derwent Wood, R.A.'. The artist is putting his skills in the service of the military.

In all three photographs representing Wood and the soldier, the artist is the only active person. Even when Wood is not actually painting, he is the one holding the mask and examining it. The first photograph (not

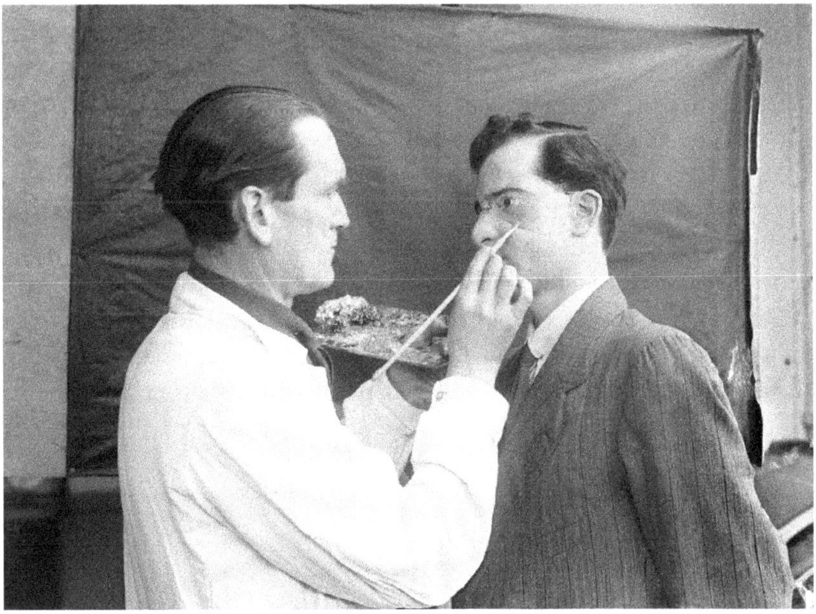

Figure 11: Horace Nicholls, 'Painting the plate' © IWM (Q30457).

reproduced here) is representative of the relationship between *gueules cassées* and the rest of the world: the mask is positioned between the two men, like a filter through which Wood sees the other man. The disfigured man is a 'work in progress', as shown in the photograph that pictures Wood painting the mask positioned on the face (Figure 11). This procedure aims to find the right shade of paint so that the mask will blend with the patient's skin colour. The artist is almost painting directly onto the man's face, as if giving him human features again. The last photograph presents the artist examining the plate; the patient is standing beside him but is not looking at the result, just as he had not looked at the mould earlier. The power is again in the hands of the artist who gives life to a plate, a composite of human flesh and inanimate material, sometimes made of the very metal which had caused the destruction of the face.

The more theatrical connotations of facial masks, plates and attachments are obvious in the last two photographs of this series. Such a dimension was perceived by surgeons themselves, for instance by the American Fred Albee, who wrote that 'Hundreds of soldiers who would otherwise have been too revolting to appear on the street, were restored to something like their old appearance by papier-mâché noses; rubber ears, coloured like flesh and almost as pliable [...]'.[20] The photograph featuring the moulds and plates at different stages shows the practical steps of making such items but at the same time it also makes the mask look like a prop. The theatrical effect is increased by the fact that there is no human being represented alongside these objects. The last photograph does not focus upon the technical and artistic process; rather it represents, again like theatre props, a collection of glass eyes, noses, ears and other attachments destined to be fixed upon faces (Figure 12).

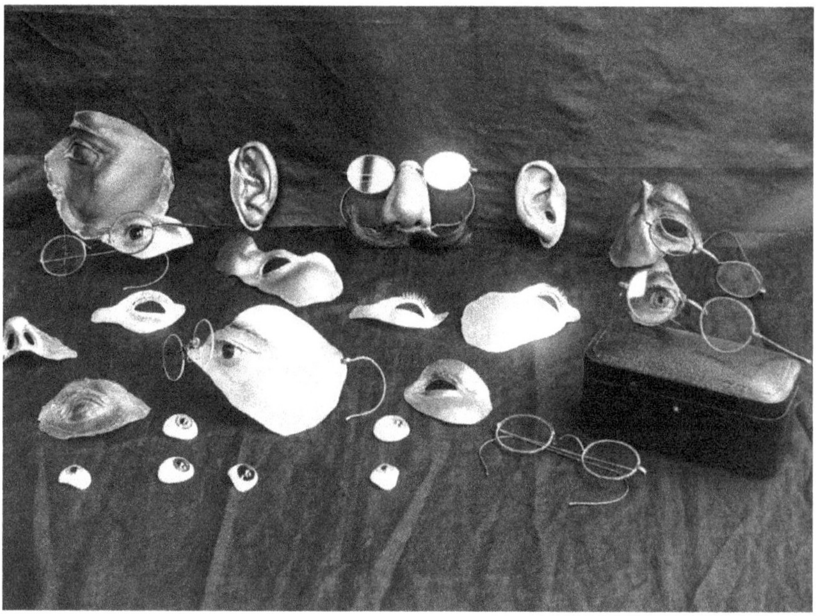

Figure 12: Horace Nicholls, 'Repairing war's ravages: renovating facial injuries. Various plates and attachments in different stages of completion' © IWM (Q30460).

20 Albee, *A Surgeon's Fight to Rebuild Men*, p. 108.

These inanimate objects highlight the fact that masks often looked unnatural and failed to convey emotion since 'Unlike a living face, with its infinite variety of response, the tin mask remained capable only of the one expression imposed by the artist'.[21] Artists themselves acknowledged the limitations to their work, Wood declaring 'I have to call attention at the outset to two important points: no attempt is made in any of my contrivances for the alleviation of the sufferings of the wounded, to restore functioning or to produce a cosmetic effect by plastic methods'.[22] Thus, although at first sight masks may have facilitated relationships with society, the limits of these 'props' were obvious as soon as the man tried to communicate with other people. In contrast, plastic surgery aimed to restore function and enable patients to express emotion.

Medical photographs were taken by professional photographers who worked in the hospital wards where patients were treated. In her discussion of visual representations of mutilation and restoration, Ana Carden-Coyne underlines the fact that 'Clinical photography was used extensively in the First World War and it enjoyed the reputation of a precise science'.[23] Photographic representations of facially injured soldiers were no exception to this rule. Medical photographs mostly represent *gueules cassées* during their treatment, which sets them apart from official photographs. The latter largely focus upon facially disfigured men towards the end of their treatment or those who are having masks fitted. Whilst literature indicates that *gueules cassées* felt uncomfortable at being photographed in social situations, the abundance of medical photography suggests that they did not have a choice, or responded favourably given the 'clinical' context in which medical photographs were taken. Indeed, in hospital wards, everyone was disfigured and photographers – who were sometimes the ward orderlies themselves – were used to seeing wounded men. The close relationship between photography and surgery led to the establishment of a photographer's studio alongside an artist's studio at the Queen's Hospital, Sidcup.

21 Nicolson, *The Great Silence*, p. 67.

22 Wood, 'Masks for Facial Wounds', p. 949.

23 Carden-Coyne, *Reconstructing the Body*, p. 95.

The patients' willingness to pose may be partially attributed to the purpose of medical photography. Its main function was to provide an illustrated record of the treatment and surgical operations performed. As plastic surgery was a fast-developing discipline, photographs enabled practitioners to share their techniques; they had a didactic function as well as a political and documentary purpose, as they served as proof of the progress made. Those with access to the photographs mostly belonged to the medical profession and the circulation of these pictures remained limited. However, with the publication of treatises on plastic surgery (for instance by surgeons Harold Gillies in English and Erich Lexer in German), more people came across these images. The selection of subjects was not dictated by the same concerns as with official photographs: clinical photographers did not shy away from showing severe wounds since they made the case more interesting from a scientific point of view.

Clinical photographs are usually part of a series of at least two pictures (before and after surgery, or sometimes between operations). In medical treatises, several photographs taken at different stages are placed side by side, accompanied by technical explanation and sometimes sketches or drawings. Clinical images are mainly close-ups of the face of a patient whose expression is neutral, consistent with the scientific purpose of these pictures. The camera angle and lighting effects place the focus upon the wound rather than upon the face as a whole. The soldier's pose sometimes looks unnatural since his wound is what has to be most visible, while in reality *gueules cassées* tended to avoid drawing attention to their scars.

During the war, clinical photographs were taken in France, Germany and Great Britain. Harold Gillies included many photographs in his 1920 medical treatise *Plastic Surgery of the Face*. So did Erich Lexer, in *Wiederherstellungs-Chirurgie*, published in Germany the same year. Medical photographs were also taken in France: over a hundred prints of patients treated by the French surgeon Hippolyte Morestin are still in existence.[24] In the introduction to *Plastic Surgery of the Face*, Gillies acknowledges the valuable work of the photographer:

24 Wellcome Library archives, iconographic records, for instance references 569937i, 570112i, 570414i, 570415i, 570434i.

> The majority of the photographic figures in the book have been prepared by Mr Sidney Walbridge. Their excellence speaks for itself, but gives no idea of the time and care this late N.C.O. has devoted to ensuring that they shall be an honest and true record. He has had to suborn his art to this end, sternly suppressing the temptation to manipulate the lighting or retouch the negatives.[25]

Photography is identified as an art and the assumption appears to be that as such it can be deceptive. However, the scientific purpose of medical photographs requires the photographer to fight this tendency of art to transform reality. This supports Sontag's observation that the public seeks 'truth' in photography and that people are suspicious if there is a 'taint of artistry'.[26] A closer examination of the visual depictions published in *Plastic Surgery of the Face* sheds light upon the differences between medical drawings and photographs, and enables us to get a better understanding of how photographic representations were used in a clinical context (Figure 13).

This set of iconographic documents juxtaposes photographs and a drawing, thereby providing an interesting contrast. The descriptions accompanying the illustrations of this case are given from the point of view of Gillies himself, which introduces a human element to this scientific textbook. The fact that the patient's eyes are hidden on the photographs suggests that he wanted his anonymity to be preserved; however, the sketch makes them clearly visible, which implies either that their form and expression were deliberately changed, or that drawings were regarded as a form of art less likely to represent reality. The absence of identification of the patients in medical treatises leaves, according to Sontag, more room for manipulation: not only is it impossible to check that they were actually injured in the war, and that before-and-after photographs actually represent the same men, but it is also difficult to determine their national origins. The anonymous individual patient, like the Unknown Soldier in the Tomb, becomes a symbol for all disfigured men.

The short description (see p. 195) that accompanies these case notes does not jeopardize the patient's anonymity: the only element given is the man's military rank, and his age or name, for instance, are not specified. Only

25 Gillies, *Plastic Surgery of the Face*, p. xi.

26 Sontag, *Regarding the Pain of Others*, p. 23.

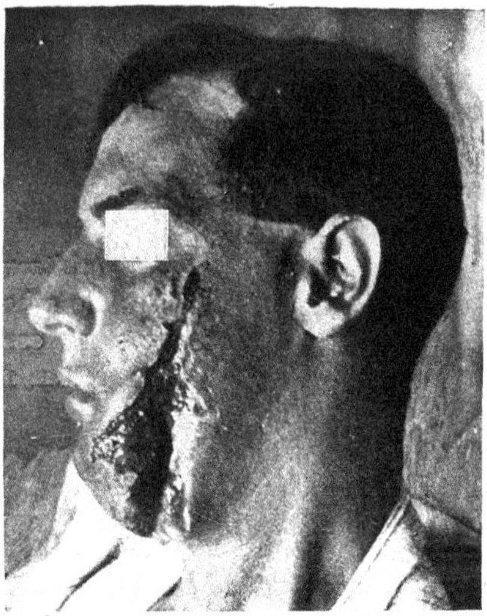

FIG. 15.—On admission 10 days after wound. Lower facial paralysis

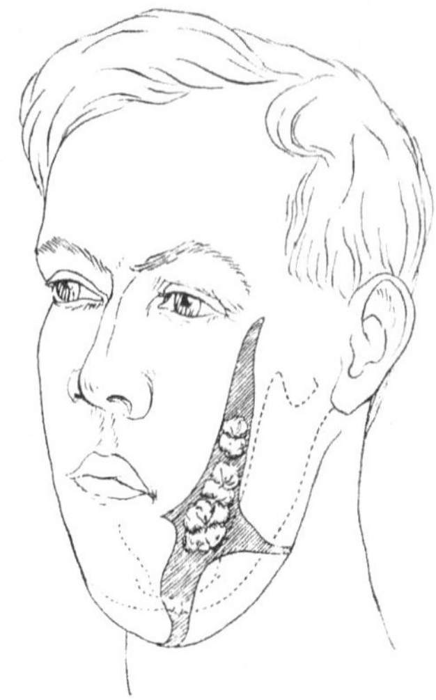

FIG. 16 represents fat flaps rolled in towards the centre of the depression.

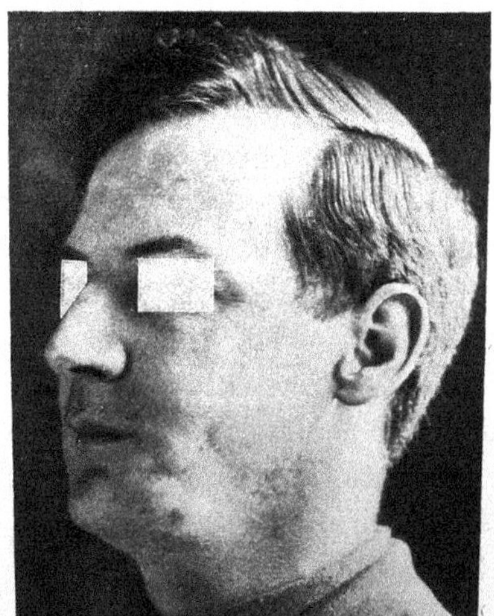

FIG. 17.—*Result.*—Note: the smudge beneath the chin was a result of shaving, and has been removed on the print. There was no appreciable facial paralysis at this stage.

Figure 13: Case 37 in Harold Gillies, *Plastic Surgery of the Face* (London: Frowde, 1920).

his origins ['the Dominions'] are later given; the date and place where he received his wound remain unknown. In the last paragraph, which does not offer any technical information and could therefore be considered as useless in such a scientific text, Gillies's voice is heard again, relating the unhappy conclusion of this successful treatment: 'The final history of this gallant officer from the Dominions is pathetic. Soon after being posted back to duty he volunteered for foreign service again, was shot through the knee-joint and died of wounds in the same Casualty Clearing Station as that which received him when his face was wounded.'[27] The officer's bravery is not denied, yet his circumstances of death suggest that the surgeon's efforts were to some extent wasted.

Such a detailed account of the destiny of a patient is not a common feature of Gillies's book, as the surgeon usually limits his case studies to scientific considerations. These are not restricted to the description of technical prowess: Gillies also considers practical challenges following his patients' discharge, such as their ability to chew. He was not only concerned with the artistic quality of his workmanship, but also interested in the patients' quality of life. Interestingly, some of the photographs included in his book show patients smiling. A happy face was not something unusual in photographs taken at the time – one smiles for the camera and therewith eternity – but this attitude is still striking when it comes to medical photographs of *gueules cassées*. These images point to the surgeon's achievements in terms of functional and psychological reconstruction. More than the soldier's looks, his ability to move his muscles in a natural manner bears testimony to the doctor's skills. Beyond the aesthetic and practical dimensions, these photographs also convey the message that with their new face, veterans can lead a normal life. The damage inflicted to their bodies has been cured owing to scientific and technological advances; medicine has triumphed over war. Whether this smile is a true expression of the patient's relief, an automatic response to the presence of a camera or an attitude they were asked to adopt by the medical photographer cannot, of course, be ascertained.

27 Gillies, *Plastic Surgery of the Face*, p. 42.

Medical photographs were shown in temporary and permanent exhibitions in war and post-war years in France (Val-de-Grâce museum) and in Great Britain (Sidcup, Manchester). Like official photographs, clinical photographs in an exhibition told a story. They were integrated into a narrative of restoration and constituted a visual proof that 'nothing more wonderful has been given to humanity than this triumph of man's science over man's malignity'.[28] Such belief in the goodness of science is opposed to the 'evil' of mankind, a contrast often thematized in the interwar years. This frame of interpretation also serves to justify the display of photographs, which are presented as evidence for its claims. A 1918 article published in the *Manchester Guardian* thus reports on exhibits from the Jaw Centre (Fallowfield, Lancashire) shown to the general public at the Disabled Service Men's Exhibition. Describing the photographs, the journalist writes:

> Some of the photographs would not have been allowed publicity in the good days before we had of necessity accustomed ourselves to the contemplation of the horrible. But here they serve a purpose.
>
> They depict not isolated cases, but a large class of injuries which is daily being replenished from the battle fronts, and they show, fortunately, that the men who suffer can be saved from intolerable disfigurement.[29]

The shock effect of photographs is not denied, as images and objects are described as 'painful to look at'.[30] However, the emphasis is upon the message of hope that they convey.

Medical photographs were also used to further political stances, especially anti-war propaganda. This is particularly the case in Germany, where pictures of facially wounded men taken at the Westdeutschen Kieferklinik (Düsseldorf) and the *Charité* hospital (Berlin) featured prominently in Ernst Friedrich's 1924 pamphlet *Krieg dem Kriege!*. This pacifist manifesto, published five years after the Versailles peace treaty, signals a different use of photographic representations of *gueules cassées* in defeated Germany.

28 'Face Restoring: Wonders of War Surgery', LMA H02/Y01/05, p. 61.

29 'Facial Wounds: Merciful Work of Modern Surgery', *The Manchester Guardian*, p. 3.

30 Ibid, p. 3.

The author, a Socialist militant and founder of the Anti-War Museum in Berlin, addresses not only his fellow countrymen, but also people from France, the Netherlands and from English-speaking countries by including parallel translations in his pamphlet.[31] This work is therefore anti-war in its content but it also aims to bring former enemies together by a shared topic. The title *War against War!* echoes the poster made in 1922 by the Frenchman Théophile Steinlein, also titled *Guerre à la Guerre*, and it highlights that Friedrich himself is on the warpath against 'all war profiteers and parasites, [...] all war provokers'.[32] In order to fulfil his goal, Friedrich turns to photography to present 'a picture of War, objectively true and faithful to nature, [...] records obtained by the inexorable, incorruptible photographic lens', the impact of which upon viewers means that 'not a single man of any country whatsoever can arise and bear witnes [*sic*] against these photographs, that they are untrue and that they do not correspond to realities'.[33] Friedrich acknowledges in his 'concluding remarks' that the documents presented are of predominantly German origin, although he does not wish to single out his fellow-countrymen as being the most apt to cruelty.[34] He even calls for readers to send him material from other countries, to be included in a future edition and in his museum collection.

Friedrich arranges the documents, or rather his 'evidence' for the case for pacifism, in chronological order. They are concerned with 'education' for war, the experience of the front and life after the war. Photographs of facially disfigured soldiers are included in the last part of the book. This section contrasts the effects of war upon the 'ruling class' and upon 'proletarians', in Friedrich's terminology.[35] Several maimed veterans (most of

31 Ernst Friedrich (1894–1967) was arrested in 1933 and the Anti-War Museum was closed. After his release, Friedrich moved to Belgium, then emigrated to France, where he opened a centre promoting peace and international cooperation. The Anti-Kriegs Museum was reopened in 1982 in Berlin. <http://www.anti-kriegs-museum.de/english/history.html> [accessed 18 August 2015].

32 Friedrich, *War against War*, p. 23.

33 Ibid, pp. 22–23.

34 Ibid, p. 249.

35 See in particular Friedrich, *War against War*, pp. 196–99.

them amputees) are shown, but the number of pictures of facially injured men is greater than that of other wounded soldiers: the twenty-four photographs of servicemen with facial wounds make up ten percent of the documents contained in the book. This quantitative difference reveals their importance, as does the fact that one of these photographs features on the original cover page. These images contrast with official portrayals of the banality of war, as displayed elsewhere in the book.

The captions in the section on 'The Visage of the War' are mostly free of irony, as if Friedrich found these photographs self-explanatory and saw no reason why he should add anything to their already powerful impact. Out of the twenty-four photographs, only three feature non-factual captions. The first one represents a disfigured man who has lost his eyes. The other two (one front and one side view) come last in the section and are displayed on two pages facing each other (Figure 14).

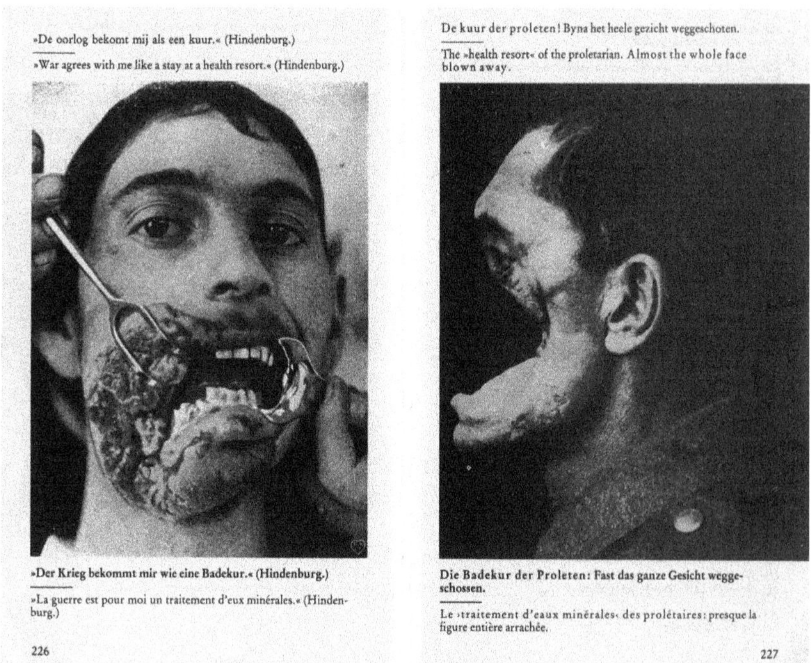
»De oorlog bekomt mij als een kuur.« (Hindenburg.)

»War agrees with me like a stay at a health resort.« (Hindenburg.)

»Der Krieg bekommt mir wie eine Badekur.« (Hindenburg.)

»La guerre est pour moi un traitement d'eux minérales.« (Hindenburg.)

226

De kuur der proleten! Byna het heele gezicht weggeschoten.

The »health resort« of the proletarian. Almost the whole face blown away.

Die Badekur der Proleten: Fast das ganze Gesicht weggeschossen.

Le ›traitement d'eaux minérales‹ des prolétaires: presque la figure entière arrachée.

227

Figure 14: Ernst Friedrich, *Krieg dem Kriege!*, pp. 226–227.

Both photographs picture severely wounded men. While the first man's features are still recognizable, and his ongoing treatment is suggested by the presence of medical instruments, the viewer's imagination cannot fill the vacuum in the second soldier's face.

The first caption is a quotation by the German Field-Marshal Paul von Hindenburg, also translated into English: 'War agrees with me like a stay at a health resort'.[36] The contrast between the destructive effects of the conflict upon this anonymous soldier and the beneficial virtues attributed by one of the top German generals to war is striking, illustrating the gap between military leaders who directed operations and the soldiers who fought them. This discrepancy is further emphasized in the second caption which, taking up the same topic, reads 'The "health resort" of the proletarian: Almost the whole face blown away'.[37] It alludes to a belief that guided the first few years of the conflict: that the war was the maker of men, who were becoming too soft and thereby decadent in peacetime.

The men in these last two photographs are not identified, unlike some of the others. Overall, twelve photographs are accompanied by information regarding the subject's name, age, rank, professional occupation or nature, date or place of injury. Tellingly, facially wounded soldiers are the only people who are identified in Friedrich's book, apart from prominent political leaders such as Wilhelm II or the Crown Prince. On a practical level, such information might not have been available for other, non-medical, photographs. Yet also, the identity of *gueules cassées* was challenged by their wounds to such an extent that Friedrich felt the need to dwell upon what made them human, i.e. their names and their past. Details regarding the number of operations they have undergone are also sometimes included.

The journalist and satirist Kurt Tucholsky offers a glimpse of the reception of the book in a brief reference that consciously avoids reviewing the document:

36 Ibid, p. 226.

37 Ibid, p. 227. Photographs of this patient at different stages of his plastic reconstruction by Joseph are to be found in Natvig, *Jacques Joseph*, pp. 116–18.

> The photographs of the battlefields – the slaughterhouses of the war – and the photographs of the war mutilated are some of the most appalling documents I have ever seen. There is no criminology treatise, no publication that equals them in barbarity, truthfulness and instruction.
>
> The evil conscience with which officers and nationalists of all kinds conceal, and of course must conceal, the true face of war from us, demonstrates what they have to fear from such publications. Written texts fail to convey this. No writer, not even the greatest, can match the weapon of the image.[38]

Tucholsky's choice of words is striking since he argues that the images will impact upon the reader far more than any written contribution ever could. The effect of photographs and more generally the ability of visual representation to convey the horror of war is underlined.

In Friedrich's book, captions that do not give details about the men represented on the photographs are generally more descriptive. They nevertheless bear a strongly emotive tone, as made clear by the use of exclamation marks and qualifiers such as 'gruesomely disfigured' and 'unhappy'.[39] The number of surgical operations and references to the man's inability to eat add to this sense of bleakness. Photographs of patients undergoing treatment are particularly shocking, especially those representing surgical instruments such as forceps in use. A caption specifies that 'many operations have to be carried out in full consciousness (without any narcotic or anaesthetic)'.[40]

38 'Die Fotografien der Schlachtfelder, dieser Abdeckerein des Krieges, die Fotografien der Kriegsverstümmelten gehören zu den fürchterlichsten Dokumenten, die mir jemals unter die Augen gekommen sind. Es gibt kein kriminalistisches Werk, keine Publikation, die etwas Ähnliches an Grausamkeit, an letzter Wahrhaftigkeit, an Belehrung böte.
Das böse Gewissen, mit dem Offiziere und Nationalisten aller Art verhindern und natürlich verhindern müssen, daß das wahre Gesicht des Krieges bekannt werde, zeigt, was sie von solchen Veröffentlichungen zu befürchten haben. Geschriebene Bücher schaffen es nicht. Kein Wortkünstler, und sei er der größte, kann der Waffe gleichkommen', Kurt Tucholsky, 'Waffe gegen den Krieg' (1926), in *Kurt Tucholsky: Gesammelte Werke*, ed. by Mary Gerold-Tucholsky and Fritz J. Raddatz, 10 vols (Reinbek by Hamburg: Rowohlt, 1975), IV (1925–1926), p. 360.

39 Friedrich, *War against War*, p. 207.

40 Ibid, p. 225.

This information, placed beneath a photograph representing what looks like a painful procedure, provokes the viewer's empathy and horror.

Although some of the men agreed to have their photographs taken, Friedrich specifies that many refused, '[fearing] that their relatives who had not seen them again, would either collapse at the sight of their misery, or would turn away forever from them in horror and disgust'.[41] This refusal indicates their struggles to cope with their wounds. It is also telling of their worries at how their relationships with the others, especially their families, will evolve as a result of their disfigurement. These 'unseen' photographs widen the perspective of horrors into the unknown. Friedrich assumes that disfigured men expect to live 'cut off from the world [dragging] on their existences far from their families and friends and relatives, in the hope that they may perhaps after years again acquire the appearance of human beings'.[42] In fact, the section on facially disfigured soldiers does not include any pictures representing them in a social situation (even with fellow patients), or at work (unlike other maimed German veterans, or representations in British and French arts). The final photographs and captions are pessimistic as to the possibilities of facial reconstruction and ultimately, of social reintegration. Indeed, while most of the photographs show patients under treatment – and therefore leave room for hope – the very last picture in the section is that of a soldier whose wounds are apparently cured and who is still missing most of his face. The next section is devoted to pictures of cemeteries, as if the next step after disfigurement is death. Photographs are, then, included in a narrative that evolves towards death, that is, in the opposite direction from visual narratives found in France and Great Britain, which are overwhelmingly stories of individual and national reconstruction.[43]

41 Ibid, p. 211.

42 Ibid, p. 219.

43 Even in the 1932 French publication *Nous Voulons la Paix*, which features photographs of French facially injured soldiers, the tone remains positive as the focus is on national and international efforts to maintain peace. *Nous Voulons la Paix: Concentration des Efforts Universels des Forces Pacifistes* (Paris: SRIP, 1932).

Since the First World War, photographs of disfigured combatants have been mainly used as illustrations of either the horrors of the First World War or as signs of scientific progress. Thus, the 2007 National Army Museum 'Faces of Battle' exhibition was presented by the BBC as '[revealing] a hidden side to the horror of World War I'.[44] The 2014 *Gueules Cassées: Scars from the Great War in Contemporary Art* exhibition at the Mainz Kunsthalle makes the link with contemporary medical practice and political agenda:

> Severely injured servicemen and women from the Iraq and Afghanistan war theaters are given medical treatment at the local military hospitals. Our present-day 'gueules cassées' are directly nearby, yet unlike the battle-injured from the First World War, their modern counterparts are shielded from public view and rendered invisible for propaganda reasons.[45]

At the Val-de-Grâce museum in Paris, in the very building where French disfigured soldiers were treated, the work of plastic surgeon Hippolyte Morestin in the First World War is still presented as a landmark in the development of military surgery. Throughout the century, images of disfigured soldiers have rarely been shown and discussed outside the context of war and medicine.

Art and medicine: The double purpose of medical drawings

At the Queen's Hospital, clinical photographs were used alongside drawings by British artist Henry Tonks (some of which are included in Gillies's medical treatise), and technical sketches by Gillies himself. In France too, doctors

44 'In pictures: Faces of Battle', BBC News, 2009, <http://news.bbc.co.uk/1/shared/spl/hi/picture_gallery/07/magazine_faces_of_battle/html/1.stm> [accessed 18 August 2015].

45 *Les Gueules Cassées: Scars from the Great War in Contemporary Art*, Kunsthalle Mainz, February-June 2014, <http://www.kunsthalle-mainz.de/en/exhibitions/past/les-gueules-cassees/> [accessed 18 August 2015].

and artists joined forces to restore the faces of injured soldiers. Sculptor Robert Wlérick and award-winning painter Jean Dupas worked with Dr Gabriel Moure in Bordeaux whilst Raphaël Freida joined Albéric Pont in Lyon. Freida's drawings are not on public display and they have rarely been studied; yet the comparison between his works and Tonks's sheds a new light upon these visual representations. No evidence of similar collaborations between artists and surgeons can be found for Germany, where historical documentation focuses upon the work of surgeons (such as Erich Lexer and Jacques Joseph) with no mention of sculptors, photographers or artists contributing to the reconstruction of wounded faces. Medical drawings are visual representations of an unconventional nature and have a double role: they combine a medical function with a clear artistic purpose.

Henry Tonks (1862–1937) trained as a surgeon before he undertook an artistic career at the turn of the century. Having become a member of the Slade School of Fine Art, he returned to the practice of medicine during the First World War and started working with Harold Gillies.[46] The pastel drawings he made of patients were informed by his knowledge of the human body, acquired during his medical studies. Tonks enjoyed the artistic challenge and in a letter to his friend D.S. MacColl he casually writes:

> I am doing a number of pastel heads of wounded soldiers who have had their faces knocked about. A very good surgeon called Gillies, who is also a champion golf player, is undertaking what is known as the plastic surgery necessary. It is a chamber of horrors, but I am quite content to draw them, as it is excellent practice.[47]

The Australian Daryl Lindsay also created visual depictions of Sidcup patients and the later contribution of another artist, Sidney Hornswick, is acknowledged by Gillies: 'Latterly, [Tonks's] work has been ably carried on by Mr Sidney Hornswick, who, on his own initiative, has considerably improved and standardised methods of recording flap operations.'[48]

46 John P. Bennett, 'Henry Tonks and his Contemporaries', *British Journal of Plastic Surgery*, 39 (1986), 9–33.

47 Tonks, quoted in Pound, *Gillies*, p. 30. Dated from April 1916.

48 Gillies, *Plastic Surgery of the Face*, p. x.

The Frenchman Raphaël Freida (1877–1942) was conscripted into the medical services and assigned to Albéric Pont's *Centre Maxillo-Facial Pour les Mutilés de la Face* in Lyon. There, Freida produced drawings of facially wounded soldiers almost exclusively, and compiled over twenty of them in an album destined for publication (1917–1919). Although this project never came to fruition, it raises questions about the artist's motivations and the reasons why this book was never published.

Both Tonks and Freida had a medical background, although it was only a short experience in Freida's case. The techniques they and their colleagues used were conventional – pastel drawings, pencil drawings, watercolours – yet the setting in which these works were realized and the purpose they fulfilled make them unique. They are both artistic and scientific. Their medical interest lies partly in the fact that they give a better idea of the skin and flesh colours than clinical photographs, which were black and white. Gillies acknowledges the value of Tonks's contribution in his preface:

> Not a small feature in the development of this work is the compilation of case records. The foundation of the graphic method of recording these cases lies to the credit of Professor H. Tonks (Slade Professor), many of whose diagrams and photographs of his remarkable pastel drawings adorn these pages.[49]

The artistic, perhaps even aesthetically pleasing, dimension of Tonks's pastels is suggested by the verb 'adorn'. This close collaboration between artists and doctors is further confirmed in Freida's dedication of his album to the surgeon Albéric Pont. The usefulness of these artistic works for treatment is also explained by the aesthetic dimension of maxillofacial surgery, as opposed to many other medical specialties. Like drawings sketched in court-rooms, medical drawings fix on paper what most people will never see first-hand. The scientific and artistic qualities of these representations cannot be separated, echoing the holistic nature of plastic surgery itself.

49 Ibid, p. x.

Tonks's works have been the object of scholarly discussion since the 1980s.[50] The drawings examined here aim to add to the existing debate through a comparative study with Freida's works, and by drawing parallels with other visual arts, especially photography.

The documentary dimension of these images is emphasized by the fact that they are close-ups of the men's faces (Figures 15 and 16).

Despite Tonks's medical background, critics disagree in their assessment of the scientific accuracy of his pastels. Whilst John Bennett, a surgeon himself, underlines the 'mastery of technique which records traumatised tissues; scarring, oedema, salivary fistulae', critic Tom Lubbock notes 'pictorial uncertainties' and warns against 'Tonks's vagueness and our ignorance', which may make these pastels 'a lesson in vagueness and its risks'.[51] In contrast, Freida's technique involves clearer line work. His drawings, however, represent fewer extensive injuries and some of them show bandaged heads rather than wounds. As in clinical photographs, the angle chosen highlights the wound. Some of Tonks's works are in fact limited to the wound itself, and the soldier's face remains invisible.[52]

In general, little detail about the patient is available. Whilst photographs are usually carefully annotated, medical drawings often remain unidentified: we are confronted with a medical case rather than a person. The man's shoulders and torso are often absent in Tonks's pastels, strengthening the impression that the patient is reduced to a disfigured face. When more of his body is represented, he is wearing the standard blue uniform, whereas Freida's drawings systematically represent the upper part of the body, revealing military uniforms and on occasion medals.

In comparative studies of photographs and drawings, critics often emphasize the merits of the latter. Freeman judges that 'skin tones, mass,

50 See, for instance, the articles by Freeman, 'Professor Tonks', and Bennett, 'Henry Tonks and his Contemporaries'.

51 Bennett, 'Henry Tonks and his Contemporaries', p. 14; Lubbock, 'Doing Damage', p. 61.

52 See *Detail of surgical treatment to reconstruct a facial injury*, pastel by Henry Tonks. London, Royal College of Surgeons, RCSSC/P 569.72 21.

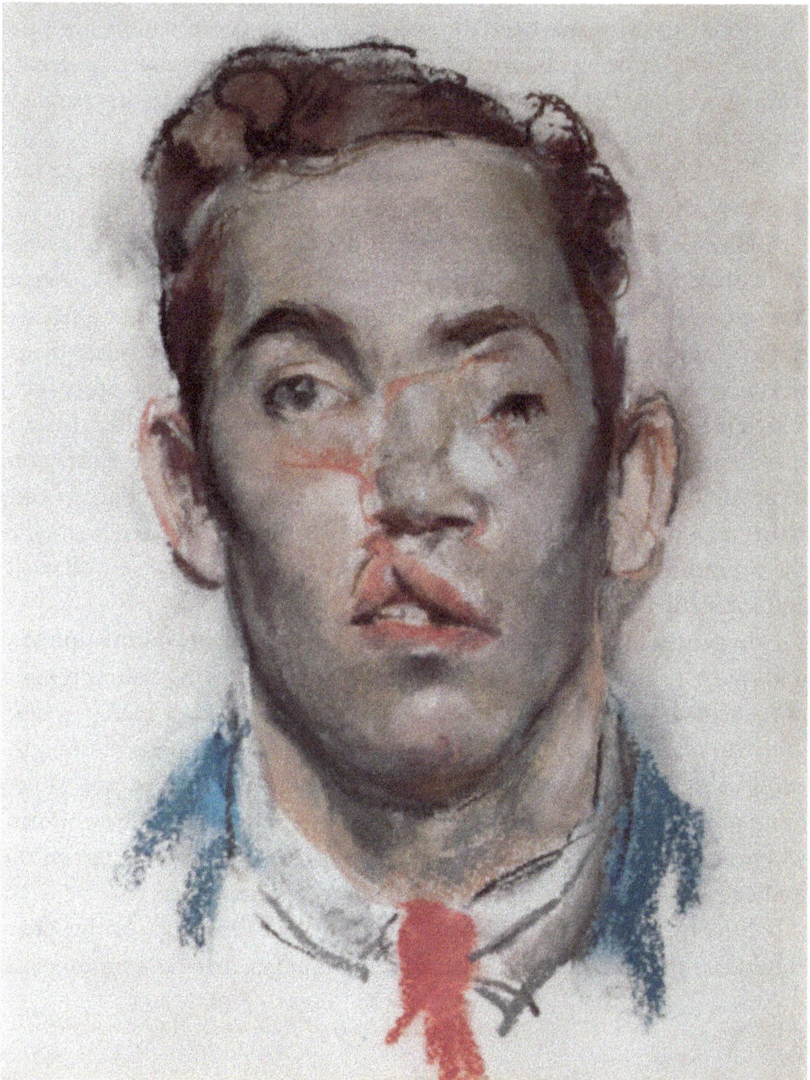

Figure 15: Henry Tonks, Portrait of a wounded serviceman
© Royal College of Surgeons of England, London.

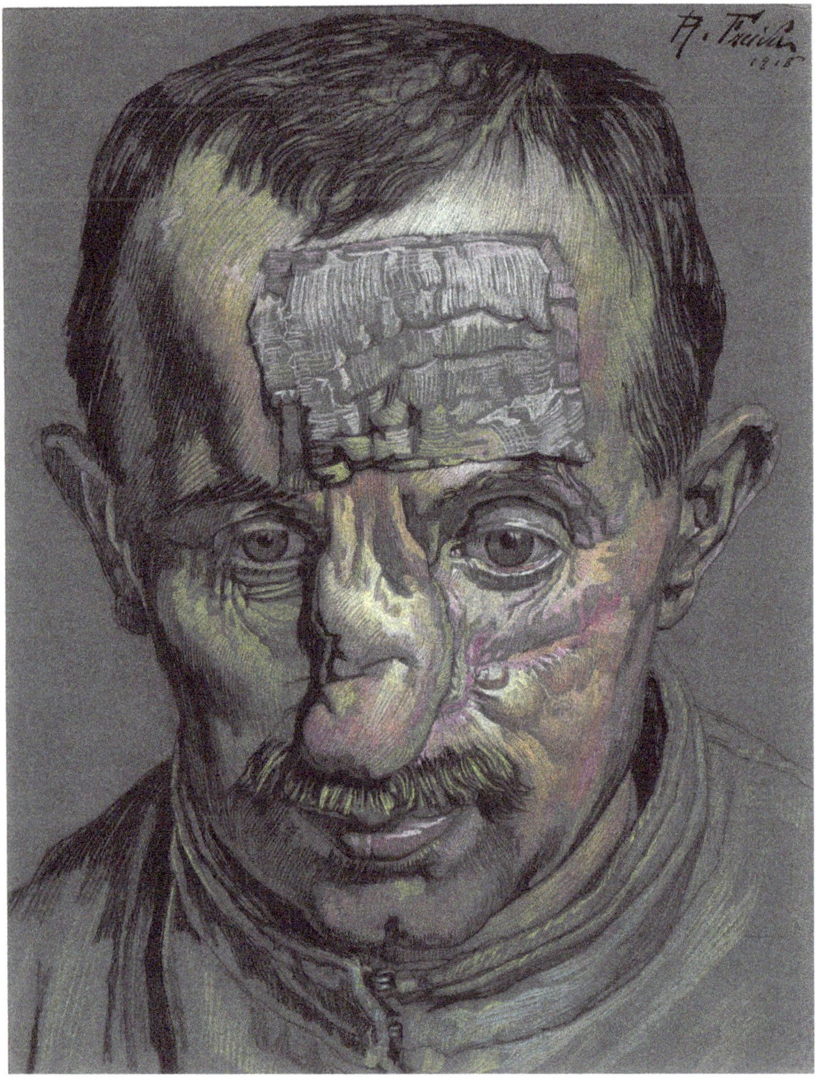

Figure 16: Raphaël Freida, unidentified soldier

shape and colour all appear, all of them beyond the reach of the camera.'[53] Paintings and drawings suggest a greater degree of the artist's personal engagement, in contrast to the mechanical recording process that photography was often perceived as representing. To a greater degree than photographs, medical drawings re-humanized patients, not only in the eyes of the viewer but also in the eyes of the wounded themselves, as suggested by the experience of the twenty-first-century disfigured patients who took part in the *Saving Faces* project. Medical psychologist Paul Ferrand explains that 'Looking at the portraits enables patients [...] to adjust psychologically to their new appearance [...] Whilst [standard photographs] captured the physical characteristics of the patient they did not capture the patients' personality.'[54] The sitters were often reluctant to be photographed but found sitting for the artist a cathartic, even therapeutic, process. The relationship established by Mark Gilbert with them may be very different from the one between soldiers and artists in wartime; nevertheless, this does suggest another facet of the close relationship between art and medicine in the First World War.

Gilbert's portraits often include paintings of the patient before and after surgery, much like the photographs and pastels realized by First World War artists. Tonks's before-and-after pastels, like photographs, testify to the achievements of the surgeon, the pastels emphasizing the change to an even greater extent since they do not show intermediate stages (Figures 17 and 18). Although not all of Tonks's drawings were paired, they had a function as records of the treatment. In contrast, Freida does not appear to have produced before-and-after sets for his album. This was not due to a lack of time (the book features portraits made over several months, in 1917 and 1918); rather, it suggests that Freida put less emphasis upon the documentary aspect of his works. An overview of some technical features is further evidence for this: whilst most of Tonks's sixty-nine pastels and ink-and-pen sketches were made on light paper backgrounds, Freida largely used charcoal, pastels and watercolours on blue or red Canson Kraft paper (Figures 19 and 20).

53 Freeman, 'Professor Tonks', p. 289.

54 Farrand, 'Portraiture as Therapy'.

Freida's dark background prevents him from making full use of colours; the game of shadows and light is, however, more visible in his portraits. In contrast, Tonks's light colours are more realistic and create a warmer atmosphere. Most scholars and critics posit an emotional involvement on the part of the artist, and a powerful impact of the works upon the viewer. Bennett even judges that the worth of Tonks's pastels lies in their subjective nature: 'They are of more impact than photographs because the artist has, in a sense, instilled his sympathy and understanding into the record'.[55] The degree of the artist's engagement in the surgical treatment and psychological recovery of patients is obviously hard to assess but Tonks and Freida nonetheless spent a significant amount of time in the soldiers' presence.

In some of their drawings, Tonks and Freida represent the patient looking in a different direction: his gaze does not meet the onlooker's. There is no 'point of entry', thereby to some extent contradicting Helmers' descriptions of Tonks's images as 'gateways' introducing the viewer to the subject's suffering.[56] The depiction of physical and psychological suffering is defined as the prevailing quality in these portraits: 'In the eyes of those portrayed, the expression of pain, anxiety, resignation and anguish makes them one of the most moving and impressive records of human disfigurement which have been handed down to us'.[57] The validity of this statement could be questioned in the light of the documentary function they fulfilled and the absence of emotions represented. Tonks's pastels were on display as part of the maxillofacial hospital museum collection; they were not widely disseminated, however, even after the war, and did not feature in a later Tate Gallery exhibition (1936) alongside some of his other works.

Tonks was approached by the British propaganda services during the war but he was not keen to let his pastels be used in public documents. In a letter to the Ministry of Information, he writes: 'The pastels which I have done are of wounded soldiers with face injuries. They are, I think,

55 Bennett, 'Henry Tonks and his Contemporaries', p. 15.

56 Helmers, 'Iconic Images of Wounded Soldiers', p. 197.

57 Bennett, 'Henry Tonks and his Contemporaries', pp. 14–15.

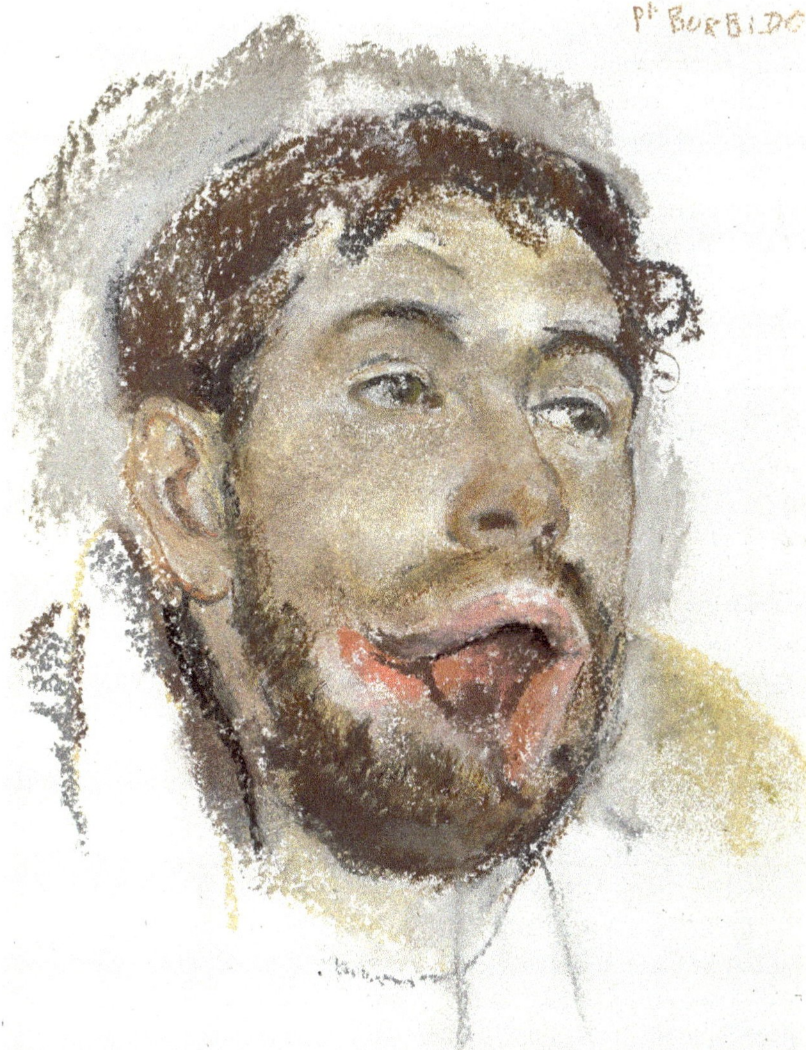

Figure 17: Henry Tonks, Portrait of Private Harold Burbridge, 1917

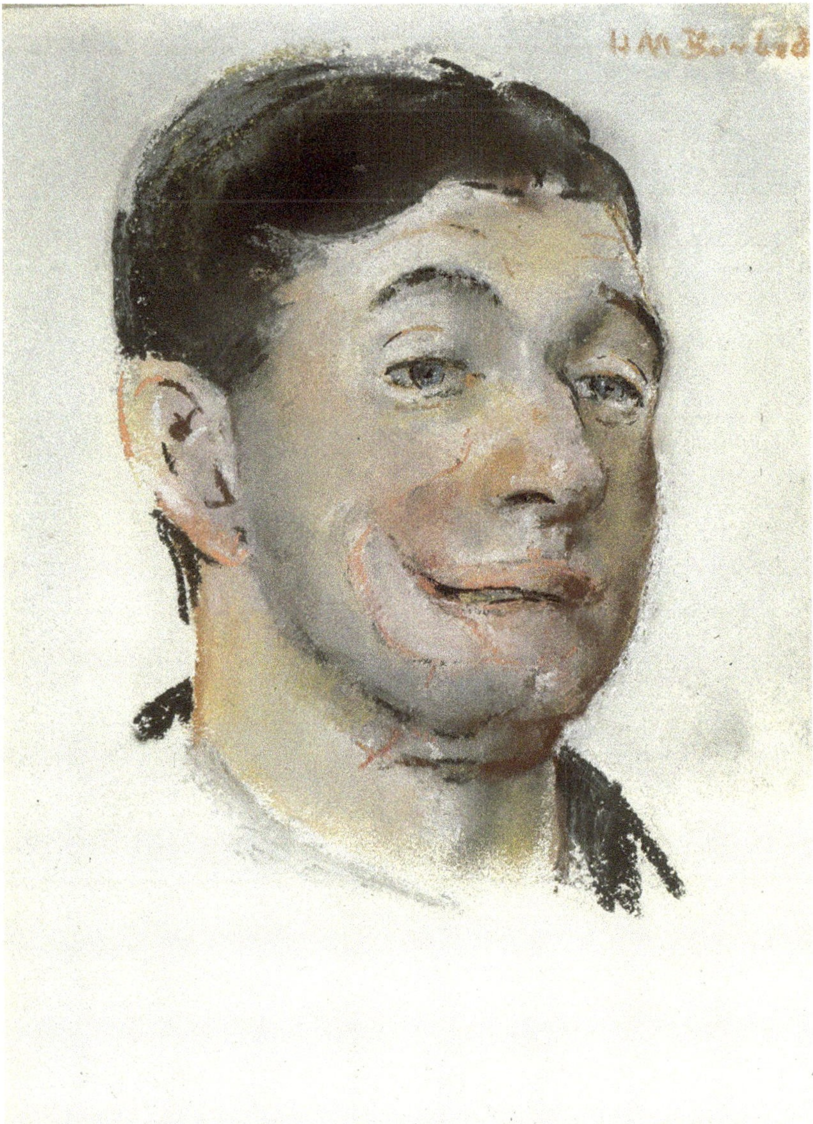

Figure 18: Henry Tonks, Portrait of Private Harold Burbridge, 1918
© Royal College of Surgeons of England, London.

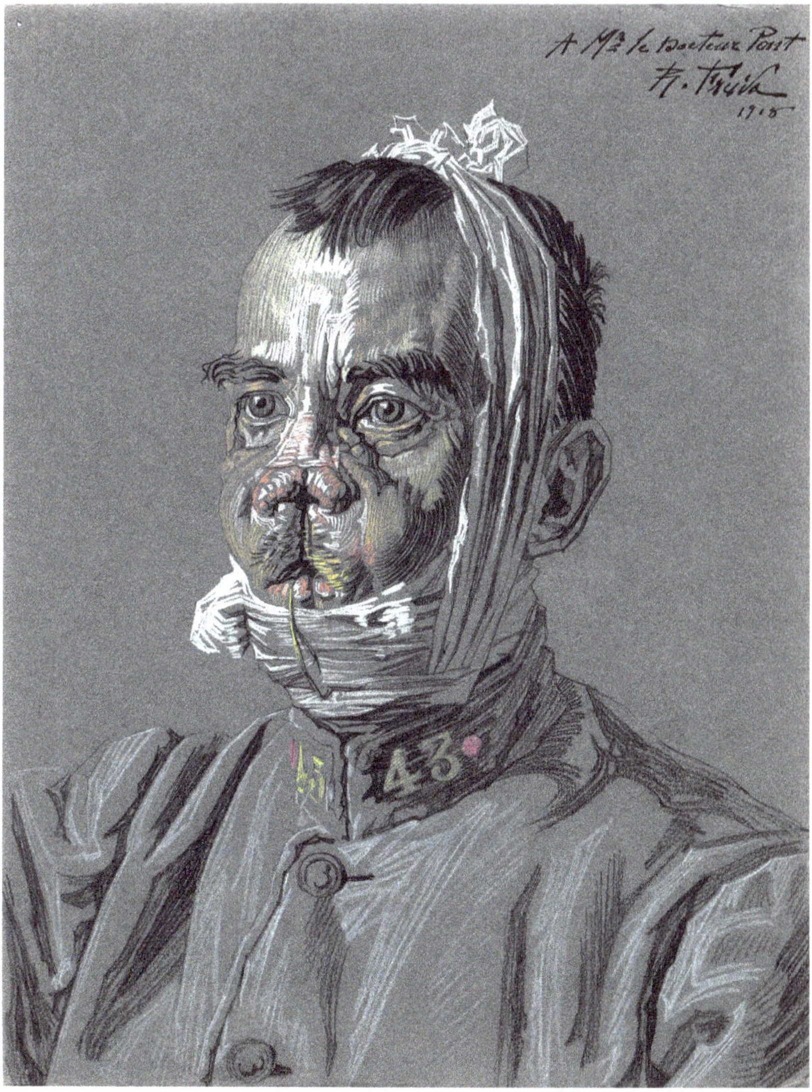

Figure 19: Raphaël Freida, Portrait of a wounded soldier
© Musée du Service de Santé des Armées au Val-de-Grâce, Paris.

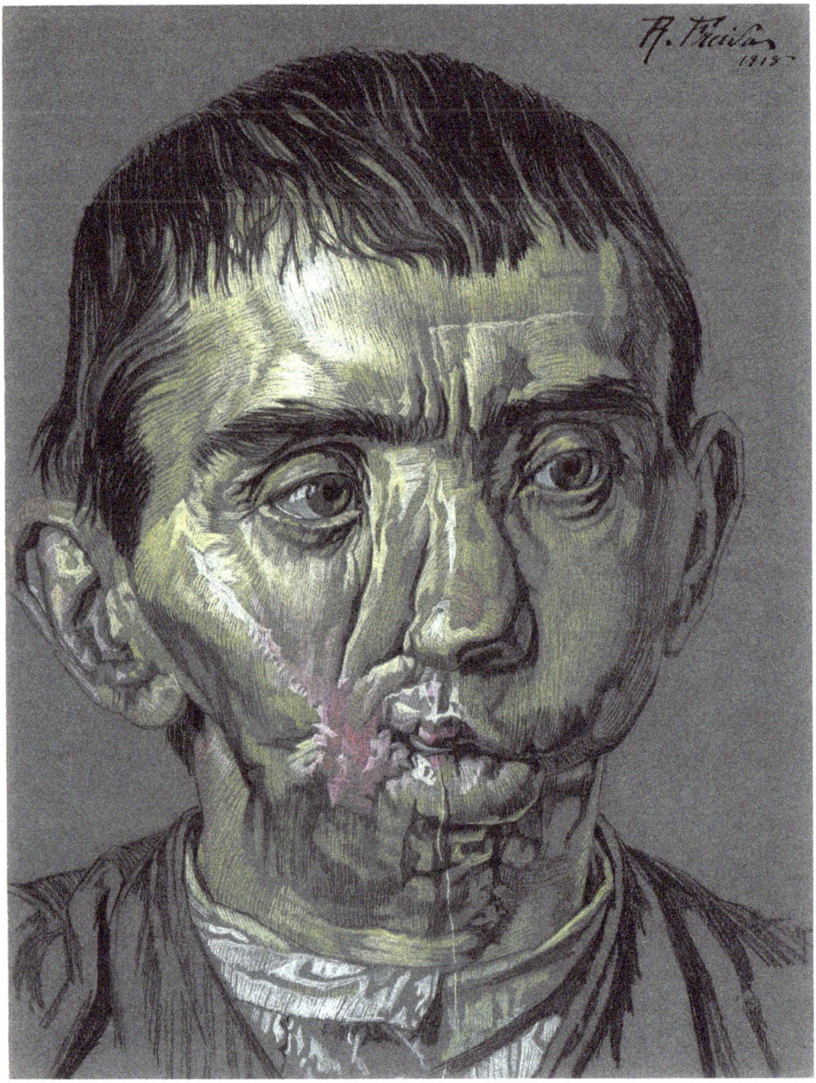

Figure 20: Raphaël Freida, Portrait of a wounded soldier
© Musée du Service de Santé des Armées au Val-de-Grâce, Paris.

rather dreadful subjects for the public view'.[58] This reluctance contrasts with Freida's wish to publish some of his drawings. Whilst in Tonks's case, the artist himself was the one reluctant to confront the general public with his works, in France Freida was keen to disseminate his artistic depictions. A difference in terms of the authorities' attitude to visual representations and censorship policies is a possible explanation for this difference. Another hypothesis is the later date of Freida's endeavour. Indeed, at a time when war pensions were discussed in the French Parliament (in 1919), the publication of visual representations may not have been desirable. Another possible factor is the propagandistic use to which the British authorities considered putting the pastels, whereas in Freida's case he himself had prepared the book, which was descriptive more than argumentative. Tonks disliked the fact that his works were on display in the hospital museum, describing the visitors' interest as 'morbid'.[59] In contrast, Freida was keen to show his works to the French public. This greater willingness to see and show *gueules cassées* in France reflects the later developments in France, not least with regard to the visibility of veterans through the organization they founded, the *Union des Blessés de la Face*, discussed in Chapter 3.

More time-consuming to make than photographs, drawings rarely trace the reconstruction process in the same way as medical photography. This discrepancy accounts for the feeling of an absence of progress in the works. Yet regardless of these documentary qualities, medico-artistic representations appear to be another area in which the violence of war has given rise to progress and innovation. The usefulness of these works is indeed signalled by the fact that similar techniques were used during the Second World War. For example, one of these later artists was Diana 'Dickie' Orpen, daughter of First World War artist William Orpen, who trained at the Slade School under Tonks. Diana Orpen (1914–2008) drew in the operating theatre at the Plastic and Jaw Centre, St Albans, and she

58 Henry Tonks, quoted in Bennett, 'Henry Tonks and his Contemporaries', p. 15.

59 Henry Tonks, Letter to MacColl, p. 128.

produced more than 2,700 works during the Second World War.[60] Her work, as well as Mark Gilbert's, testifies to the close and lasting relationship between art and maxillofacial surgery.

Essays that discuss the reception of medical drawings such as Tonks's posit that they provoked both repulsion and compassion in the viewer, although no contemporary account actually records these reactions.[61] For war artists, *gueules cassées* are subjects with whom they can experiment and develop their skills. Tonks himself described his work at Sidcup as 'excellent practice' in his letter to MacColl.[62] Drawings were less widely disseminated than photographs and, whilst some were interpreted in a positive light, they largely present disfigured soldiers as victims, all the more so since most of them depict men before the end of their treatment.

The wealth of medical drawings that represent facially injured soldiers testifies to the visibility of the soldiers, at least in the medical sphere. This variety in terms of the visual representations of *gueules cassées* is indicative of different ways in which people tried to capture the experience of facial disfigurement. Medical drawings, like photographs, form part of a wealth of visual documents that defy categorization: they are partly private, partly public, partly scientific and partly artistic. These works bear testimony to the visual impact of facial injury and to the importance of the onlooker's gaze. Through the eyes of the painter, the viewer is given more than the wounds to see. Drawings and pastels may not unfold as detailed a narrative as photographs, nor give as realistic a portrait; yet they offer a more human image of disfigured men, mediated by the artist and their perceptions.

60 Dickie Orpen drawings, British Association of Plastic, Reconstructive and Aesthetic Surgery <http://www.bapras.org.uk/about_us/our_archives/archive_news/dickie_orpen_drawings> [accessed 11 April 2014].

61 See, for instance, Lubbock, 'Doing Damage', and Chambers, 'Fragmented Identities'.

62 Tonks to MacColl, quoted in Chambers, 'Fragmented Identities', p. 588.

Isolation or integration: Images of facially injured soldiers in interwar arts

Works by Tonks and Freida remained unseen for decades and have only recently been shown to the wider public. In contrast, paintings by contemporary artists such as Otto Dix and George Grosz were produced with the intention of being looked at and engaged with at the time. The apparent absence of (at least existing) medical drawings in Germany contrasts with the predominance of other works of art in the country featuring *Menschen ohne Gesicht* [men without faces]. Such paintings and drawings are more 'conventional' artistic representations insofar as they do not have a scientific purpose, and they often convey a political message.

In French and British arts, works representing *gueules cassées* are placed in the continuity of medical representation: they speak of physical and social rehabilitation. They were integrated into discourses of individual and national reconstruction insofar as they convey the suggestion that just as facially injured soldiers can overcome their trauma, so can the rest of society. In her study of masculinity, Amy Lyford goes as far as saying that the rehabilitation of the male body and psyche, and the restoration of the traditional image of male heroism, were presented as 'the prerequisites for national renewal'.[63]

In this spirit, John Hodgson Lobley (1878–1954) painted soldiers at The Queen's Hospital, Sidcup. In his capacity as an official war artist, Lobley, a Slade School student, was commissioned by the Royal Army Medical Corps to the maxillofacial centre where he painted rehabilitation workshops. These four oil paintings represent the dental mechanics' class, the carpenters' shop, the commercial class and the toy makers' shop. Lobley's paintings had a propagandistic function insofar as they aimed to shape society's perception of injured veterans. They also showed the efforts made to enable soldiers – at Sidcup and elsewhere – to be re-trained and to contribute to the nation's economy despite their wounds.

63 Lyford, *Surrealist Masculinities*, p. 11.

Whilst medical painting and photography focus upon specific individuals, these paintings represent groups of men in training, apparently not posing for the artist. Lobley's works do not single out individuals, nor do they highlight their disfigurement. All men wear the customary blue suits (or white coats in the dentist mechanics' class) and the technique used by Lobley does allow the viewer to clearly distinguish wounds or scars. Were it not for the bandages some of them are wearing, they could be any men at work. *The dental mechanics' class* pictures several men in profile, sitting in a row, bent over workbenches. They are visibly concentrating on what they are doing, although the exact nature of the work is unknown. What is emphasized in this painting is not what wounded soldiers are learning, or the result of their efforts, but the fact that they are working, as part of a group, and under circumstances to which the onlooker can relate. This is only the first step towards a wider economic and social reintegration. *The commercial class* (Figure 21) produces a similar effect; the students this time

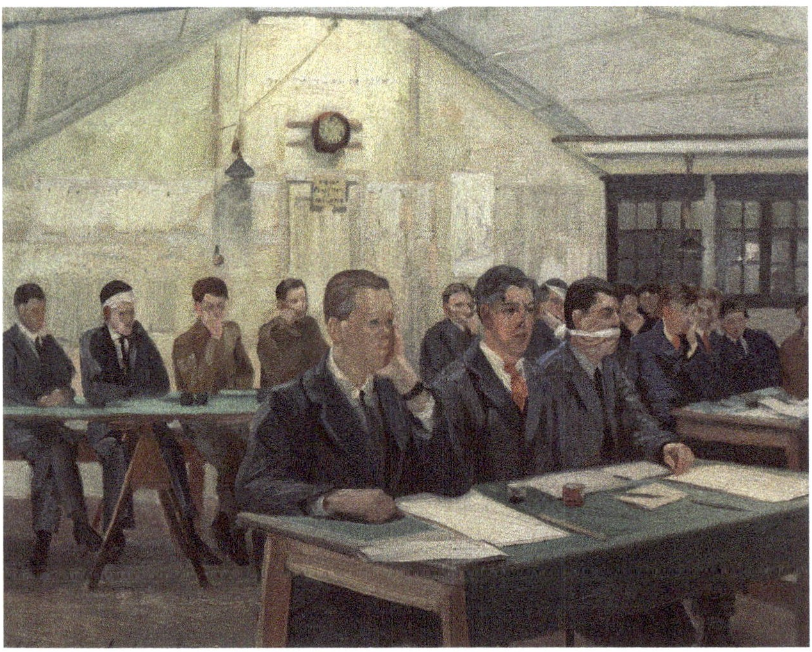

Figure 21: John Hodgson Lobley, *The commercial class* © IWM (ART 3767).

simply listen. This painting shows men from a different angle, rendering their bandages more visible although the patients in the foreground do not have any apparent injuries. They appear to be able to concentrate and learn this new trade – their facial wounds have not impeded their intellectual ability. *The carpenters' shop* (Figure 22) and *The toy makers' shop* represent men actively involved in manual activities. Artefacts bearing testimony to their efforts are pictured: a table in the carpenters' shop and a stuffed teddy bear in the toy makers' shop.

The context in which these paintings were realized is of interest, especially with regard to the contemporary commissioning of Nicholls as an official photographer in Wood's studio, and the presence of other artists at The Queen's Hospital, such as Tonks. The choice to depict injured soldiers as men in professional training, rather than as patients, indicates the

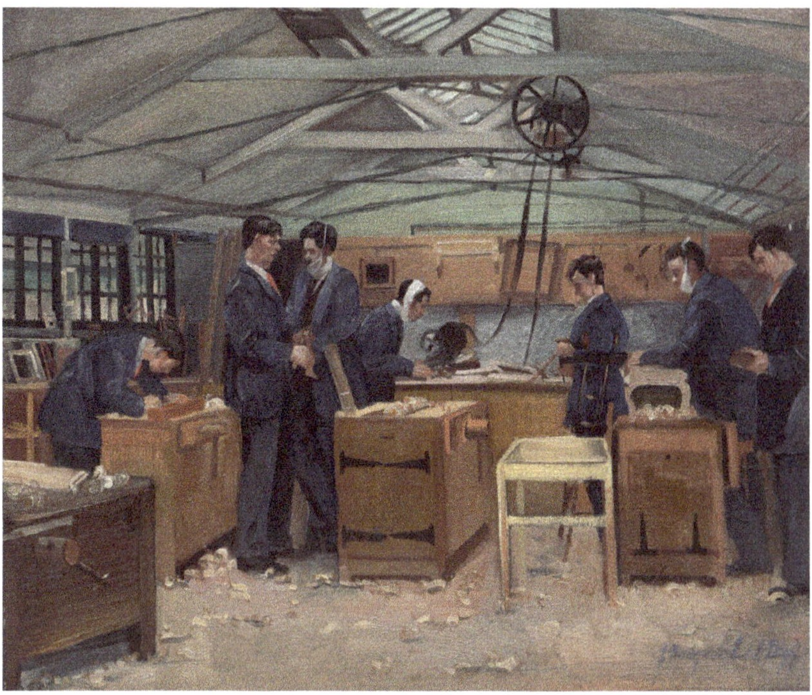

Figure 22: John Hodgson Lobley, *The carpenters' shop* © IWM (ART 3728).

positive discourse that authorities sought to promote through these images. Although the men are wounded, they are preparing for their return into employment. They are presented as active, even during their treatment in hospital, getting ready to reintegrate into civilian society.

Lobley's artistic choices – the subdued tones and blurred lines that do not draw attention to the wounds and scars, the individual men who can hardly be identified – combine with the reassuring message of men at work conveyed in these paintings. They fit in with official discourse and point not to the destructiveness of war, but rather to men's ability to overcome their trauma and make a productive contribution to post-war society. These images speak of re-integration; the sense of disintegration shown in other artists' work is counteracted. The fact that the wounded men are painted at work links them with the 'real', outside world. As such, they are propaganda material and they evidence the trend in Great Britain to represent facial injuries as curable and the future of disfigured men as normal. In contrast, in French and German arts, *gueules cassées* were singled out and appear to be polarizing figures hailed or reviled in triumphant and defeated nations. Jean Galtier-Boissière's *Défilé des Mutilés*, for example, shows the 14 July 1919 march in Paris. It features several facially injured soldiers, this time in a more formal, military context (Figure 23).

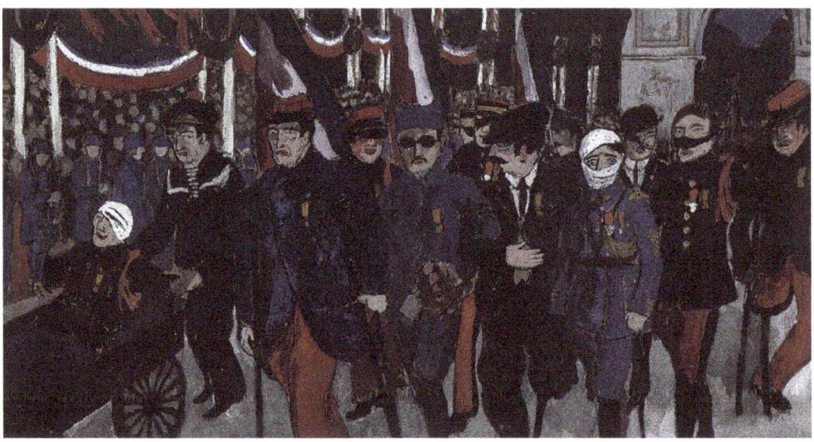

Figure 23: Jean Galtier-Boissière, *Défilé des Mutilés*. Reproduced courtesy of the Bibliothèque de Documentation Contemporaine Internationale, Paris.

An eyewitness of the war, the French artist Jean Galtier-Boissière is better known for his writings (*La Fleur au Fusil* records his war memories) and his instrumental role in setting up one of the most popular French soldiers' newspapers, *Le Crapouillot*. His *Défilé des Mutilés, 14 Juillet 1919*, is an oil painting depicting French mutilated soldiers in their army uniforms, walking under the Arc de Triomphe and surrounded by a crowd. The presence of French flags and tricolour banners increases the sense that the nation is paying homage to and celebrating its heroes. There is a stark contrast between the faceless spectators in the background and the rows of maimed veterans, represented in more detail. Most of them suffer from several injuries, their amputated legs and wounded faces standing out. Two of them, in the second row, seem to have swollen, red scars leaving them permanently disfigured while the bandages worn by two other soldiers in the front row imply that they are still undergoing treatment. Several men are wearing black patches over part of their face. Their disfigured bodies, as well as the fact that most of them cannot walk without a support, hardly make them proud war survivors.

This painting suggests that the presence of facially injured servicemen was acceptable in a context such as a military march. They belonged to the military world, and to wartime. The soldiers and the public remain separate, the latter being the ones gazing and the former the ones under the gaze. This encounter is between two groups, not between individuals, and it is to some extent staged by the authorities, who decided to have wounded servicemen parading at this march devoted to the celebration of victory. They embody the human cost of this victory and remind the onlookers of their debt.

The posture of the men depicted in the *Défilé* painting differs from that of most of George Grosz and Otto Dix's soldiers: despite their maimed features, the French veterans are marching down the famous avenue, holding their heads high. Galtier-Boissière's choice to represent the victory march reveals the will to honour the 'war heroes' whilst at the same time wanting to forget about the 'war to end all wars'. Mutilated veterans, and *gueules cassées* especially, were regarded as particularly evocative of war memories. The situation in which Galtier-Boissière chose to represent them – that of the nation celebrating the men who made victory possible – integrates them into a narrative of successful reconstruction. French society is ultimately pictured as united and victorious.

Galtier-Boissière and Lobley overall participate in a positive discourse about the role and place of facially injured men. In contrast, artistic representations produced in Germany picture isolated figures and difficult interaction with society.

Works by Otto Dix (1891–1969) include several representations of facially disfigured men. His personal experience of the front adds authenticity to his art: he volunteered in 1914 and served for four years, taking part in the Battle of the Somme and receiving a wound in 1918.[64] He went on to become a prominent artist in Weimar Germany, contributing to the Dadaist, Expressionist and New Objectivity movements, and he denounced contemporary society and its perceived depravity in his work.[65] The representation of soldiers and veterans suffering from facial injuries in Dix's oeuvres suggests that they were a common sight, or at least that they made a powerful impression upon the artist. The paintings discussed here were all produced after the conflict (Figure 24).

Transplantation (known in English as *Skin Graft*) is one of the fifty images in the portfolio *Der Krieg*. Published in 1924, this collection of etchings, aquatint and drypoint benefited from the support of the organization Never Again War.[66] The etching shows a patient in hospital, as suggested by his clothes, the frame and the bedding in the background. His face, the dominant focus of the picture, is extensively damaged. Although

64 Dietrich Schubert, *Otto Dix* (Leck: Clausen & Bosse, 1996; Hamburg: Reinbek, 1980), pp. 21–29.

65 Rainer Metzger, *Berlin, Die Zwanzigerjahre: Kunst und Kultur 1918–1933* (Vienna: Christian Brandstätter, 2006), pp. 111–13 and p. 179.

66 The *Nie Wieder Krieg* movement included prominent representatives such as Kurt Tucholsky and artist Käthe Kollwitz, whose poster *Nie Wieder Krieg* was produced the same year Friedrich published his pamphlet. A discussion of Dix's works is to be found in Heather Hess, German Expressionist Digital Archive Project, *German Expressionism: Works from the Collection* (2011), <http://www.moma.org/collection_ge/object.php?object_id=63267&curated=1> [accessed 18 August 2015].

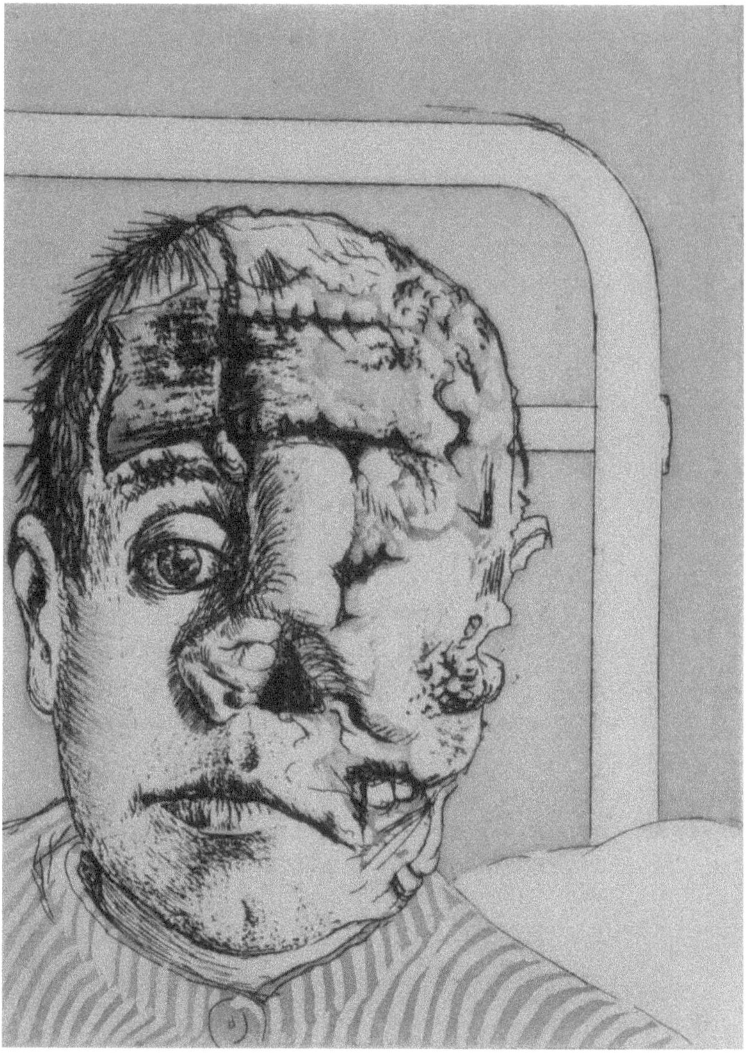

Figure 24: Otto Dix, *Transplantation* (1924)
 Digital image, Historial de la Grande Guerre, Péronne.

no direct reference to the war is made, the theme of the portfolio permits the assumption that he is a wounded soldier. The title refers to a surgical procedure, then a new development, but there is no emphasis upon the human dimension. Other pictures in *Der Krieg* have titles pointing to a particular situation, such as *Verwundeter*, *Fliehender Verwundeter*, *Sterbender Soldat*, *Toter* (Injured Man, Injured Soldier Trying to Escape, Dying Soldier, Dead Man). Unlike *Transplantation*, they do not refer to an act, but to a scene. In the latter, the loss of individual identity for facially injured men is emphasized.

The man's face occupies most of the picture and it stands out against the austere background. His eye stares straight at the onlooker, providing a visual point of entry. The face is depicted with documentary accuracy, as opposed to the simplicity of the other elements represented. The plain and well-delineated shapes of the objects in the background and of the patient's clothes, contrast with the chaos of the face, which gives the impression of a patchwork of pieces 'transplanted' from elsewhere on the body. The damaged side of the face is at the centre of the etching.

The most distinctive characteristic of this visual representation is the duality of the face, half intact and half mangled. Perfectly recognizable human features are visible: ear, eye, mouth and hair. They allow for a comparison that strengthens the sense of loss. The nose and forehead are damaged but identifiable. The viewer involuntarily searches for similar features between the two halves. This division of the face into two very distinct halves, one intact and one damaged beyond recognition, is also to be found in *Kriegsverletzter* [War Invalid], a watercolour based upon photographs, made by Dix in 1922.[67] This portrait depicts a wounded soldier wearing a hospital shirt, the right hand side of his face a gaping wound. The vivid colours used to paint the wound make it all the more conspicuous against the softer shades of the rest of the painting. While the patient in *Transplantation* has distorted features, swollen flesh and scars, the wound of Dix's earlier *Kriegsverletzter* is a big hole; half of the face is characterized by the absence of any human features.[68] In contrast with this damaged side,

67 This watercolour is in a private collection and was reproduced with permission in the catalogue of the 1992 Dix's retrospective exhibition: *Otto Dix: 1891–1969*. Tate Gallery exhibition catalogue (London: Tate Gallery Publications, 1992), p. 140.

68 It is interesting to note that Dix chose to paint the wound at this early stage. The American surgeon Albee notes that 'a scarred face is small matter compared with a

the other half is intact and the man's features are well delineated. There is no emotion on display. Dix used photographs taken in war hospitals to paint mutilated men; this medical background accounts for the similarities between these paintings and some clinical photographs and drawings, such as the empty background. Whereas the title *Transplantation* points to a scientific procedure, *Kriegsverletzter* points to the man, as if the facially wounded soldier was representative of all *Kriegsverletzte*.

The combination of intact and damaged features is a recurring motif in artistic and literary depictions, for instance in Vicki Baum's description of Doctor Otternschlag in her novel *Menschen im Hotel* [*Grand Hotel* in its English translation].[69] The disfigured veteran is in effect a problematic living embodiment of death, a transgressive presence in a society struggling to mourn, heal and forget. This combination of death and life echoes medieval representations of the dance of death (a theme explicitly chosen by Dix in another etching from *Der Krieg* portfolio). In *Transplantation*, the personified death and its victim are two facets of the same person.

The man's hospital clothes in both *Kriegsverletzter* and *Transplantation* remind the viewer of a prisoner's uniform. This impression is reinforced by the metal frame of the bed in the background of *Transplantation*. These elements evoke confinement and underline the situation of the wounded man, trapped in his own disfigured body. There is, however, an element of hope: the setting – a hospital – implicitly refers to treatment and the possibility of restoring the patient's features. Moreover, *Transplantation* explicitly refers to scientific progress, suggesting that the disfigured man may benefit from this medical technique.[70]

Other works by Dix also represent facially mutilated veterans, individually or in groups, although they are never in direct interaction with

---

gaping hole where a nose or a mouth has been', underlining the impact of missing features (*A Surgeon's Fight to Rebuild Men*, p. 110).

69 Vicki Baum, *Grand Hotel*, trans. by Basil Creighton (London: Geoffrey Bles, 1930), first published under the title *Menschen im Hotel* in Germany, 1929. This work will be discussed in more detail in the next chapter.

70 Dennis Crockett, *German Post-Expressionism: The Art of the Great Disorder, 1918–1924* (University Park, PA: Penn State University Press, 1999), p. 97.

civilians. *Die Skatspieler* [The Skatplayers] (Figure 25) depicts injured men in a more secluded environment, playing cards.

This work, a combination of oil paint and collage, underlines the destruction caused by war and features a Dadaist component noted by Dietrich Schubert in his study of the life and work of Otto Dix.[71] The three veterans represented are all maimed; not one limb appears intact. However, this does not prevent them from playing cards. The multiplicity of injuries and mutilations gives an almost comical effect to the scene through its hyperbolic dimension. Bright colours and the technique of collage highlight the fragmentation of the body caused by the war. The prosthetics, very similar to the legs of the chairs, evoke the ambiguous relationships between man and machine: the latter tore flesh apart during the war, and yet helped to reconstruct the body after the conflict. *Die Skatspieler* can be understood as a reflection of a dysfunctional post-war society that 'kills time' for want of a productive occupation – here by playing cards as soldiers did in the trenches.

This scene does not single out facial disfigurement; rather it places it within a wider range of war injuries. Nevertheless, in the midst of this accumulation of wounds, facial injuries still stand out, their composite aspect and the presence of metallic prostheses attracting the viewer's attention. It is upon the metal jaw of one of the men that Dix added a photograph of himself, along with the words 'Unterkiefer: Prothese Marke: Dix. Nur echt mit dem Bild des Erfinders' [Lower jaw: prosthesis trade mark Dix/ Only authentic if featuring the picture of the inventor]. Eyes, jaws, noses and ears are deformed or absent, preventing the veterans from showing emotions, and probably also from communicating efficiently. The man on the left especially has amidst his scars an unnatural smile fixed upon his face. The overall impression is one of suffering and isolation from the rest of the world, a far cry from the heroism the military background of the veterans, one of whom has been awarded the Iron Cross, could suggest. Although the war is over, they have not found a place in post-war society. This composition also features a satirical element, as suggested by Carol

71 Schubert, *Otto Dix*, p. 41.

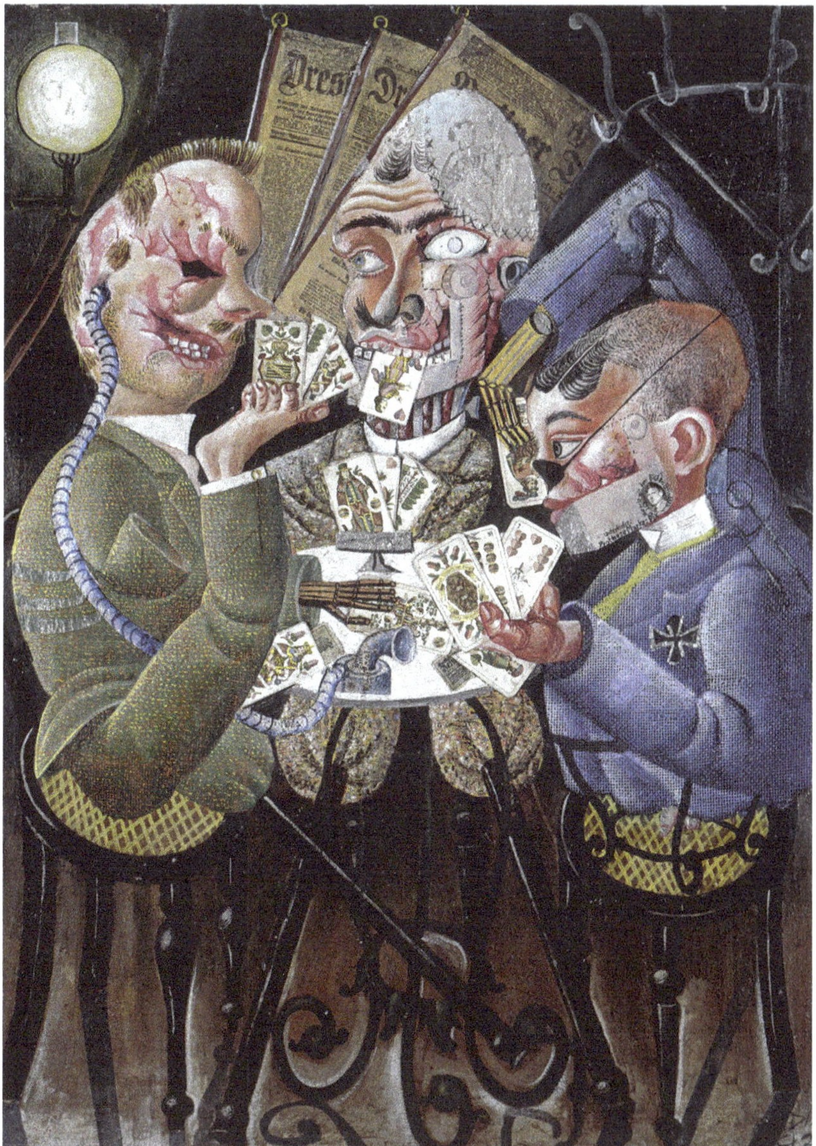

Figure 25: Otto Dix, *Die Skatspieler* (1920)

Poore. In her study of disability in the Weimar Republic, she interprets the *Skatplayers* as 'monstrous holdovers of an authoritarian system, […] still dyed-in-the-wool militarists [who] keep on playing their game the way they have always played it'.[72] These men embody fractured times, the unsettled dimension of this period highlighted by the element of chance or gamble at work in card games. The newspapers in the background provide their only link with the day-to-day affairs of the rest of the world. Two years after the end of the First World War, these men are hardly heroes; they function, according to Ashley Bassie, 'as an accusation and a warning against militarism', the utilization of the figure of the maimed veteran pointing towards the purposelessness of war.[73]

A similar sense of irony can be found in Dix's *Die Kriegskrüppel* [War Cripples] (1920), which portrays legless ex-servicemen parading in front of a shoe shop (Figure 26).

Despite the impact of war upon their bodies they still march in military formation, at regular intervals and with heads held straight (except for the shaking, probably shell-shocked soldier). This work is based upon an oil-painting exhibited at the Erste Dada-Messe in Berlin in 1920 and entitled '45% Erwerbsfähig' [45 per cent fit to work], ironically pointing toward the ways in which German authorities assessed the usefulness of mutilated veterans.[74] This capitalist view of mankind makes no allowance for the pain of the veterans, nor for their courage, although it was officially recognized by military decorations. It is hardly surprising that this picture was interpreted as '[humiliating] and [making] a laughing stock

72 Carol Poore, *Disability in Twentieth-Century German Culture* (Ann Arbor: University of Michigan Press, 2007), p. 32.

73 Ashley Bassie, *Expressionism* (London: Parkstone Press, 2008), p. 121.
See also Otto Friedrich's analysis that argues the defeat led German people to feel that men had fought, suffered and died in vain. Otto Friedrich, *Before the Deluge: A Portrait of Berlin in the 1920s* (New York: Harper Collins Publishers, 1995).

74 This was already thematized in 1916–17 by George Grosz in *Die Gesundbeter*.

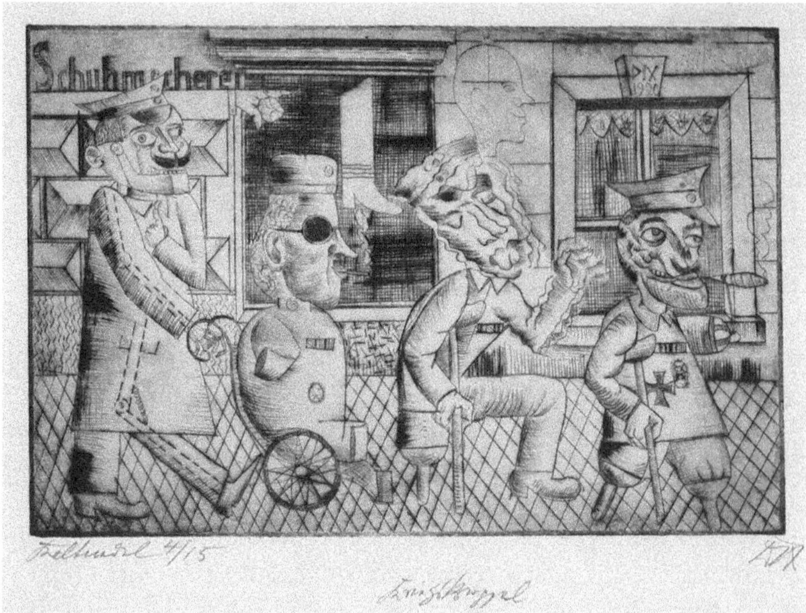

Figure 26: Otto Dix, *Kriegskrüppel* © DACS 2014. Digital image, The Museum of Modern Art, New York/Scala, Florence.

of the German soldier' and subsequently 'it was one of the first works to be confiscated by the Nazis'.[75]

Dix thus pictures facial injury as a commonplace at the front as well as in post-war life. But although disfigured men are physically present on the street, they remain 'outsiders'.[76] French and British visual arts had a more inclusive approach and showed the veteran's body in a process of reconstruction within the wider frame of society, whereas Dix's treatment highlights the veterans' isolation and Germany's military and moral defeat.

75 *Otto Dix: 1891–1969*, Tate Gallery exhibition catalogue (London: Tate Gallery publications, 1992), entries by Keith Hartley and Sarah O'Brien Twohig, p. 101.

76 Steve Plumb, *Neue Sachlichkeit, 1918–33: Unity and Diversity of an Art Movement* (Amsterdam: Rodopi, 2006), p. 27.

Even in works by George Grosz (*Das Gesicht der herrschenden Klasse* [The face of the ruling class]) and Max Beckmann (*Der Nachhauseweg* [The Way Back]), which represent injured German soldiers in a social context, the interaction between ex-servicemen and their surroundings is not pictured as smooth and serves instead as political criticism. Galtier-Boissière's *Défilé des Mutilés* depicts facially injured soldiers marching in the parade's front row and suggests that the general public acknowledged their sacrifice; in contrast, works by German artists emphasize the difficulty, even hostility, faced by mutilated veterans in polarized interwar Germany.

George Grosz (1893–1959) had a more limited experience of army life than Dix, and his time was mainly spent in hospitals. Martin Kane underlines the growing hatred of man that Grosz developed during this period, and the mental breakdown he suffered, which led to his permanent discharge in 1917.[77] The influence of Grosz's initially Marxist political allegiance is felt in his post-war works, in which facially injured men feature. Like Dix, Grosz often harshly portrayed contemporary German society, and especially the big city.[78]

Grosz's series of 57 caricature-syle drawings entitled *Das Gesicht der Herrschenden Klasse* was published in 1921 and it is characteristic, as Peter Gay observes, of the artist's political 'propaganda against fat industrialists and war profiteers'.[79] In showing the 'face of the ruling class', Grosz also depicts their 'victims', in this case First World War veterans. Two of these drawings represent soldiers with visible facial wounds, although they are not the only apparent injuries. Both scenes take place on the street and picture veterans as separated from the rest of the population. In 'Etappe Gent' (Figure 27), three wounded soldiers appear to be interacting together but outside any relationship with the rest of society. Their posture suggests that they are standing still, unlike other passers-by who are in movement. The man in the middle of the drawing – the only one who is not painted in profile –

77 Martin Kane, *Weimar Germany and the Limits of Political Art: A Study of the Work of George Grosz and Ernst Toller* (Tayport: Hutton Press, 1987), pp. 16–20.

78 Metzger, *Berlin*, pp. 81–83.

79 Gay, *Weimar Culture*, p. 112.

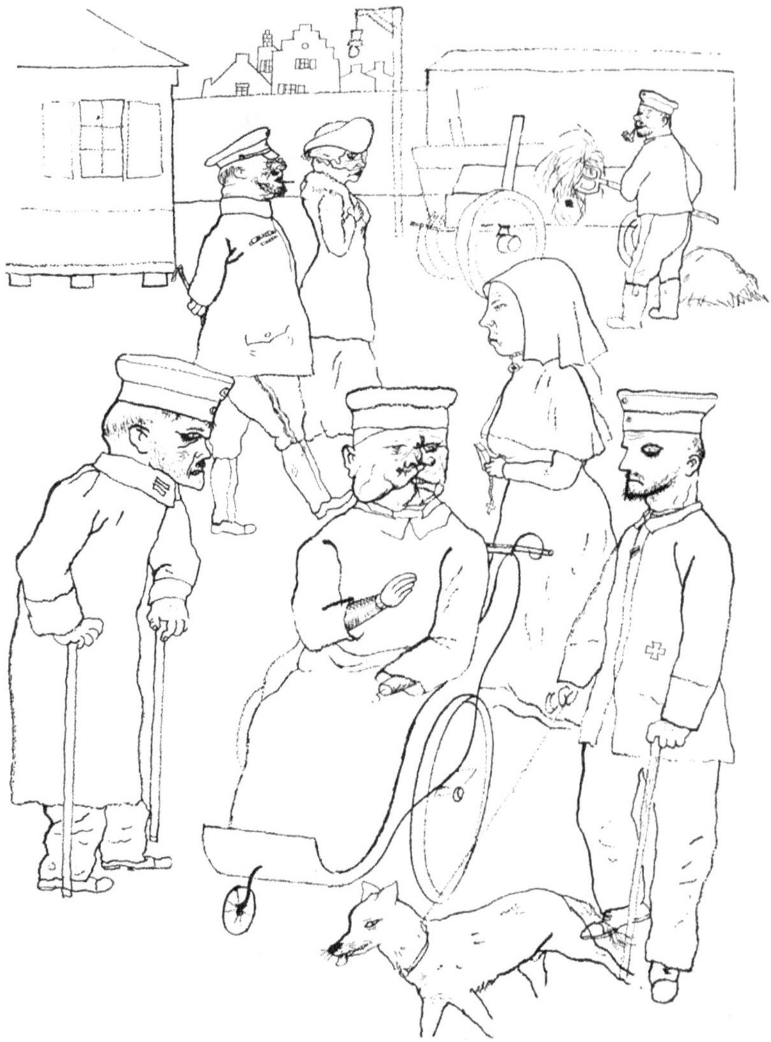

Etappe Gent 31

Figure 27: George Grosz, 'Etappe Gent!', *Das Gesicht der herrschenden Klasse* © Estate of George Grosz, Princeton, NJ/DACS, 2014. Digital image, The International Dada Archives, University of Iowa Libraries.

presents several mutilations, including facial injuries. The accumulation of disabilities as well as his central place in the picture make him stand out. Although his mouth is distorted, he looks like he is trying to communicate with the blind soldier on his left. 'Des Vaterlandes Dank ist euch gewiss!' [You can be certain of the gratitude of the Fatherland] portrays a German beggar in his uniform, wearing his medals; despite these outward signs of his military achievements, he is in a position of inferiority. Having lost his legs, he is sitting on the pavement, immobile, whilst other people are walking past, some of them ignoring him, others staring. His missing nose is covered with a black patch, the dark square in the middle of his face drawing attention to the absent feature. The indifference shown by passers-by highlights the irony of the title, which reminds the viewer of the respect and thankfulness soldiers had been promised, an irony also highlighted by Friedrich and Roth. This drawing, like 'Etappe Gent', emphasizes the broken relationship between society and veterans – largely, Robert Whalen argues, due to the state's intervention.[80] In contrast, Max Beckmann's *Der Nachhauseweg* pictures a civilian in direct physical contact with a wounded veteran (Figure 28).

This lithograph is one of a series of eleven works entitled *Die Hölle* [Hell], published in 1919. Beckmann's depictions of destroyed bodies are informed by his visit to Berlin, as well as his own experience as a medical orderly during the war. A recognized artist before the war, the years 1914–18 profoundly influenced him: 'His drawing became deliberately distorted; it remained realistic enough to convey the dreadful scenes he had witnessed – the wounded and dying soldiers, the corpses.'[81] In *Die Hölle*, Beckmann represents a society falling to pieces. Like Dante journeying through the circles of suffering of Hell, Beckmann depicts himself and his family going through the afterworld created by the aftermath of war. In it, familiar places and objects such as an attic and his son's toy are in effect a torture chamber and a grenade respectively. The sense of safety and familiarity has been lost and in its place stand the chaos and danger of post-war Germany.

80 In his essay, Whalen argues that the German authorities' control over the support of war veterans, by suppressing private initiatives, in effect isolated ex-servicemen from the rest of society. Whalen, *Bitter Wounds*.

81 Gay, *Weimar Culture*, p. 114.

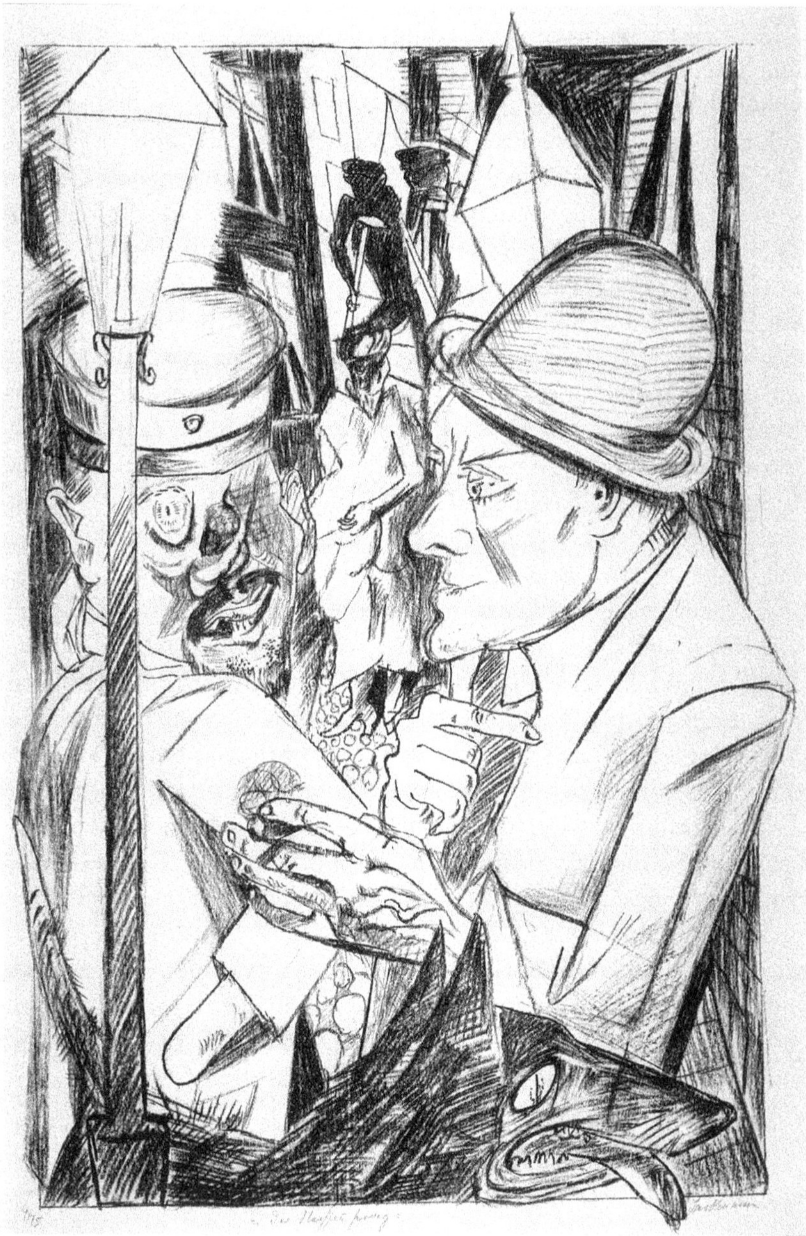

Figure 28: Max Beckmann, *Der Nachhauseweg* (1919) © DACS 2014. Digital image, The Scottish National Gallery of Modern Art.

Der Nachhauseweg is the second plate in this series and it portrays a civilian, possibly Beckmann himself, looking at a wounded soldier. This scene is taking place out on the street: buildings can be seen in the background and a lamp post shines in the foreground, drawing the viewer's attention to the disfigured veteran's mangled body. His posture, half-turned, and his eye staring at the onlooker, make him stand out.

Like Grosz's and Dix's veterans, Beckmann's ex-serviceman presents multiple injuries. His features are still recognizable but one half of his face is missing. The left eye is altogether absent, what stands in the middle of his face bears only a vague resemblance to a nose, and the mouth is distorted. The other man however does not shy away from the veteran's unsightly appearance but looks – as if into a mirror – straight at him, even whilst the disfigured man confronts him directly with the mangled side of his face. This work represents the presence of disfigured and disabled ex-servicemen in interwar society as disturbing. They not only bear the imprint of death, but they are also embodiments of hopelessness: for the nearly-dead of the war the future was Hell. The return home, which should be a happy experience, turns out to be an unpleasant confrontation with unfamiliar figures, accompanied by the looming ghosts of war. The situation of facially disfigured veterans as observed by Beckmann is thus much more sombre than the image given by Lobley and Galtier-Boissière.

Beckmann's lithograph features other characters: a man walking on crutches is visible in the background, although his body remains completely in the shade, whilst the lit form of the woman standing in front of him reveals her exhausted features and undressed body. The presence of the prostitute, although she is not in direct contact with any of the protagonists, raises the question of the visual representation of relationships between disfigured veterans and women. Whilst the profession of the woman pictured in *Der Nachhauseweg* is uncertain, Dix openly identifies the woman in *Dirne und Kriegsverletzter* as a prostitute (Figure 29).

The man is wearing a hospital uniform, which suggests that he is still in treatment; the gaping wound from his cheek to his mouth is further evidence of his condition as a patient. The damaged side of his face is in the middle of the picture, the prostitute almost leaning against it. Her emaciated body and her tired eyes, which her make-up cannot conceal, make her look unattractive. Both she and the man return the viewer's gaze

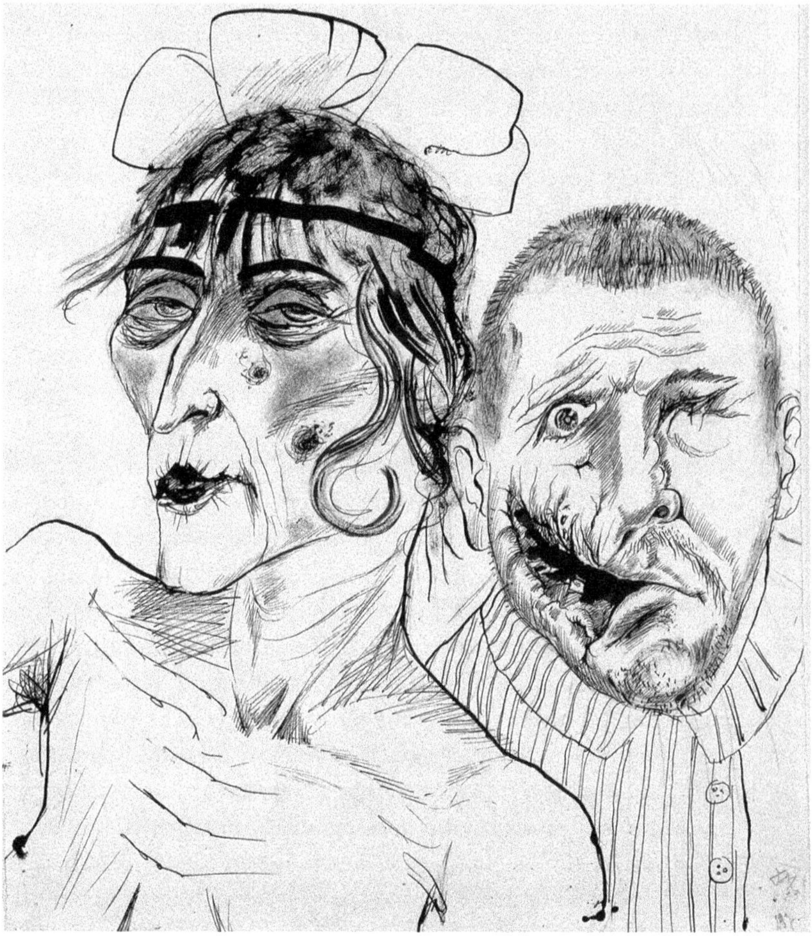

Figure 29: Otto Dix, *Dirne und Kriegsverletzter: Zwei Opfer des Kapitalismus* (1923) © DACS 2014. Digital image, LWL-Museum für Kunst und Kultur (Westfälisches Landesmuseum), Münster.

and their postures suggest no intimacy between them. Both are nameless casualties of the state, 'victims of capitalism', and both represent whole groups of people who have, to some extent, lost face.

The idea that mutilated veterans, and facially disfigured men especially, would not attract women because of their injuries, is a recurring motif in literature, too.[82] Facial injuries represent a challenge to the victim's masculinity not only in terms of his social role as the family breadwinner, but also in his more intimate life, as he could perceive himself as robbed of prospects of marital happiness. Dix's picture points to this justifiable fear of being rejected by women, described in literature as all the more cruel for men whose desires have not disappeared with the loss of their face. This work emphasizes the disfigured man's status as a victim. Both he and the prostitute bear physical marks upon their bodies. The coupling of these outcasts – products of a society which has used them but does not want to acknowledge them – bears similarities to Grosz's use of mutilated veterans and underlines that the only really ugly face is that of capitalistic society. This indictment is further echoed in Friedrich's pamphlet published one year later, in which he urges his readers: 'Kämpft gegen den Kapitalismus – und Ihr kämpft gegen jeden Krieg!' [Fight against capitalism and you will fight against every war!][83] Far from being heroes, facially injured men are presented as misfits.

Summary

What journalist Robert Blatchford could not put into words, artists attempted to capture in photographs, drawings and paintings. Two different narratives emerge, however: in Germany, the figure of the facially disfigured soldier or veteran appears to be consistently deconstructed and emphasis

82 Characters in Dumas's and Henri Galis's novels both confess to having paid women for sex (Pierre Dumas, *L'Homme qui Mourut Deux Fois* (Paris: Editions Delmas, 1943) and Henri Galis, *Mon Visage Fait Horreur: Confession d'une Gueule Cassée* (Paris: Les œuvres libres, 1929)). The more recent novel by Dugain, based upon his grandfather's story and adapted for a film, also pictures *gueules cassées* visiting a brothel (Dugain, *La Chambre des Officiers*). There, the matron is unsure if she will find a woman for them.

83 Friedrich, *War against War*, p. 11.

is put upon the soldier's physical brokenness as well as upon his isolation from the rest of society – unless he himself represents society's flaws (for example in *Die Skatspieler*). Even in depictions of patients in hospital, the injured man is not positioned in a process of therapeutic reconstruction; rather these artistic depictions are a statement of the degraded humanity of these individuals, and beyond this, of society as a whole. Furthermore, the disfigured soldier is represented as integral to the war and post-war experience – he is the 'true face of the war' and therewith becomes part of a political agenda in the defeated country.[84]

In contrast, the visual representations of France and Great Britain present facially wounded men in social contexts, and although they are never pictured in direct interaction with their surroundings, no conflictual relationship between the soldier and society is expressed. The focus is not upon the soldiers' wounds, which are seldom apparent. Rather, their maimed bodies are pictured in movement: their injuries have not robbed them of their dignity, diminished them or hindered them, but on the contrary, they are outward signs of courage. This positive message conveyed by French and British artistic representations insists upon the possibility of reintegration, turning *gueules cassées* into examples of successful physical and social reconstruction, and figures of national pride.

84 The National Socialist Party's victory in 1933 marked a change in the ideological representations of veterans, although the political treatment of disabled ex-servicemen (presented by the new regime as the 'first citizens of the Third Reich') did not necessarily reflect an evolution in popular perception (See, for example, James Diehl, 'Victors or Victims: Disabled Veterans in the Third Reich', *The Journal of Modern History*, 59: 4, 705–36, p. 727, and Niall Barr, 'The Legion that Sailed but Never Went: The British Legion and the Munich Crisis of 1938', in Julia Eichenberg and John P. Newman, eds, *The Great War and Veterans' Internationalism* (Basingstoke: Palgrave MacMillan, 2013), pp. 32–52, p. 38).

CHAPTER 5

Describing the 'Unspeakable'? *Gueules Cassées* in Literature

Visual representations only ever provide snapshots of society, albeit often complex ones; literature, on the other hand, allows for the exploration of a whole narrative. Whilst novels may not be able to convey the visual significance of facial disfigurement, they nonetheless provide valuable insight into the emotional and social journeys of facially disfigured soldiers. Literature ultimately reflects, and to some extent shapes, society's perception of *gueules cassées*.

This chapter examines the strategies used to depict facial injury and disfigurement in literature, and explores the psychological and social implications of wounds as described through this medium. It provides a further insight into the destinies – both real and imagined – of *gueules cassées*. Whilst the narratives explored here may differ in their depictions of the protagonists' reintegration, they nevertheless each highlight the powerful role of society in this process. The variations observed in visual arts regarding the symbolism of facially injured soldiers, as explored in the previous chapter, are reinforced in these literary accounts.

Four primary literary works provide the focus for this chapter, with additional references made to other novels of lesser relevance to the study. One was written by a German-speaking author (Vicki Baum's *Menschen im Hotel*, studied here in its English translation) and is set in interwar Berlin. The three other key texts are French and were written by Renée Girard (*La Vie Intime d'une 'Gueule Cassée'*), Henri Galis (*Mon Visage Fait Horreur: Confession d'une Gueule Cassée*) and one better-known author, Jean Renaud (*Gueules Cassées*). This discussion is not intended to be literary criticism; rather, it draws upon the texts to investigate yet another historical form of representation of, and response to, the presence of facially disfigured veterans. Of prime importance will be the concept of representing in literature what was deemed to be 'indescribable', namely the experience of war and facial disfigurement; the evolution of relationships between veterans and society as described in fiction; and, by extension, what these narratives of successful or failed reintegration say about post-First World War societies.

The figure of the facially wounded soldier in interwar literature

The year 1929 can be seen as a threshold in the history of literary representation of the war in general and of facially injured soldiers in particular. Most novels featuring *gueules cassées* were published in 1929 or later, thus indicating that the tenth anniversary of the Armistice and the Treaty of Versailles marked a turning point. This ten-year literary gap is to be considered alongside the real-life media coverage of facially disfigured soldiers. By the mid-1920s, the interest in veterans that newspapers and magazines had previously shown had mostly dried up, apart from the work of the *Association* in France. Related articles published in Germany and Great Britain were mostly scientific publications or newspaper contributions concerned with treatment and life in maxillofacial hospitals. They often overlooked the men's actual war experiences, and only hinted at the long-term psychological and social consequences of facial injury. This journalistic treatment in Great Britain and Germany focussed primarily on what they described as the 'wonders' achieved in hospitals, and thus virtually ceased upon the closure of the major maxillofacial centres in the early 1920s. Press publications reporting on the *Association* in France treated *gueules cassées* as a group, with very little attention paid to individual destinies (with the exception of Picot).

Antoine Prost acknowledges a greater willingness to talk about individual war experiences from the late 1920s onwards:

> It took about ten years for memories to settle, and for soldiers to begin evoking their war. They did so first through the most superficial aspects, the most anecdotal. It

> was only in 1931 that the most influential veterans' journal (the *Journal des Mutilés*) opened its columns to descriptions of war, for items without strong emotion, evoking rats, lice, or the rough wine.[1]

This shift, evidenced in France by the publication in 1929 of Jean Norton Cru's *Témoins*, can also be observed in literature.[2] It may be assumed that the men's destinies were by this point more or less settled; enough time had passed for fiction to start exploring the reasons for the failure or success of their reintegration. *Gueules cassées* were by then a sight common enough to no longer be regarded as a threat, but their status as 'walking reminders of the war' was still sufficiently powerful enough for writers to choose them as characters for their novels.

Differences between countries are noticeable in the literary treatment of disfigured soldiers; France leads the way with the greatest number publications featuring them. Furthermore, in French literature, a facially injured soldier tends to be the main character, with the story centring upon his life, whilst the place of disfigured veterans in the few existing British and German works is more marginal. In France, even in cases in which his facial injury plays no significant part in the plot, the term *gueule cassée* may yet appear in the title, as if it had become a catchphrase.[3] One hypothesis accounting for this proportionally greater emphasis in France is that facially wounded soldiers had a visible presence in the public sphere thanks to the *Union des Blessés de la Face*. Their visibility in the media during the fundraising campaign for the *Maison* in the second half of the 1920s further contributed to a greater symbolic investment in *gueules cassées*. Thus, in France, facially injured soldiers were not an unusual figure in interwar literature.

1 Prost, *In the Wake of War*, p. 13.

2 Jean Norton Cru, *Témoins-Essai d'Analyse et de Critique des Souvenirs de Combattants Edités en Français de 1915 à 1928* (Paris: Les Etincelles, 1929).

3 See, for instance, Jean Renaud, *Gueules Cassées* (Paris: Les Etincelles, 1929) and Max Barthélemy, *Mémoires d'une 'Gueule cassée'* (Nevers: Imprimerie de la Nièvre, 1930). Both titles have the phrase 'gueule cassée' but the narratives mainly describe the lives of the soldiers before their injury.

Putting loss and pain into print

Vicki Baum's *Menschen im Hotel* is one of the author's most famous works and also one of the first great successes of the publishing house Ullstein in Berlin (along with Remarque's benchmark anti-war novel *Im Westen nichts Neues*, published the same year). Set in a luxurious Berlin hotel, Baum's novel explores the atmosphere of the German capital in the 1920s. The publication of an English translation the following year, the production of a Hollywood film based upon the story in 1932 and later re-editions of the novel are all evidence of its success, both in Germany and abroad. The facially injured character, veteran Doctor Otternschlag, does not take centre stage, although he is introduced first. Rather he forms part of the array of fates that characterize post-war society.

French novels that are actually centred upon *gueules cassées* did not meet with such success. Only one of them, *Mon Visage Fait Horreur: Confession d'une Gueule Cassée* by Henri Galis (1929), was published in more than one edition. It first appeared in a volume containing several other stories, edited by the French publishing house Fayard, as part of a collection called 'les oeuvres libres'. The latter featured only unpublished literary works of fiction or real stories, designed to be a 'faithful reflection of modern life' while avoiding political bias.[4] Galis's narrative was included in a set of stories entitled 'La bibliothèque du combattant' (The combatant's library); however, the greatest battle faced by Galis's hero was not the war but the fight to re-appropriate his damaged face and his life. This novel, which focuses upon the main character's post-war years, was published again in 1930 by Les Etincelles, the publishing house that was to release Renée Girard's *La Vie Intime d'une 'Gueule Cassée'* the following year. Les Etincelles, which also published Norton Cru's *Témoins* in 1929, seems to have specialized in individual accounts of the war, whether fictional or real.

4 'reflet fidèle de la vie moderne', Foreword to *Les œuvres libres*, July 1921, <http://www.archive.org/stream/lesoeuvreslibres00pari/lesoeuvreslibres00pari_djvu.txt> [accessed 18 August 2015].

Neither Galis nor Girard were well-known writers and they do not appear to have published any other works, unlike Jean Renaud. His *Gueules Cassées* was also released in 1929 by Les Etincelles. Jean Jacques Ernest Renaud (1880–1952) was a prolific author who had already written several novels by the time his *Gueules Cassées* was published. His literary works draw upon his own experiences as a military officer in the French colonies and on the Western front during the First World War. His right-wing political stance led him to join forces with the industrialist and politician François Coty, to whom the novel is dedicated. Together they founded the far-right league *Solidarité Française* in 1933. In spite of his political involvement, Renaud's novel remained relatively obscure. Featuring *gueules cassées* was therefore by no means a guarantee of success for literary works in the 1920s and 1930s, as can also be verified in the case of Max Barthélemy's *Mémoires d'une 'Gueule Cassée'*. This book, presented as a copy of the notes made by a soldier, narrates the man's experience of war. Contrary to what the title implies, these memoirs stop on the day that the soldier is wounded. This shows the fundamental 'turning point' nature of an injury to the face, and also indicates that the phrase *gueule cassée* was thought to sell well.

Prefaces

Novels featuring facially disfigured soldiers frequently feature prefaces, which allow insight into the author's motivations. Renaud's takes the form of a long dedication, in which he expresses his admiration for Coty's patriotic values. To Renaud, Coty shares with *gueules cassées* an admirable readiness for sacrifice.[5] This parallel raises questions, since the industrialist and politician himself did not go to the front, and actively defended fascist ideas in the 1920s, during a time when the *Association* was criticizing people who had benefitted financially from the war without taking part in it. Renaud's text exemplifies the political appropriation of the phrase *gueules cassée*, and

5 Renaud, *Gueules Cassées*, p. x.

also extends its use to include civilian heroes, thus suggesting that the term itself had in France become a positive and wide-ranging symbol.[6]

Renaud's praise of the *Poilus* is paradoxically accompanied by an underlying criticism of war itself.[7] The author manages to reconcile these two somewhat opposing views by distinguishing between the soldier and the man. The soldier is envisaged from a traditional heroic perspective and is presented as proud of bearing scars that, like military decorations, show the sacrifice he has made for his country. In contrast, the man longs for the end of the conflict and for a return to normality, both politically and physically. In Renaud's novel, pride always prevails over shame and the soldier has the upper hand. This may be accounted for by the fact that the author himself served in the army, and that his main character is a professional soldier, not a conscripted civilian. In spite of this contextual grounding, the fictional nature of this work is clearly indicated on the cover page: it is a novel, albeit a 'roman vécu' [real-life novel]. These extra-diegetic elements contribute to making the story appear realistic: Renaud, unlike other writers (such as Girard), cannot be criticized for not being able to understand what life in the trenches was like, having himself fought in the Great War. In spite of this personal involvement, the story is not presented as particularly important to him: he mentions that the manuscript of the novel was discovered by chance, years after it was written. The ten-year gap appears to be a coincidence. On the other hand, this anecdote might aim to conceal the fact that the date of publication was strategic on the part of either the publishing house or the author.

In Max Barthélemy's preface, the author presents his work as a real-life account obtained from an injured combatant. Although the latter survived his wounds, he refused to tell Barthélemy extra information or to fill in the gaps created by the loss of some of his notes. The reason given for this refusal is the narrator's lack of trust in his own memory; this attitude is presented by Barthélemy as testifying to the man's honesty. In this preface, and throughout the novel, the *gueule cassée* comes across as a heroic but

6 Renaud, *Gueules Cassées*, p. x.

7 Ibid, p. xii.

humble patriot, who did not intend his notes to be published. Barthélemy decided to share them for a specific purpose: to remind a forgetful society of the 'real face' of war so that 'those [who will read these startling facts] will never feel the desire to re-live them one day'.[8] The facially wounded soldier is here associated with a plea against war and his memories are presented as revealing the true nature of war, in a fashion somewhat reminiscent of Ernst Friedrich's endeavour to show 'the face of war'.

Henri Galis's preface also indiactes the goals he ascribes to his writing. The novel is dedicated 'Aux hommes', which may refer to males (and therefore implicitly to soldiers), or may embrace mankind as a whole. This suggests that the message conveyed has a universal appeal, reinforcing the image of the *gueule cassée* as a symbolic figure. Whilst the author may at first appear unconcerned by the identity of his readers, he goes on to imagine their expectations and advises those in search of 'pleasant fictions' or of 'imaginary misfortunes' against reading his book.[9] Galis then narrows his target audience down to those who are able to feel 'manly pity'.[10] The term seems paradoxical, especially in the context of post-war years that saw men reasserting their social status, which had been questioned both on the front (machines taking over men) and at home (with the emancipation of women). It also contradicts the testimonies of real-life *gueules cassées*, who did not want to inspire pity. Galis's initial warning does not include any explicit reference to facial disfigurement, although from the title *Mon Visage Fait Horreur: Confession d'une Gueule Cassée* (My Face Inspires Horror: Confession of a Gueule Cassée) the reader is conscious of this theme. A 'confession' suggests an intimate link between the recipient and the narrator; in the novel, Galis invites his readers to meet the veteran in what is presented as a challenging encounter.

Finally, Renée Girard's preface serves to defend her credibility as a female author writing about men wounded in the war. The fictional nature

8 'ceux qui [liront ces faits saisissants] n'éprouveront plus jamais le moindre désir de les revivre un jour', Barthélemy, *Mémoires d'une 'Gueule cassée'*, pp. 7–8.

9 'agréables fictions', 'malheurs imaginaires', Galis, *Mon Visage Fait Horreur*, p. 29.

10 'pitié virile', Ibid, p. 29.

of the story is clear; however, the author states that she has secured the approval of real-life *gueules cassées* before publication, thus strengthening the link between story and reality. Contrary to Galis's more general 'Aux hommes', Girard's initial dedication explicitly refers to facially injured soldiers. This choice highlights the author's respect for and even admiration of the veterans, as do the terms she uses with regard to them ('respectfully' and 'Facially wounded' instead of the more colloquial 'gueules cassées' used in the title).[11] By describing the support the novel obtained from members of the *Association*, Girard anticipates any criticism against her possible lack of understanding or unfaithful rendering of physical and psychological struggles. Like the other prefaces, hers has a eulogistic tone and functions as a form of tribute paid by the author to the sacrifice of *gueules cassées*.

The literary treatment of the figure of the facially injured soldier

The presence of facially injured soldiers was not limited to the war literature. Only Renaud and Barthélemy devote a significant part to the military achievements of their main character. Barthélemy focuses entirely upon the narrator's war; the fact that the hero was wounded is mentioned only in the last few pages. This account provides little insight into the life of the narrator after his injury; rather the fact that he is a *gueule cassée* is described as giving more credibility and value to his war memoirs. Renaud also insists upon the wartime experience of Lieutenant Jacques Rey who, having been taken to hospital, is reunited there with an old friend, the narrator Paul Dambre. The narrative is partly made up of the officer's *carnets*, which are said to have been written at the front.

Galis, Baum and Girard focus upon the years following the conflict. They represent the disfigured man in a civilian context as he is faced with the situations of everyday life. In Baum's novel, issues such as friendship, love and adultery are addressed, as well as money (and the lack thereof),

11 'Respectueusement' and 'Mutilés de la face', Girard, *La Vie Intime d'une 'Gueule Cassée'*, preface.

adventure and boredom. In *Mon Visage Fait Horreur*, Galis portrays his hero François's relationships with his former fiancée and with his mother, and his difficulties in finding a new goal for his life. In contrast, Girard's novel is a conventional love story with a happy ending in which love brings the facially injured man back to life. More than the patriotic values of the war hero, it is his female companion's strength of character that is highlighted. This 'lighter' treatment of facial disfigurement, as well as the happy ending to the story, makes it stand out from other contemporary literary works. The sentimentality of this approach does not contradict the author's admiration for real-life *gueules cassées*, and neither did it stop her from securing their support for her book. The fact that facially disfigured soldiers started to feature in popular literature indicates that their presence within French society was well acknowledged and widely accepted.

Two trends in the literary treatment of disfigured soldiers can therefore be observed. On the one hand, the fact that facially injured soldiers featured in popular literature reflects a positive sense of trivialization: they are presented as ordinary people. On the other hand, their achievements and their patriotic sacrifice – sometimes their tragic fates – are also extolled. Literary representations of *gueules cassées* thus oscillate between heroicizing wounded combatants and highlighting the subsequent banality of their destiny. This literary treatment echoes the variety of the representations of disfigured men in the press and in their own newspapers and bulletins.

Representing the indescribable

In literary accounts, facial wounds and disfigurement are often only briefly described, and this depiction usually occurs in a similar context and fashion. Literature nevertheless gives access to the memories associated with the injury, which were sometimes difficult to verbalize, as shown in previous chapters. Whilst the debate about 'unspeakability' has focussed primarily upon the Holocaust, the three main meanings of this word, set out by

Thomas Trezise, can also be applied to facial injuries.[12] Indeed, literary accounts point to the difficulty of verbally expressing the nature and consequences of wounds, to the inherently 'bad' (moral or aesthetic) quality they convey and their transgressive dimension, and to a 'profanation' of the sacred, in this case the human body.[13] The visual disruption triggered by disfigurement challenges the writer who attempts to represent it. This section explores the strategies used by authors to describe 'the indescribable'.

A realistic setting

One key shared feature of literary representations of *gueules cassées* is their intentionally realistic dimension. Baum's *Grand Hotel* is usually associated with the Excelsior Hotel in 1920s Berlin. Likewise, Girard, the author of *La Vie Intime d'une 'Gueule Cassée'*, takes great care to anchor her narrative in a reality that the reader would be able to relate to. References to dates and places are specific and match historical events and existing locations, whilst characters are identified by their full names.[14] Accurate references to extra-diegetic elements are not the only strategy used by writers to give a realistic atmosphere to their narratives. Galis, on the other hand, goes to the other extreme: under the pretext of preserving people's anonymity, he does not specify the full name of the main character, who is always designated as 'François' (no surname), as if there was a risk that he could be identified. In addition only initials are used for most other characters,

12 Trezise differentiates between three different senses of the word 'unspeakable': firstly, the idea that what is unspeakable is 'verbally unrepresentable'; secondly the accompanying sense of moral, aesthetic or social judgement (the 'bad' or 'objectionable' quality of the unspeakable); thirdly the almost 'sacred' dimension that (Thomas Trezise, 'Unspeakable', *The Yale Journal of Criticism*, 14 (2001), 39–66 (p. 39)).

13 This function of the skin as identity and boundary is also examined in reference to Tonks's pastels by Chambers, 'Fragmented Identities', pp. 593–96.

14 See, for instance, references to streets in Paris (avenue Kléber, rue de la Croix Nivert, avenue de Wagram, rue Férou, rue de Vaugirard), shops and cafés (*Maison de la Gerbe d'Or*, *Café de la Rotonde*, *Restaurant Maire*).

for instance, 'M. et Mme D … -R …' or 'M. V …'. The context in which François tells his story – he is confessing to a prison chaplain – also suggests a confidential and realistic setting for the narrative.

Paul Dambre, the narrator of Renaud's *roman vécu*', also claims to have received the testimony of a facially injured soldier, this time not in jail but in hospital. The narrative is divided into five main parts: the first and the last sections are shorter and narrated from the point of view of Dambre, while the three central ones are 'notes' written by the wounded protagonist, Jacques Rey. Rey's writing tells of the wounds he received on the Western front. These notebooks, which are presented as authentic documents, provide a realistic atmosphere, as do several parentheses, notes and footnotes evidencing the genuineness of the documents.[15] At the beginning of chapter 20, another comment states that the notes contained in this part of Rey's journal (allegedly written during Rey's time on the front) had to be re-arranged because part of the writing was stained with blood and was illegible.[16] Likewise, chapter 24 contains two supposedly authentic letters, said to be found amongst Rey's notes.[17]

In addition to these 'material' resources of 'authenticity' in Renaud's novel, the narrator's own comments are also used to convey a realistic impression. Dambre asserts at the very beginning that although the conflict is still going on, a long time has passed since the events related, which makes him, he claims, less biased. This assertion of reliability is further emphasized by the overriding reason the narrator gives as to his motivation for telling the story: duty.[18] Not only does Dambre feel he owes this to his dead friend, but he sees in Rey's story the epitome of a more general type of man.[19] The narrator repeatedly claims that he is speaking the truth, even if it does not show him in a favourable light. Moreover, the fact that the author was a military officer himself suggests that his narrative is a reliable

15 See Renaud, *Gueules Cassées*, pp. 98–99, p. 131 and p. 132.

16 Ibid, p. 131 and p. 142. A similar statement is made by Max Barthélemy about the testimony of his main character (Barthélemy, *Mémoires d'une 'Gueule Cassée'*).

17 Renaud, *Gueules Cassées*, p. 169.

18 Ibid, p. 1.

19 Ibid, p. 9.

source. In this narrative as well as in others, the disfigured combatant is presented as the embodiment of real-life soldiering experience and sacrifice.

The presence of a 'mediator'

The presence of a narrator in novels featuring *gueules cassées* heightens their realistic dimension, as his voice appears to be more detached and more reliable than that of the wounded man. Even when the moment of the injury and the patient's feelings are described from the point of view of the disfigured man himself, none of the novels under discussion are purely first-person narratives. The presence of a 'mediator' between the reader and the wounded man is a recurring feature.

In Baum's *Grand Hotel*, Otternschlag's face is illuminated from different angles. The presence of the narrator can be felt: the depiction starts with a comment clause ('His face, it must be said, […]'), the remaining part of his face is compared with that of a 'Jesuit', and the nickname the German veteran gives to his wound when alone is revealed ('a Souvenir from Flanders').[20] Otternschlag's mutilated face stands in contrast with another hotel personality, a noble-turned-thief, whose looks appeal to the others, particularly women.

In Renaud's *Gueules Cassées*, the importance of the narrator is evidenced by the fact that he is the first protagonist to appear and it is through him that the wounded soldier is first introduced. The narrator presents his act of writing not as a creative process but as a transcription of memories, which his sense of duty demands. His previous acquaintance with the wounded soldier implies that he is well placed to assess the difference between the 'old' Rey and the new, post-injury Rey. The fact that the narrator Paul Dambre is at first unable to recognize his friend is indicative of the complete change in his appearance.

There is no pre-existing relationship between the narrator and the facially disfigured man in the other novels, although instances of previous

20 Baum, *Grand Hotel*, p. 3.

contact can be found in Girard and Galis. In the latter a first-person voice, which is expressed in the title *Mon Visage Fait Horreur: Confession d'une Gueule Cassée*, prevails in the narrative itself, although the form it is given – a confession – leads to occasional interventions by the priest. The story of the disfigured soldier is largely narrated from the veteran's point of view but it is framed within two contextual descriptions by an external narrator, who also gives the reader an insight into the chaplain's thoughts. A previous encounter between the priest and the prisoner is mentioned: the priest, who was then serving as an ambulance man, transported the wounded soldier after his injury in 1917. Galis's narrator performs similar military duties as Dambre in Renaud's novel: both take part in the conflict, but are in the business of curing soldiers, not killing them. The priest has seen many wounded men, but transporting François from the battlefield remains a lasting memory.

The second, post-injury encounters between Dambre and Rey, and the priest and François, contain similarities: they both take place in a secluded environment. In Renaud's novel, they meet at the hospital where Rey was taken. In Galis's novel, François is in jail and the priest comes to visit him to receive his confession. While the narrator is free to come and go, the wounded man is physically constrained in the ward or prison cell. This physical imprisonment mirrors the sense of confinement experienced by the disfigured man, who feels as if his old, unchanged, self is locked inside in a body that does not belong to him.

Although the initial reunions between the narrator and the *gueule cassée* are coincidental, the following meetings happen by the initiative of Dambre and the priest, not the disfigured men. This interest may be a form of morbid fascination, as mentioned by Tonks with regard to the visitors at Sidcup museum. It may also be the result of the narrator's will to physically or spiritually help the *gueule cassée*. In both cases, the disfigured man is in a position of inferiority and appears to be condemned by an illness or by the law. A difference is noticeable, however, in the reactions of Rey and François towards their interlocutors: whilst Rey welcomes Dambre's offer of help, François initially rejects the priest's. By the end, however, both narrators have been entrusted with a physical document (a photograph in François's case and notebooks in Rey's), which is material evidence of the facially disfigured man's wrongdoing (mostly adulterous conduct). The *gueule cassée* has trusted the narrator; the reader is now invited to do the same.

In Girard's *La Vie Intime d'une 'Gueule Cassée'*, the focus is upon Paule's thoughts. The plot centres upon the love story between this young woman and a facially injured veteran, Gérard Thiercelin. It brings female patriotism and self-sacrifice to the forefront. Here again, the presence of Paule functions as a filter between the wounded man and the reader. There is a pattern of repeated encounters between Paule and Thiercelin. The story, set in the late 1920s, commences on a highly symbolic date: 11 November 1928. It ends nine months later, in August 1929, when the pregnancy of the main female character is announced. Although the two main characters meet for the first time on the day of the military march, Paule remembers having seen Thiercelin before, in a film.[21] Again, she is the one who takes the initiative. In an attempt to trace him, she goes to see an old friend of her father's and convinces him to take her to the mansion where Thiercelin lives. The plot, as indicated in the title, consists of a conventional love story, and the central chapter of the novel is, once again, a confession (it is even titled 'Confession'). The female character and the facially injured soldier confide in each other, this chapter marking the beginning of the ex-serviceman's redemption. Confession is thus a recurring theme that bears witness to a close relationship between the narrator-confessor and the disfigured veteran. It also suggests that, in the world of fiction at least, *gueules cassées* managed to verbalize their experiences.

The confessions also have an impact upon the person who hears them. Dambre is still haunted by Rey's narrative years later, when he starts telling the story. His own emotions are explicit, especially his guilt at not telling Rey's wife what he read in his friend's *carnets*. This narrative is therefore also a form of confession for Dambre. He now wants to unburden his conscience of what he was unable to tell the widow, although he says that duty

21 This reference, probably to *Pour la Paix du Monde*, is evidence of the author's awareness of the work of the UBF and it is possible that Girard took inspiration from real-life stories.

is his main motivation: his aim is to honour Rey and his comrades. This religious dimension to Dambre's narrative, close to expiation, is emphasized by his own description of his endeavour as 'a deep and religious homage', and his attitude towards the writing Rey entrusted to him as one of contemplation.[22] Likewise, Paule is moved by Thiercelin's story, and the priest in Galis's novel is described as having changed after his encounter with the prisoner: he has become more withdrawn and he avoids talking about his experience on the frontline. The priest has also taken a controversial stand on some doctrinal matters such as divine justice.[23] In terms of the impact upon the *gueule cassée*, the only confession that has a positive outcome is the one made to Paule: the woman is the only person who is able to lead her interlocutor to 'redemption', understood here as reintegration within society. Where religion (represented by the priest in Galis's novel) and medicine (in the person of the doctor-narrator Paul Dambre in Renaud's narrative) have failed, love seems to overcome.

Facially disfigured veterans appear never to be fully in charge of the narratives, echoing their lack of control over their lives. Their wounds deprived them of the future they had imagined; correspondingly, they are not permitted to write their own stories in literature. Although none of the characters in these literary works has lost his speech, it is as if they could not speak for themselves. The figure of a second protagonist who acts as an intermediary is a recurring pattern: the mediator 'guides' the exploration of both the impact of the wound (and of war itself) and particular personal contexts. The presence of a mediator is indicative of the difficulty in accessing the disfigured man; it is as if the breach in his flesh had exposed him, and the protective presence of a narrator between him and the reader is required. Facially injured veterans rarely appear to be on their own, except in the German narrative. This echoes the isolation of German mutilated men that can be observed in the visual art.

22 'Un hommage profond et religieux', Renaud, *Gueules Cassées*, p. 27, p. 31, p. 34.

23 Galis, *Mon Visage Fait Horreur*, pp. 111–12.

Literary descriptions of the injured face

Literary descriptions of the physical damage done to soldiers' faces are brief, as if writers did not want to dwell upon these sights. Depictions of mangled faces emphasize either their unnatural, inhuman aspect, or depict them as absent altogether. The importance of the disfigurement to the soldier's face is evidenced by the fact that even his close friends almost fail to recognize the wounded man. Paul's first reaction upon seeing Rey is one of incredulity: 'Jacques Rey? It's impossible! Jacques Rey? That? That trooper in rags? That man with a face disfigured by monstrous scars? [...] I looked at him but I could not understand, I could not believe what I was seeing'.[24] The use of 'ça' ['that'], a pronoun that generally designates an undetermined object, is telling: the army officer's human status is threatened. This dehumanization, also a salient feature in some journalistic accounts of the maimed face, is further emphasized a few paragraphs later when the face is described as 'monstrous'.[25]

As shown in Chapter 2, newspaper articles highlight the horrifying nature of facial injury; so does the nurse who takes care of Rey. Having rejected his request to be given a mirror, she describes the face to him: 'You would only see an awful assortment of colours from the iodine solution, the vaseline and the picric acid ....'[26] Although two months have passed, his face still has no semblance to that of a normal human being. The nurse's choice of the adjective 'awful' is far from comforting but Rey is not distressed at this description, probably because it does not tell much about the face itself, but more about what has been put on to it, the external ointments. The nurse constantly changes the subject from his damaged face to the luck he has had to recover from his more serious thigh wound.

24 'Jacques Rey? Ce n'est pas possible! Jacques Rey? ça? Jacques Rey, ce troupier hailloneux? Cet homme au visage mutilé par des cicatrices monstrueuses? [...] Je le regardais sans comprendre, surtout sans croire', Renaud, *Gueules Cassées*, p. 3

25 Ibid, p. 4.

26 'Vous ne verriez qu'un affreux bariolage de teinture d'iode, de vaseline et d'acide picrique ...', Ibid., p. 147.

When Rey finally sees his face, he is shocked: 'I held the mirror. For one or two seconds, I closed my eyes, then I suddenly opened them and I saw … Ah! … what I saw …'.[27] At this point he is unable to put what he sees into words; the only way he can refer to himself is by using the informal demonstrative pronoun 'ça': 'And 'that' is what I have become? That is what war turned me into?' The use of this pronoun by the wounded man himself introduces a distance between the speaker and the object referred to; this discrepancy is even greater considering that the narrator is talking about his own face.[28] He does not recognize it as his own.

If Rey does not manage to describe his face, François's reaction upon seeing his for the first time is more detailed: 'half of my face was nothing but a heap of pallid and purple flesh, featureless, in which the burst eye was like a seal in the horrible and hollow socket'.[29] This description emphasizes the lack of harmony between the two sides of the face. As in visual representations, the focus is upon the half that has been destroyed. The coexistence of an undamaged part of the face with the other, unrecognizable part appears frequently in both visual and literary works. Baum's description includes elements of the remaining half of the face, unlike Galis's. This only serves to emphasize the contrast between the two:

> His face, it must be said, consisted of one-half only in which the sharp and ascetic profile of a Jesuit was completed by an unusually well-shaped ear beneath the sparse grey hair on his temples. The other half was not there. In place of it was a confused medley of seams and scars, crossing and overlapping, and among them was a set glass eye. 'A Souvenir from Flanders', Doctor Otternschlag was accustomed to call it when talking to himself.[30]

27 'J'ai pris la glace. Une seconde, deux peut-être, j'ai fermé les yeux, puis, brusquement, je les ai ouverts et j'ai vu … Ah! … ce que j'ai vu …', Ibid, p. 163.

28 'Et c'est "ça" que je suis devenu? C'est ça que la bataille a fait de moi?', Ibid, p. 161.

29 'La moitié de mon visage n'était plus qu'une masse de chair livide et violette, sans traits, où l'œil crevé marquait, comme un sceau, un enfoncement horrible', Galis, *Mon Visage Fait Horreur*, p. 44.

30 Baum, *Grand Hotel*, p. 3.

The emphasis here is upon facial emptiness. Rather than being described as different from the other, or disfigured, the injured half is characterized by absence. Unlike François in Galis's novel, Otternschlag does not cover – or hide – his face. This choice, as well as the way he cynically names his wound, suggests that the German doctor has managed to live with it, although the psychological damage and the sense of loss are obvious. Remarkably, he presents himself in one of the most frequented places, the hotel's entrance hall, seeing and being seen. As such, the entrance hall marks a threshold between belonging and exclusion.

The absence of human traits is also visible in Girard's description of Thiercelin's face:

> In the first row, the president of the *Gueules Cassées* was surrounded by two or three disfigured veterans whose faces were presenting to the fearful gaze of the spectators nothing but a heap of shapeless flesh, which science had tried to repair using grafts, thereby attempting to replicate what nature does so perfectly well.[31]

This passage echoes the depiction of Otternschlag's face as a 'medley of seams and scars'. Amongst the disfigured men, one is singled out as 'the tallest and certainly the most awfully disfigured'.[32] After this first comparison, the narrator describes the man's figure, hair and eyes rather than focusing upon the damaged face, which is only mentioned in passing. The first depiction of Thiercelin's face is brief and it is included in a more general description of his body, clothes and manners. It is given from the point of view of the female spectator:

> Judging from the visible scars, Paule guessed that his jaw must have been shattered; his nose and his upper lip were grafts that, although successfully executed, remained very visible; his chin was almost gone and the lower part of his face was shapeless.

31 'Au premier rang, leur dévoué président était entouré de deux ou trois blessés de la face dont le visage n'offrait plus aux regards pleins d'effroi qu'une masse de chairs informes, que la science s'était efforcée pourtant de réparer au mieux par des greffes humaines, en tentant de se rapprocher de ce que la nature réussit si parfaitement bien', Girard, *La Vie Intime d'une 'Gueule Cassée'*, p. 14.

32 'Le plus grand et certainement le plus affreusement mutilé', Ibid, p. 14.

> His mouth was fixed in a horrible grin, showing teeth that were too white and too new; the left ear had been ripped to shreds. Thankfully the eyes were intact; his forehead, which gave him an air of intelligence and energy, had also been spared.[33]

This description stands out from others as it makes it clear that the disfigured soldier underwent surgical operations. They did not, however, result in a complete restoration of the man's face: his fixed expression looks unnatural. But unlike Otternschlag and François, who lost a whole side of their face, the upper part of Thiercelin's face has been spared. The fact that his two eyes have not been damaged seems to give him an advantage; his first 'discussion' with Paule is in fact limited to visual communication. An account of his injury, given from the disfigured man's point of view, highlights the speech problem resulting from the injury to his mouth:

> He had moved his hands across his face, realising that his nose was missing and his chin was hanging miserably, his jaw fractured.
>
> He must have spat his teeth out and, mad with horror, he had tried to cry, to shout for someone, but his tongue full of holes simply disappeared into the hole where his palate was partly gone![34]

In spite of the extent of this initial damage to his speech organs, no later mention is made of any sort of speech difficulties in the novel. The consequences appear to be aesthetic, not functional. His abilities to communicate

33 'Il avait dû avoir la mâchoire fracassée, autant que Paule pouvait en juger, par les cicatrices très apparentes; son nez et sa lèvre supérieure étaient des greffes humaines, merveilleusement réussies, mais visibles à n'en pas douter; son menton avait presque disparu, le bas de son visage était informe. La bouche avait un rictus affreux, découvrant des dents trop blanches, trop neuves et l'oreille gauche était comme déchiquetée. Les yeux, par bonheur, étaient intacts; le front intelligent, plein d'énergie, avait également été épargné', Girard, *La Vie Intime d'une 'Gueule Cassée'*, pp. 14–15.

34 'Ayant promené les mains sur sa face, il chercha en vain son nez et son menton pendait lamentablement, la mâchoire fracassée. Il avait dû cracher ses dents et, fou d'horreur, il avait voulu crier, appeler, mais sa langue perforée en plusieurs endroits se perdait dans le trou vide de son palais, en partie emporté!', Girard, *La Vie Intime d'une 'Gueule Cassée'*, p. 115.

have not been permanently impaired, yet he chooses to withdraw from society until a woman brings him out of his seclusion.

Thiercelin, like Otternschlag, does not hide his face from the view of other people. François, on the other hand, covers his damaged features, as shown in the very first description of his face (given from the priest's point of view): 'A piece of black taffeta was covering almost half of his face: part of his forehead, his left eye and the upper part of his cheek'.[35] The brevity of this initial description leaves room for the reader's imagination, simultaneously indicating the main character's unwillingness to expose his face. Hiding the wound can be regarded as an understandable protective gesture; yet it also echoes his failure – or refusal – to overcome his disfigurement. His facial covering symbolizes covered feelings. More than his physical appearance, it is his forced emotional distance and eventual rejection that lead to his engagement to Gisèle, the young woman he loves, being broken. François's choice to hide his wounds can be interpreted as evidence that, being convinced that people cannot understand him, he does not want to force others to confront his disfigurement.

The man in the mirror: The psychological consequences of facial disfigurement

Even if *gueules cassées* could successfully hide their injuries, they could never hide from the reality of their disfigurement. The brevity of the accounts describing the appearance of wounds highlights the fact that the context and consequences of a facial injury matters just as much as its visual impact. Unlike visual representations, literary accounts allow for an exploration of a man's psyche in the long term.

Renaud's narrative suggests that soldiers particularly feared facial injury. Rey spends a long time in hospital undergoing treatment before he is allowed to see his face. Ignorance about the extent of his wound causes

35 'Un bandeau de taffetas noir lui couvrait près de la moitié de la face, une partie du front, l'œil gauche et le haut de la joue', Galis, *Mon Visage Fait Horreur*, p. 32.

him great worry: although he is portrayed as a brave officer throughout, the thought of resembling some of his disfigured comrades, whom he finds 'monstrous', is a source of anxiety.[36] He goes further: by his own admission, life is not worth living with a maimed face: 'I shiver at the thought of looking like them; I would never have the courage to live to be an object of pity or terror ....'[37] At first, Rey is relieved to be alive but as time goes by and he is not permitted to see his face, he starts to wonder. The psychological impact of his wound, as opposed to his severe thigh injury, is highlighted:

> I nearly died of this wound [to his thigh], yet I morally suffer more from that other one, the one that burns my cheekbones, my nose, my lips. That one is, the doctors say, only superficial, and yet it is the only wound that worries me.[38]

In spite of the reassuring discourse of the medical staff, he perceives that an important change has taken place. The face, previously a familiar sight, has become 'the unknown'. The soldier's worries are sometimes justified, as shown in François's reaction upon seeing his image for the first time:

> I screamed. I quickly repositioned the cloths onto my face and ran away through the park.
>
> For several hours I wandered through the ravaged woods, the flowerbeds turned to shrubbery, the grass-covered paths. I heard the lunchtime bell ring and then almost immediately after, or so it seemed, the dinnertime bell. Someone called out my name for a long time, I hid under acacia trees. [...] At dusk, I finally went back. I saw my mother standing on the front steps, waiting for me, immobile and pale like a statue.[39]

36 Renaud, *Gueules Cassées*, p. 147.

37 'Je trembe à l'idée de leur ressembler; je ne me sentirai jamais le courage de vivre pour n'être qu'un objet de pitié ou d'horreur ...', Ibid, p. 147.

38 'J'ai pourtant failli mourir de cette blessure [to his thigh]: j'en souffre moins, moralement surtout, que de celle qui me brûle ... aux pommettes, au nez, aux lèvres, et qui n'est, paraît-il, que superficielle, pourtant elle seule m'inquiète.', Ibid, p. 146.

39 'Je jette un grand cri. Je rajuste les linges sur ma face, et je m'enfuis dans le parc. J'errai plusieurs heures à travers les bois ravagés, les massifs changés en halliers, les allées tapissées d'une herbe tendre. J'entendis sonner le clairon du repas de midi, puis presqu'aussitôt, me sembla-t-il, le clairon du repas du soir. Quelqu'un m'appela longuement, je me cachais sous des acacias. [...] Enfin, à la tombée de la nuit, je

François is horrified by his own appearance. The title *Mon Visage Fait Horreur* can thus be interpreted as referring not only to other people, but also to the disfigured man himself. François sees his professional career as an artist and his matrimonial plans thwarted; and more than this, his very identity is at stake. This is evidenced by the fact that, while the priest's name is given from the start ('Abbé S …'), it is only much later that we learn that the main character is called François, as if his identity no longer depends upon his name but rather upon his physical appearance.

The disfigured men's difficulty in accepting the changes to their appearance is highlighted throughout these texts. The doctor who treats Thiercelin in Girard's novel expresses concern towards his patient's psychological condition. He judges that nothing can be medically done to help Thiercelin, and that his injury is the cause of depression: 'he has become mistrustful, his spirits are very low, he is bitter and irritable … he struggles mentally and I believe he suffers from acute neurasthenia. The wound to his soul seems incurable ….'[40] The fact that some writers chose to describe the face only as half damaged can be regarded as an external, visible embodiment of the interior conflict raging between the *gueule cassée*'s appearance and his psyche. The remaining half reminds the wounded man of who he was before the war; it points to his past and evokes the future he could have had. The disfigured half is a constant reminder of the war that changed the man (a 'Souvenir from Flanders' as Otternschlag calls it) and an obstacle to interaction with other people.

Another telling element observed in literary descriptions is the comparison of the damaged face with a mask that the wearer is unable to get rid of. François, who hides his wounds behind a scarf, sees himself as already wearing a mask: 'My ugliness was like a carnival costume I could not take off, and the piece of cloth covering my forehead was stuck on it like a grotesque

---

rentrai. J'aperçus, debout à la première marche du perron, ma mère qui m'attendait, immobile et pâle comme une statue', Galis, *Mon Visage Fait Horreur*, pp. 44–45.

40 '[Il] est devenu farouche; son moral est déplorable, il est aigri, ombrageux … [il] souffre moralement, je le crois atteint de neurasthénie aiguë; la plaie de son âme me semble inguérissable …', Girard, *La Vie Intime d'une 'Gueule Cassée'*, pp. 37–38.

Harlequin's mask'.[41] The disfigured face is not perceived as his own; it is an external object that hides his true and unchanged self. Likewise, Rey refers to 'the mask war has given [him]' and expresses his desire to hide it from the sight of others.[42] This mask can evoke various emotions. François regards it as a prop reducing him to Harlequin, nothing but a ridiculous character. In contrast, Paule sees Thiercelin's courage reflected in his 'horrible mask, which forever bore the mark of heroism and bravery'.[43] Rey struggles to reconcile his ambitions and his vision of war with the actual impact of the battle upon his body, and he cannot imagine that his 'mask' will provoke any response but pity:

> I would have preferred any kind of mutilation to facial disfigurement. A man is still a man, even if he is missing a leg or an arm. But with a mask like mine, he is only a creature full of pain, suffering from the pity he sees in the eyes of people too afraid to look away, suffering from the embarrassed silences and awkwardness …[44]

Coping with facial injuries

In narratives of soldiers' post-injury lives, literary works describe different ways in which the men try to cope with their disfigurement and its repercussions. Otternschlag resorts to morphine in order to relieve his physical pain and fall into oblivion and, like François, he becomes obsessed with tragic

41 'Ma laideur était pour moi un déguisement de carnaval impossible à dévêtir; et le bandeau de mon front s'y collait comme le masque grotesque d'un Arlequin', Galis, *Mon Visage Fait Horreur*, p. 71.

42 Renaud, *Gueules Cassées*, p. 162.

43 'Masque horrible, qui portait pour toujours la marque ineffaçable de l'héroïsme et de la vaillance', Girard, *La Vie Intime d'une 'Gueule Cassée'*, p. 13.

44 'J'eusse mieux aimé n'importe quelle mutilation, plutôt que celle du visage. L'homme reste un homme avec un bras ou une jambe en moins, tandis qu'il n'est plus, avec un masque comme le mien, qu'une créature douloureuse qui souffre de toutes les charités devinées au fond des regards qui n'osent pas se détourner, comme elle souffre de toutes les gênes qui créent du silence ou du malaise …', Renaud, *Gueules Cassées*, p. 162.

stories. This fascination can be seen as an attempt to make sense of their wounds by setting them against greater distresses. The responses of François and Otternschlag to the sufferings endured by others differ, however. The German veteran, whilst reading the newspapers, is described as not having

> found anything to satisfy him. A typhoon, an earthquake, some petty war between blacks and whites. Arson, murder, political strife. Nothing. Too little. Scandals, panic on the Bourse, colossal fortunes lost. What did it matter to him? How could it affect him? Ocean flights, speed records, sensational headlines. Each page screamed out louder than the last till finally you heard none of them. The noise and bustle nowadays made you blind and deaf and deadens all sensations.[45]

While Otternschlag's perceptions have been minimized, François's are exacerbated. The latter develops an obsession for pain, but unlike Otternschlag he does not feel immune to suffering:

> The idea of all the suffering on this earth haunted me. I started to look at the world from a different, unique angle. All my reflections brought me back to pain, which seemed to be the centre of everything. [...] The thought of universal suffering is the only one that truly fills you with despair. I suffered through a thousand other people. My own unhappiness seemed to grow bigger as it was fuelled by other people's sufferings and I reproached God with not only my woes, but the woes of the whole of humankind, even of the whole of Creation.[46]

François is simultaneously attracted and repelled by the suffering of others. It does not alleviate his own pain, and it fuels his anger. These tragedies add to his torment, rather than freeing him from it. He reproaches God with allowing this to happen. References to religion are rather frequent in this context, and can be interpreted as another way of trying to make sense

45 Baum, *Grand Hotel*, p. 8.

46 'L'idée de la souffrance répandue sur le globe me hanta. Je me mis pour ainsi dire à regarder le monde sous un angle nouveau et unique; et la douleur, où me ramenaient toutes mes réflexions me parut le centre de tout. [...] Le sentiment de la souffrance générale est seul vraiment désespérant. Je souffrais dans mille individus. Mon malheur semblait s'élargir et s'accroître dans tous les malheurs et je reprochais à Dieu non seulement mes maux, mais tous les maux de la terre, et la création même.', Galis, *Mon Visage Fait Horreur*, pp. 84–89.

of the wounds. In contrast, Paule and her husband regard the mutilation suffered by Thiercelin as a blessing, since it brought them together. This is also the case for Rey and his mistress: they are reunited following the officer's injury. But Rey's disfigurement can also be interpreted in the opposite way and be seen as a punishment for adultery. Facial wounds can lead to the fall of an apparently righteous man: François becomes a rapist and a murderer following his injury. In his own words, his disfigurement may be a punishment for his participation in the war: 'I wondered if I deserved my disfigurement, if it was a divine punishment, and I thought about what the reason might be. Had I not taken part in the war? Had I not killed?'[47] From this religious perspective, a spiritual solution appears to be the way for *gueules cassées* to come to terms with their injuries. However, François's confession fails to lead him to redemption. While verbalizing emotions is nowadays regarded as therapeutic, soldiers who returned from the battlefield then often found themselves unable to put their experiences into words.[48] François finally gives in to the chaplain's insistence: his confession exposes his misdeeds but also seeks to prove that religion is powerless to save him. The fact that the priest finally gives up on him and finds himself changed by having received this confession seems to prove that François was right.

The ultimate solution for *gueules cassées* to escape the prison of their bodies appears to be death. Narratives featuring facially injured soldiers include multiple references to death as the only way out of a life that is not worth living. Otternschlag has a supply of syringes and ampoules of morphine, which makes him relish the feeling of being in control of the time of his death: 'You cannot really put up with all the pain that being

47 'Je me demandais si je ne méritais pas ma difformité comme une punition divine; et j'en donnais d'étranges motifs. N'avais-je pas fait la guerre? N'avais-je pas tué?', Ibid, p. 74.

48 This inability or unwillingness to talk about what he saw on the front is also experienced by Paul Bäumer, the hero of one of the most successful war novels, Remarque's *All Quiet on the Western Front* (pp. 107–28).

on this earth entails unless you know that at any moment you can make an end of it. Life is a miserable sort of existence, believe me'.[49]

For men who lost control of their bodies and lives, to choose the time of their death is a desperate attempt to regain power over their destiny. Otternschlag goes as far as to describe himself as being already dead, and only awaiting the final blow:

> I am a suicide, you must understand. As a rule you only see suicides after the event – when they have already turned on the gas or pulled the trigger. I, as I sit here, am a suicide before the event. To put it in one word, I am a living suicide – a rarity, you will agree. One of these days I shall take ten of these ampoules out of this box and then I shall be a living suicide no longer.[50]

Otternschlag does not perceive himself as truly living, which may explain why he remains an observer, on the outside of the events. But when he is given the opportunity to take his own life, he finds himself unable to do so.

François also tries to commit suicide, but his project is thwarted by the unexpected arrival of his ex-fiancée. Love and death are inextricably linked, the latter always prevailing over the former. What should have been the climax of the main character's emotional and physical rehabilitation – intercourse with his ex-fiancée – takes place in a tomb. Death, which François desires more than anything else, is delayed several times, first by his own inability to kill himself, then by the jury's refusal to condemn him to capital punishment. He later tries to jump from a window, again failing to put an end to his life once and for all.

Whilst the priest wants to absolve him, François judges himself beyond all hopes of rehabilitation. He is not described as a criminal, maybe because he has not yet been tried, or maybe to put greater emphasis upon his confinement: he is a prisoner more than he is a murderer. It is only at the very end, in a final account of what happened to François and to the chaplain after the trial (narrated by a different narrator), that François is referred to as a murderer. The use of this term at that particular moment is all the

49 Baum, *Grand Hotel*, pp. 247–48.

50 Ibid, p. 249.

more striking as the jury has declared him not guilty. In spite of this verdict, he is put in a mental hospital. This paradox is another illustration of the tensions between freedom and confinement experienced by facially disfigured soldiers.

Thus, whilst actual descriptions of physical injury may be brief, literary works extensively describe the inner torments experienced as a result of disfigurement. Various attempts to change do not alter the veteran's perception of himself and of his future, nor do they free him from his own physical prison.

Facing the world

Literary narratives explore the post-war experience of facial disfigurement from the point of view of the *gueule cassée*; they also provide insight into other people's feelings. They sometimes cover extended periods of time, depicting the journeys of the veterans and the people around them. Whether the stories have a happy or a tragic ending, they stress the powerful role of society in determining the fates of disfigured men.

The rejection of other people

Gueules cassées are usually represented as standing apart from the rest of the world, and even as deliberately isolating themselves. Rey's first reaction is aggression: he resents the doctor, the nurse and his mistress – who came every day to visit him in hospital – for not confronting him with the truth. He is then overwhelmed by grief, but even in this state of sorrow he ignores the words of comfort offered to him by others. He is particularly angry at his mistress, whom he accuses of having lied to him by not telling him how serious his injury was. He seeks to displace his shame and fear. When his irritation subsides, and although he is grateful to her for having stayed with him, he tries to dismiss her. In an attempt to preserve his own feelings, he urges his mistress to leave, persuaded that even if she is not quite repelled by him now she will soon stop loving him. This pattern – a disfigured man rejecting others before they can reject him – is frequently found in literary works, and reflects real-life stories such as that of the Corporal and his fiancée Molly.[51]

Upon his discharge from hospital, Rey avoids contact with the rest of the world and chooses to isolate himself. Likewise, François avoids the company of other people, even the young boy who brings him his meals and shops for him. His reunion with his fiancée Gilberte does not live up to his expectations:

> As soon as I saw her, more beautiful and loveable than ever, my heart stopped and I displayed an indifferent attitude. A strange and hypocritical mixture of modesty, timidity and probably also of fear that she would not love me anymore, seized me and for the rest of our meeting I spoke to her lightly, pretending that I was unconcerned.[52]

Driven by the fear that she might not love him anymore or that she will marry him out of pity, François feigns indifference towards her. He keeps her at a distance in order to avoid being hurt and, for the same reason, he later calls off their engagement. From this moment onwards, François begins to isolate himself. The broken engagement marks his giving up all claims upon his old life: his facial disfigurement has robbed him of his future.

In literature, the powerlessness felt by disfigured veterans leads them to cut themselves off from the rest of the world. Thiercelin decides to live a secluded life in a mansion with other wounded veterans, this house being in all likelihood the *Maison des Gueules Cassées* in Moussy. Some men are pictured as unaware that they are keeping other people at a distance. Thus,

51 This case, reported by Catherine Black (Black, *King's Nurse – Beggar's Nurse*, p. 89) is described in Chapter 2.

52 'A peine je la vis s'avancer au détour de l'allée, plus belle et plus aimable que jamais, mon cœur s'arrêta, et je pris une attitude indifférente. Par une bizarre hypocrisie, où il entrait de la pudeur, de la timidité, et sans doute aussi la crainte de n'être plus aimé, j'affectai de l'aborder d'un air distrait et de lui parler d'un ton léger, dont je ne me départis pas durant toute notre conversation', Galis, *Mon Visage Fait Horreur*, p. 46.

Otternschlag's paradoxical isolation – he spends most of his time sitting in the hotel lounge, without getting involved in what is going on around him – is described as an involuntary attitude:

> When he paid he put the money on the plate, not into the boy's hand. He always set a distance between himself and others, though he was not aware of it. The half of his mouth that was still intact even smiled after a fashion as he unfolded the papers and began to read. He expected something that never came, just as no letter, telegram or call ever came; he was dismally alone, empty, cut off from life.[53]

The constant activity and life in the lounge contrasts with Otternschlag's immobility and solitude. He is alone in the middle of the crowd. The social and emotional emptiness of his life echoes the physical emptiness of part of his face. His repeated enquiries at the hotel reception about a letter, a telegram or a call underline his loneliness. Although he is not completely passive – he intervenes to help another visitor, Kringelein, for instance – the German doctor seldom acts to improve his own condition. Whilst Kringelein obtains a better room, Otternschlag remains in the same ordinary room he has occupied for ten years, 'partly because he is staying en pension, partly because his means were moderate, chiefly, however, because he was too apathetic to demand a better'.[54]

The fear of being rejected that *gueules cassées* experienced thus accounts for their indifference, sometimes even their hostility, towards the outside world. It is a way for them to retain some control, but more importantly it is a means of self-preservation: they reject other people out of fear that they might be rejected themselves. This safety mechanism was often observed in real life, and was described in nurses' accounts as discussed in Chapter 1. The distance between veterans and others after their return, whether suffered or sought, reflects and fuels the extra-ordinary representations of *gueules cassées*.

53 Baum, *Grand Hotel*, p. 7.

54 Ibid, p. 13.

Responses of strangers

The disfigured man's attitude of rejection and isolation is based upon the presupposition that other people will react negatively to him. The reaction of passers-by is telling of society's perception, since their encounters with *gueules cassées* are unexpected and their responses less guarded. Given that they do not know the injured man personally, they are also less likely to try to hide their feelings. In Girard's novel, pity is repeatedly mentioned as people's first reaction. Strangers are described as looking at Paule and Thiercelin with pity or horror. At the opera, the couple overhear two young men talking about the disfigured veteran:

> 'Can you see, this guy is so bashed up?!' 'Poor devil', the other replied, 'he had his face smashed-up'. Gérard, who had heard, turned white. Paule impulsively moved forward and tapping the shoulder of the young man standing closer, she whispered, 'You are right, my friend, but it is precisely to enable your generation to live in peace that this man has sacrificed his face. He is a war hero'. Startled, the two young men came back and, spontaneously and respectfully, extended their hands to shake Gérard's.[55]

The young people's first reaction is pity, but once Paule has drawn their attention to the reason behind her fiancé's disfigurement and the implications for them, they show respect. In doing so, Paule echoes the voice of real-life *gueules cassées*, who, in their newspaper *La Greffe Générale* and through the UBF, expressed their wish not to be pitied, but respected.

Like Picot, Thiercelin does not mind being the centre of attention; rather it is the nature of strangers' reactions that upsets him. Rey in Renaud's novel also appears to tolerate the gaze of others, but reacts strongly when

55 '"Dis donc, t'as vu le type s'il est amoché?" L'autre répondit: "Ce pauvre diable, il s'est fait casser la 'g …'". Gérard, qui avait entendu, changea de couleur. Impulsive, Paule fit deux pas en avant et, touchant du doigt l'épaule de celui qui était le plus près d'elle, elle lui dit à voix basse: "Vous avez raison, mon jeune ami, mais c'est justement pour que votre génération connaisse des jours plus tranquilles que monsieur a sacrifié sa figure: c'est un héros de la guerre". Un peu interdits, les deux jeunes gens revinrent sur leurs pas et, spontanément, en silence et avec respect, ils tendirent la main à Gérard, l'un après l'autre', Girard, *La Vie Intime d'une 'Gueule Cassée'*, pp. 158–59.

shown pity. During a walk with his mistress, he notices people staring at him: 'When we sat down I noticed, without embarrassment, that people were staring at me'.[56] It is the words spoken by a young woman to her boyfriend that make him uncomfortable: 'My God, if you were like him. Poor man. And this is what war is like'.[57]

This reaction is indicative of the feelings triggered by the sight of facially wounded men: they are immediately associated with the war. It is no surprise given that the scene occurs during the conflict, but the association remains strong after its cessation and highlights the status of *gueules cassées* as reminders of war. Although Rey is not affected by the curiosity of onlookers, he reacts strongly to the woman's commiseration: 'I did not shudder but I felt cold, and suddenly everything around me started looking gloomy, grey and dirty'.[58] The woman's comment triggers a change in the way he perceives the world. Whilst just moments before he was enjoying the sun shining upon his damaged face, the surroundings now seem bleak to him. Of all the reactions, he finds that the most unbearable is pity:

> Walk amongst your fellow countrymen and hear them express their pity. Listen, however painful it is, because tomorrow, the day after tomorrow, in one or two years' time, when the illusions have faded, whatever you say and do, whatever words are used to describe the beauty of heroic wounds, they will remain wounds and only wounds.[59]

During the war at least, facial wounds were seen as epitomizing patriotic sacrifice. Reflecting upon his return to Paris immediately after the war, wearing his soldier's uniform, François too feels that passers-by respect

56 'Au moment où nous nous sommes assis, j'ai remarqué, mais sans en éprouver de gêne, qu'on me regardait à la dérobée', Renaud, *Gueules Cassées*, p. 178.

57 'Mon Dieu, si tu étais comme lui. Pauvre homme. Et c'est ça la guerre', Ibid, p. 178.

58 'Je n'ai pas tressailli, mais j'ai eu froid, et tout m'a subitement paru triste, gris et sale', Ibid., p. 178.

59 'Marche au milieu de tes semblables et écoute l'expression de leur pitié qui te fera souffrir, parce que, demain, après-demain, dans un an, dans deux ans, lorsque les illusions seront tombées, quoiqu'on dise et quoi qu'on fasse, quels que soient les mots dont on qualifie la beauté des blessures héroïques, elles n'en sont et seront pas moins des blessures', Ibid, p. 161.

him: 'Under the blue cap, my wound seemed less terrible. I wanted to be forever a wounded combatant, walking along the streets on his way back from battle, his head covered in glorious bandages'.[60] François finds that wearing the uniform makes him less noticeable, despite his injured head, and that people's occasional stares are soothing rather than intrusive. This is no longer the case later on. The difference in people's reaction is attributed to the fact that François was at the time a soldier, proudly bearing his war wound. Once the war is over, strangers display such positive responses only in specific circumstances, namely situations in which facially disfigured veterans are clearly identified as ex-combatants. A form of respect and acknowledgement of sacrifice still persists, but the expression of these positive feelings is limited to contexts in which national remembrance is channelled. When Paule first sees Thiercelin, he is taking part in a march commemorating the tenth anniversary of the armistice. This context influences her perception of his face as a symbol of heroism.

In literature, the responses of strangers impact upon the way in which men cope with their disfigurement, as shown in the example of François. The only outings he enjoys are his visits to the Tomb of the Unknown Soldier. On these occasions, passers-by stop to pay homage to the veterans; this makes François feel that the *gueules cassées'* sacrifice is acknowledged and valued by fellow countrymen.[61] At a time when war memorials were beginning to be built, the symbolic value of this specific place cannot be overlooked. The parallel between the Unknown Soldier and the facially disfigured veteran is also worth noting, as if the latter was no longer identified and recognized for his want of a face.

François dreads individual attention being paid to him and to his disfigured face, but he also longs for the public to acknowledge his sacrifice. His feelings towards society are mixed; he oscillates between proud

60 'Sous le calot de drap bleu, ma blessure me semblait moins affreuse. J'aurais voulu demeurer toujours le blessé qui passe dans la rue et revient de la bataille, la tête entourée d'un glorieux pansement', Galis, *Mon Visage Fait Horreur*, p. 47.

61 Ibid, pp. 76–77.

public exhibition on commemorative occasions as part of a group, and withdrawal when he is alone:

> Entering a *metro* carriage was an ordeal. I was even dreading having to cross crowded areas and I would make long detours to avoid them. I got used to walking with my head down. I resorted to every childish trick I could think of to escape other people's curiosity.[62]

François's wish to go unnoticed in his everyday life contrasts with his choice to go to the tomb of the Unknown Soldier. Two elements appear to facilitate his interaction with society. Firstly, being part of a group who goes to the Arc de Triomphe makes him less obtrusive than taking the train by himself. Secondly, he does not dread appearing in the solemn context of military remembrance, whereas he dislikes being the focus of attention in everyday situations. Being identified as a mutilated veteran is perceived as more bearable than being seen as just any disfigured man. In the context of remembrance ceremonies, the presence of *gueules cassées* is not as transgressive as it is in daily life.

Literature evokes the positive associations of facial injury with courage and even heroism, yet most narratives nevertheless emphasize the negative reactions of strangers upon meeting *gueules cassées*. François goes even further in stating that

> Wherever I went, my presence would make people feel embarrassed. Whenever I unexpectedly came to a meeting, I could read on people's faces surprise, disgust or pity, and more frequently horror. But all of their faces reflected their secret relief at not looking like me.[63]

62 'Pénétrer dans un wagon du métropolitain était pour moi un supplice. J'en vins à redouter la simple traverse de quartiers trop fréquentés; je faisais de longs détours. Je pris l'habitude de baisser la tête en marchant, pour échapper à la curiosité du public, à quels singuliers enfantillages n'avais-je pas recours?', Ibid, pp. 72–73.

63 'Partout où je me montrais, une gêne subite paraissait. Quand j'arrivais à l'improviste dans une réunion, je lisais sur certains visages la surprise où le dégoût, sur d'autres la pitié, sur la plupart l'horreur, sur tous le secret contentement de ne pas ressembler au mien', Galis, *Mon Visage Fait Horreur*, p. 71.

While Rey deems pity to be the most likely response, and also the most difficult to cope with, François describes relief as a universal reaction; he qualifies this judgement later, however, distinguishing between adults and children. The latter's reaction is surprise and curiosity rather than horror or pity, François notes. When a child playing in a park notices the disfigured man sitting on a bench, he observes him with interest until the mother tells him off.[64] François does not seem to mind being the object of the child's attention, which is not hostile but inquisitive. Of the three people involved in this scene, the mother is the one who is uneasy.

In terms of interaction with adults, literature depicts, for example, encounters between *gueules cassées* and other soldiers or veterans. In Galis's novel, François watches the 14 July 1919 military march from the balcony of his Parisian flat. The crowds are enthusiastic and the returned combatants express their joy to be back. But when François meets them on the streets later that day, he notes the combatants' pity upon seeing him. In the middle of other people, he is more isolated than ever. Everyone, civilians and combatants alike, seems to be wondering the same thing about François: 'Who was this wandering ghost, tainting the universal rejoicing on the Paris streets, like the phantom of the dead war?'[65] The presence of the disfigured man is disturbing, for it brings back the memories of war and its horrors to people who are celebrating the victory. In blurring these boundaries, he represents a transgressive presence. Nevertheless, pity is presented as the most frequent response, although it is always described as something disfigured men despise. Literary accounts engage more strongly with representations of *gueules cassées* as victims, rather than as heroes.

64 Ibid, p. 73.

65 'Quel était ce revenant qui errait à travers la ville pour troubler le bonheur universel, comme le spectre de la guerre morte ?', Ibid, pp. 49–50.

Friendship

Some relationships with strangers develop into closer friendships. If François is ill-at-ease among war veterans, he nevertheless confesses that he feels welcome and accepted by other *wounded* war veterans:

> Since my return to Paris, it is only in the company of my old hospital pals that I have been able to forget and to enjoy brief moments of happiness. In the hospital courtyards, they were dragging their crutches next to me and sharing their hardships. The pinch of tobacco offered with a curse by a ruddy farm boy warmed up my heart more than the wordy and absent-minded pity of polite society.[66]

Other maimed soldiers are the men's new family; literature here reflects the real-life experience of members of the *Union des Blessés de la Face*. They not only share war memories, but they are also faced with similar challenges in civilian society. This choice to withdraw is presented by Girard as a way to shelter themselves from the world: 'their moral suffering was lessened and they did not have to witness the heartbreak, the instinctive fear, caused by their appearance. They no longer had to see pity and terror in the eyes of passers-by!'[67] The pensioners developed close relationships with each other and this literary account reflects, perhaps even exaggerates, the success of the Moussy endeavour. Thiercelin is well-integrated in the community: his wedding reception takes place there, amongst other facially disfigured men who are rejoicing over their comrade's departure. His marriage does not sever his links with his friends; rather to some extent his wife becomes

66 'Si j'ai pu passer encore quelques instants d'oubli et de gaîté depuis mon retour à Paris, je les dois à mes pauvres vieux compagnons d'hôpital qui traînaient près de moi sur le gravier des cours leurs béquilles et leurs rudes misères. La pincée de tabac offerte avec un juron par un garçon de ferme aux mains rouges, me réconforta mieux que la pitié verbeuse et distraite des gens du monde', Galis, *Mon Visage Fait Horreur*, p. 45.

67 'Ils souffraient moins moralement, n'avaient plus à supporter l'impression poignante, sorte de peur instinctive, que leur aspect causait invariablement et lire dans les regards qu'ils croisaient, au dehors, la pitié et l'effroi!', Girard, *La Vie Intime d'une 'Gueule Cassée'*, p. 44.

a member of this community, echoing the inclusive approach of the *Union des Blessés de la Face*.

But even the company of other wounded veterans can prove difficult to cope with, as seen in the examples of François and Thiercelin. The latter finds it sometimes hard to put up with the other pensioners. François admits that he enjoys the company of a fellow *gueule cassée*, but that he is ashamed to be seen with other disfigured men in public, except in solemn and commemorative circumstances. In literature, being with other *gueules cassées* makes the wounded man feel 'normal', but at the same time it prevents him from forgetting about his own disfigurement. This is the reason why François refuses to become a member of their organization and to move to their mansion, in spite of another wounded veteran's repeated invitations. In this respect, Galis's novel does not support the idyllic depiction of Moussy given by Girard and the UBF itself. François's one-day visit there to attend a *fête* organized for wounded veterans further confirms him in his choice. Whilst amputated soldiers celebrate outside, the house itself is silent:

> Some of the men with no lips had a perpetual, silent grin on their faces. Many had no teeth left and when they were talking, they could hardly be heard. The sounds that came out of their mouths were as deformed as their mouths themselves. Those who could no longer chew were eating gruel, gurgling like infants. Others were eating and drinking without exchanging a word, and nothing was more frightening, having just seen the noisy show that was performed outdoors, than this tragic banquet.[68]

In contrast with other maimed veterans, *gueules cassées* remain inside the house and the atmosphere is almost eerie. The hierarchy of wounds sometimes evoked in the context of war identifies facial wounds as the worst of all.

68 'Certains, n'ayant plus de lèvres, semblaient rire d'un rire silencieux, terrible. Beaucoup n'avaient même plus de dents, et, quand ils parlaient, on les entendait à peine, car il ne sortait de leur bouche qu'un son aussi informe qu'elle. Ceux qui ne pouvaient plus mâcher avalaient des bouillies d'enfants avec d'immenses gargouillements. Les autres buvaient et mangeaient sans un mot; et rien n'était plus effrayant, après le spectacle, que le calme sinistre de ce tragique banquet', Galis, *Mon Visage Fait Horreur*, pp. 79–80.

Facially injured men and their families

The responses of a facially disfigured man's relatives to the change in his appearance are described as particularly significant in literature, reflecting real-life stories. In literary fiction, relatives tend to be portrayed as those who manage to deal with their initial shock and relate to the wounded, thereby providing readers with an example of successful interaction. This participates in the construction of a story that would otherwise be very introspective and less appealing to the general public. The emphasis upon interaction also performs a didactic function in helping readers to understand the disfigured man's psyche and advising them on how to (and how not to) behave.

François's mother is the first person he sees when he wakes up in hospital. Not only has she watched over her son during treatment, but her first action upon his return to consciousness is to make physical contact with him, kissing him on the forehead.[69] He has no idea what kind of injury he suffers from and his mother's presence suggests that everything is fine. Her tender gestures remind him of his childhood, all the more so since he is treated in his own house, which has been converted into a hospital. Her behaviour is indicative of her acceptance: she is constantly at her son's bedside and appears to be relieved and even joyful. She tries to shield him by preventing him from seeing his face: 'One day, I asked her to lend me a mirror. She smiled and answered distractedly, making a joke about the little luggage she had with her'.[70] When she realizes that he knows the truth she embraces him and whispers 'My poor child!'[71] His mother's acceptance has a significant impact on François, who later moves in with her to take care of her until she dies. She is the only person whom he does not reject; nor does he reproach her for not having prepared him to face the truth. The fact that his mother accepted him without any

69 Galis, *Mon Visage Fait Horreur*, p. 41.

70 'Un jour, je demandai un miroir à ma mère. Elle me répondit en souriant d'un air distrait par une plaisanterie sur la pénurie de ses bagages', Ibid, p. 43.

71 'Mon pauvre enfant!', Ibid, p. 45.

second thoughts does not, however, prevent François from struggling with his disfigurement.

Thiercelin's mother and sister both visit him in Moussy. He kisses his mother when he sees her, and no mention is made of any repulsion on her part. He is nevertheless aware that her first reaction after his injury was sadness.[72] More insights into Madame Thiercelin's perception of her disfigured son and his future prospects are revealed through her attitude towards her daughter-in-law. She confesses to Paule that 'never would I have dared hope that my son would find such happiness', and she thanks her: 'My dear child, may God bless you for what you have done for my son!'[73] The mother harboured little hope that her son would ever get married. Her gratitude suggests that she regards Paule's marriage to the disfigured veteran to be a sacrifice more than an act of love, as if the maimed soldier was able to trigger a woman's compassion, but not her desire.

Otternschlag's experience is very different. He is haunted by a recurring dream:

> And then, two floors higher, there is Doctor Otternschlag, dreaming the dream that comes to him every week. He is going through a dream-town which he knows very well and he enters a dream-house that he has forgotten. A dream-woman lives there and she has had a dream-child while he was a prisoner of war – a horrible child of whom he is not the father. It howls in its neat perambulator whenever it sees his mangled face [...].[74]

Although his disfigurement is not described as the cause of the woman's treachery, the child's attitude is a reaction to Otternschlag's damaged face. The German veteran in Baum's novel, like the ones depicted in visual arts, is represented as betrayed and isolated.

72 Girard, *La Vie Intime d'une 'Gueule Cassée'*, p. 143.

73 'Jamais elle n'avait osé espérer un tel bonheur pour son fils', and 'Ma chère enfant, soyez bénie pour ce que vous avez fait pour mon fils!', Ibid, p. 170 and p. 176.

74 Baum, *Grand Hotel*, p. 307.

Love and romantic relationships

Acceptance by the family is presented as important, but not enough to rehabilitate a disfigured man. Love appears in literary accounts as the only way to a complete reintegration into post-war society. Most novels involve romantic relationships, and the destiny of the wounded veteran – tragic or happy – correlates with the success or failure of his love story.

Baum's novel aside, romantic relationships play an important part in these literary works.[75] Rey's mistress watches over him during his stay in hospital. While he is still unable to see his wounds, it is her reaction that he dreads the most. He wants to know how she reacted when she first saw him. The nurse's answer is ambiguous: she remains silent for a long time before telling Rey that, upon seeing him for the first time, his mistress knelt down and kissed his hands.[76] This reply relieves the wounded man's fears and appeases him. The woman he loves did not turn away. The facial injury in this novel, far from separating the couple, unites them; the woman's love is presented as the one thing that brings him through his convalescence.

Gilberte, the young woman to whom François was engaged before his injury, fulfils a similar function in Galis's novel, but the outcome of their complicated relationship is tragic. When he rejects her, she tries to convince him of her love, but in vain. François later admits that he can still feel desire. But his experiences at a brothel and with Gilberte show him that sex is not enough to make him feel 'human' again.[77] He is looking for something more than physical intercourse, as he admits after seducing – almost raping – Gilberte in his parents' mortuary vault.[78] From then on, François's life goes from bad to worse, revealing the impact of guilt and of the absence of love. As the couple are offered a chance of reunion at the end

75 In Baum's novel, Otternschlag appears to be indifferent to women, the memories of previous relationships leaving him 'without emotion, the memory occasioned only a faint creeping chill in his spine' (Baum, *Grand Hotel*, p. 8).

76 Renaud, *Gueules Cassées*, p. 148.

77 Ibid, p. 69.

78 Ibid, p. 65.

of the novel, he feels alive for the first time since his injury.[79] This possibility of a bright future is soon denied when François accidentally kills Gilberte.

Girard's novel is the only narrative that ends with the successful reintegration of the disfigured man, a happy ending that is described as the result of a woman's love. Thiercelin's decision to withdraw from society was in part the consequence of being rejected by his first fiancée. In contrast, new matrimonial prospects with Paule impact positively upon his morale and his health. Their marriage ultimately leads him to bless the wounds that enabled him to find a wife and start a family: 'I feel like myself again, I do not fear anything in life anymore!'[80] Thiercelin's feeling of estrangement from his former self because of his injury has come to an end. In this narrative, the woman's choice to marry a wounded veteran is presented as a patriotic act. In the context of the interwar years, many women found themselves alone, and the main character in this novel even admits that many spinsters would rather marry a disabled veteran than remain single.[81]

The post-war years were characterized by a shortage of men, and war pensions could be a further incentive for women to marry veterans. Literary narratives present both women who are unable – or unwilling – to pursue a relationship with their disfigured fiancés, and who engage in happy relationships. However, the one German novel analysed here suggests that to return home, and beyond this to 'normal' life, was beyond the veteran's reach. His initial betrayal by his wife further represents the 'betrayal' of a society from which he has become isolated. In contrast, in French novels, romantic love appears to be the gateway to the maimed veteran's reappropriation of his self and reintegration back into the world. Being loved, the *gueule cassée* is rehabilitated both in the eyes of other people and in his own eyes. Marriage appears to be a benchmark in the definition of 'normality' and reintegration. In turn, society, in its acceptance of its war heroes, is rehabilitated too.

79 Ibid, p. 108.

80 'Je suis redevenu moi-même, je ne redoute plus rien de la vie!', Girard, *La Vie Intime d'une 'Gueule Cassée'*, p. 188.

81 Ibid, p. 55.

Summary

Literary accounts urge the reader to go beyond the mutilated face of a veteran and to consider the psychological and social consequences of war and disfigurement. Through narratives of successful or failed reintegration, literature emphasizes the role – even responsibility – of society in helping the veteran to find a place. A tendency to 'de-heroicize' and isolate facially injured men, and soldiers in general, can be observed in the German literary tradition as in the visual arts of the time. In contrast, French novels are largely void of political criticism and give a more positive interpretation of the war and its consequences for individual combatants. However, even in accounts presenting *gueules cassées* in a more positive fashion, the injured still appear powerless to secure the maintenance or restoration of relationships. Many of them are presented as isolated and inactive by choice or by necessity, whilst society is empowered, called to remember and to act.

Conclusion

In wartime and interwar France, Germany and Great Britain, facially injured and disfigured men were a visible and recognized presence, both on the streets and in the arts. From the hospital where the wounded spent extended periods of time, to their return to civilian life, their journey testifies to the personal and collective impact of injuries to the face. Despite the desire they often expressed to go unnoticed, and thus sometimes against their own will, they became symbols of national aspiration. An exploration of their fates and representation reveals great variety in their lives: they sometimes appear as passive patients and sometimes as involved in the rehabilitation process; they are in turn unemployed and successful in a variety of workplaces; they are rejected lovers and happily married fathers; they withdraw from society and yet consciously set themselves up as examples for their fellow countrymen to follow. This study has drawn upon a wealth of sources in order to show the variety and complexity of the destinies, perceptions and representations of *gueules cassées*.

The risk of reducing facially disfigured men to one common story or symbol was already apparent in the interwar years; it is perhaps even more of a temptation today, as their absence makes it easier for us to merge all their stories into one. Since the First World War, pictures of disfigured combatants have been mainly used as illustrations of its horrors. Thus, the 2007 National Army Museum 'Faces of Battle' exhibition was presented by the BBC as '[revealing] a hidden side to the horror of World War I'.[1] Similarly, Claire Garnier, the curator of the 2012 exhibition '1917' (Metz, France), described the return home of *gueules cassées* as 'the time when the Home

1 'In pictures: Faces of Battle', BBC News, 2009 <http://news.bbc.co.uk/1/shared/spl/hi/picture_gallery/07/magazine_faces_of_battle/html/1.stm> [accessed 18 August 2015].

Front discovered the horrors of war'.[2] Likewise the premise of the 2014 exhibition '*Gueules Cassées*: Scars from the Great War in Contemporary Art' in Kunsthalle Mainz was that disfigured soldiers in Versailles embodied the 'horrors of war', this bias leading the curators to display artworks reflecting 'wounds, pain and loss'.[3] In the light of this dominant interpretative framework, the work of the French-Algerian artist Kader Attia is particularly innovative: in *Open Your Eyes*, he combines images of *gueules cassées* and images of African artwork and facial decoration to interrogate notions of beauty and identity in different European and non-European cultures.[4]

Rarely have these disfigured men been presented or discussed alongside the narratives of their lives, one notable exception being a textual-visual display of a facially disfigured soldier's life exhibited at the Hunterian Museum, London. The veteran is not reduced to his wound; rather his wound is presented as a part of his life. Almost a century after the events, there is still a temptation to isolate *gueules cassées* and to limit aspects of study to their disfigurement. The hierarchy of wounds that Kienitz suggests to be evident in interwar Germany can to some extent still be observed today. And this ranking of injuries, which she discusses in the context of Germany, is in fact also visible in the rhetoric about facial injuries in France and Great Britain, as shown throughout this book. The discourse about facially injured soldiers frequently depicted their destinies as worse than those of other veterans, and even worse than death itself.

The transgressive dimension of facially disfigured men posited in the introduction has been discussed with reference to the perceptions

2 'Le moment où l'arrière découvre les horreurs de la guerre', Claire Garnier, interview on the exhibition '1917', Alsace 20, 2012 <http://www.youtube.com/watch?v=2N7VW4Dd1U0> [accessed 18 August 2015]. The layout of the exhibition (a spiral) culminated with the display of casts of mutilated faces, thereby emphasizing these specific items, although the theme was the year '1917' more largely.

3 '*Gueules Cassées*: Scars from the Great War in the Contemporary Art', Kunsthalle Mainz, 27 February–8 June 2014 <http://www.goethe.de/ges/prj/nzv/par/en12444958.htm> [accessed 20 March 2015].

4 Kader Attia, *Open Your Eyes* (2010). It was exhibited in Germany (Kunstwerke Gallery, Berlin, 2013) and France (Musée des Ducs de Bretagne, Nantes, 2013).

of soldiers, medical staff, media professionals, writers and artists. This study has thereby revealed a tension between two major trends. On the one hand, we observe a tendency to marginalize *gueules cassées*, describing them as monsters, victims or heroes. They are presented as figures remote from normality, featuring inhuman or superhuman characteristics. On the other hand, a normalization of the figure of the disfigured man can also be found and, in some cases, explicitly claimed. The present study thus demonstrates the importance of a more nuanced portrayal of the perceptions and destinies of wounded veterans.

On a personal level, the challenges awaiting the veterans were similar regardless of the country in which they lived. The support they received from the state and the ways in which they were perceived by society differed, however. *Gueules cassées* became symbolically loaded figures in all three countries, but different aspects were emphasized depending upon national context. They were a predominant feature of German visual art, in which they often functioned as embodiments of a broken society and indictments of militarism. Their presence is more discreet in British art and society, especially after the end of the war. The existence of official photographs testifies to the possibility of them being used as propaganda tools and the building of the first central maxillofacial institution reveals a proactive approach to their treatment on the part of the government. The emphasis here was upon practical questions and a pragmatic approach was taken, under the influence of Harold Gillies, amongst others. The fact that the relationships formed at The Queen's Hospital were not maintained on a significant level after the patients' discharge, despite the provision of separate medical facilities for facially injured soldiers, confirms Cohen's view that disabled veterans were well-integrated within wider social and philanthropic networks in Great Britain. This situation accounts for the absence of an injury-specific group bringing together facially wounded ex-servicemen. In contrast to this, the current book has shed light upon the inception and development of a self-help organization in France and demonstrated the role of external and internal factors in its increase in numbers and influence throughout the 1920s and 1930s, in particular the role played by its president Yves Picot. The 'kinship' bond between *gueules cassées* described by Winter as the starting point of the *Union des Blessés de la Face* is here examined in an attempt to explain why no similar organizations emerged in other countries despite the fact that a strong comradeship between men during their treatment was observed in all three countries. In particular, the present study emphasizes the importance of charismatic individuals in the process of the reintegration of *gueules cassées* into society.

The case of facially wounded women has not been discussed here; their existence should, however, be acknowledged. Indeed, records show that there were female patients treated at the Val-de-Grâce and The Queen's Hospital.[5] The limited number of such cases and the lack of information about them do not, however, allow for a detailed analysis. Furthermore, facial disfigurement in women undoubtedly created a different set of issues – especially considering post-war demographics and gender roles – for example, the one woman described in the pages of the *Bulletin* is described as particularly 'deserving' since she lost a key female attribute: beauty. When considering those absent from this study, it is also important to acknowledge that, for the most part, only the lives of those men who 'successfully' returned home are documented. The tragic stories of those who spent the rest of their lives in psychiatric wards or chose to end their lives altogether have largely been lost, except when family members decided to investigate their fates.[6] However, the analysis of military reports and accounts by medical staff, as well as the small number of veterans who decided to live in Moussy permanently, indicate that complete withdrawal or suicide was not a very common occurrence.

5 Unidentified plaster casts at the Val-de-Grâce testify to the presence of two female patients. Andrew Bamji mentions one female case at The Queen's Hospital in Andrew Bamji, 'The Queen's Hospital and All The King's Men', paper given at the Royal Society of Medicine's History of Medicine section meeting, in Michael Smith, 'First World War Facial Injuries', *Journal of the Royal Society of Medicine*, 88 (1995), 601–02.

6 Guy Monségur thus researched what happened to his great-uncle Jean-Victor, who was facially disfigured and probably also suffered cerebral damage. His findings were published in the form of a partly imaginary narrative retracing the veteran's life until his death, alone and forgotten, in a psychiatric unit (Monségur, *Etrange et Tragique Destinée d'un Poilu*, 2004).

The present study focuses upon the period between the First World War and the outbreak of the Second World War; it is now more important than ever to acknowledge the long-term legacy of disfigured veterans of the First World War. From visual reminders of one specific war, they became generic symbols of the timeless brutality of all wars. The recent interest in popular culture in the *gueules cassées* of the First World War is indicative of their lasting iconic function; this is visible in the release of exhibitions, novels and films in all three countries since the late 1990s.[7] Most importantly, the empowerment of French veterans via the *Union des Blessés de la Face* raises questions that remain to be analysed in a broader chronological frame. The bond between members, often described as the consequence of a shared war experience, begs the question of the integration of combatants wounded during other conflicts. Indeed, the emergence of a strong sense of collective identity could have been threatened by the inclusion of soldiers injured in later wars. The fact that the *Union* welcomed servicemen disfigured after 1918, and now also supports firemen and policemen, testifies to its inclusive approach. It also shows that facial injuries have remained a powerful common denominator and that the experience of disfigurement is perceived as a 'link', regardless of the context in which it was received.

The creation in Great Britain of the 'Guinea Pig Club' – an organization that gathered airmen who had been disfigured as a result of severe burns during the Second World War – also calls for a comparison with its French precursor. This study has shown that the links between the *Union des Blessés de la Face* and veterans in Great Britain were tenuous and sometimes led to inaccurate information, such as the belief that The Queen's Hospital was a home for disfigured men. The 'Guinea Pig Club' developed in its own right but some salient features of its inception are strikingly similar to the context in which the UBF was established. The name they chose for themselves is equally humorous, if not ironic. More importantly, the role played by a small group of men in its inception, especially surgeon

7 See, for instance, Young, *My Dear, I Wanted to Tell You*; Valade, *Gueules Cassées … et alors?;* and the EU INTERREG-funded project 1914FACES2014 on the long-term cultural legacy of facial injuries in France and Great Britain.

Archibald McIndoe, parallels that of Jugon, Jourdain and Picot. Although McIndoe, like Picot, was only one facilitator amongst several men instrumental in the foundation of the club, he became its first president until his death in 1960. If he was not one of the 'Guinea Pigs' himself, his efforts to favour the reintegration of burnt airmen during their treatment at Queen Victoria's Hospital in East Grinstead made him a key protagonist in their psychological and social rehabilitation.[8] Like Picot, he acted as a spokesperson and an ambassador: both came to be 'the face' of the disfigured. In the case of the *Association des Gueules Cassées*, as in that of the 'Guinea Pig Club', there is a greater readiness to study disfigured men within a collective structure, as it presupposes that they are integrated. In contrast, individual case studies highlight the intimate relationship between personal and collective histories, as signalled by Peter Englund, a relationship which defies convenient simplifications.

8 McIndoe, with the help of the Blonds, arranged for his patients to be invited into homes in the neighbourhood so that they would not be ostracized. Details of his influence can be found on the Blond-McIndoe Foundation's website <http://www.blondmcindoe.org/sir-archibald-mcindoe.html#Blond_McIndoe> [accessed 18 August 2015].

Bibliography

Primary sources

Newspaper and journal articles

Anon., 'Albert Lebrun Visite le Domaine des "Gueules Cassées"', *Le Petit Journal*, 28 July 1933, p. 1.

Anon., Court Circular, *The Times*, 5 January 1917, p. 11.

Anon., Court Circular, *The Times*, 1 December 1917, p. 11.

Anon., Court Circular, *The Times*, 26 June 1918, p. 9.

Anon., 'Disfigured Faces Restored', *The Manchester Guardian*, 26 September 1916, p. 4.

Anon., 'Facial Wounds: Merciful Work of Modern Surgery', *The Manchester Guardian*, 18 September 1918, p. 3.

Anon., 'Generous Gifts for Frognal Hospital', *Sidcup Times*, 26 October 1917, p. 5.

Anon., '"La gueule" is Now Polite', *The Times*, London, 12 October 1920, p. 9.

Anon., 'Les "Gueules Cassées" Présentent un Grand Film Historique: "Pour la Paix du Monde"', *Journal des Mutilés*, 29 September 1927, p. 1.

Anon., '"Jig-saw", Children's Musical Play at Sidcup in Aid of The Queen's Hospital', *Sidcup Times*, 11 January 1918, p. 5.

Anon., '"The Larger Necessity": Blinded Soldiers' Children's Fund', *The Observer*, 23 September 1917, p. 11.

Anon., 'The Making of Portrait Masks by Mrs Ladd', *The First Year of the American Red Cross in France: Activities for the year ended July 1, 1918*. Washington, D.C., American Red Cross, pp. 32–33.

Anon., 'The Men Behind the Veil', *The African World*, 16 July 1921, p. 428.

Anon., 'Opening of The Queen's Hospital', *Sidcup Times*, 27 July 1917, p. 5.

Anon., 'Painters of the R.A.M.C.: New Pictures in the War Museum', *The Times*, 25 May 1920, p. 8.

Anon., 'The Queen's Hospital, Frognal, Sidcup', *The Lancet*, 3 November 1917, 687–89.

Anon., 'The Queen's Visit to Sidcup', *Sidcup Times*, 16 November 1917, p. 5.

Anon., 'Sculptor and Surgeon. How they Collaborate at the 3rd L.G.H. A Note by the C.O.', *The Gazette of the 3rd London General Hospital. Wandsworth*, I, May 1916, pp. 205–06.

Anon., 'Soldiers Craftsmen: Display of Work by Hospital Patients', *The Times*, 9 December 1919, p. 11.

Anon., 'Treatment of Disabled Soldiers: British and French Methods', *The Manchester Guardian*, 7 August 1917, p. 6.

Anon., 'The Triumphs of Sidcup', *The Manchester Guardian*, 5 November 1921, p. 8.

Bertholin, Jean, 'La Maison des "Gueules Cassées"', *Le Gaulois*, 21 June 1927, p. 1.

Bulletins de l'Union des Blessés de la Face, 1–61 (1921–1939). Paris, *Association des Gueules Cassées* private archives.

Colombier, André, 'J'accuse', *L'Actualité Cinématographique et Littéraire*, press cutting, Cinémathèque française collections, B46–137 GANCE.

Finaud, Georges, 'Les Mutilés de la Face', *Après le Combat*, reprinted in *Bulletin de l'Union des Blessés de la Face*, 8, September 1923, p. 1.

Greffe Générale, La, newspaper published by Val-de-Grâce patients, 1–8 (December 1917–July 1918). Paris, Bibliothèque nationale de France, FRBNF32783911.

Harper, Grace S., 'New Faces for Mutilated Soldiers', *American Red Cross Magazine*, November 1918, pp. 43–44.

Latzarus, Louis, 'Ils Veulent Rire', *Le Figaro*, 23 September 1917 [no page number].

Martin, Georges, '"Une Gueule Cassée" Léon Gardeblé Meurtrier de l'Ami de sa Femme Est Acquitté', *Le Petit Journal*, 7 January 1930, p. 1 and p. 3.

Queen's Hospital, The, Sidcup (June 1917–August 1929), press cuttings collection. London, London Metropolitan Archives (LMA), HO2/Y01/05.

Panter, Peter (aka Kurt Tucholsky), 'Französischer Kriegsfilm', *Vossische Zeitung*, 2 November 1927, <http://www.zeno.org/Literatur/M/Tucholsky,+Kurt/Werke/1927/Franz%C3%B6sischer+Kriegsfilm> [accessed 18 August 2015].

Plaxton, Iola 'A Wonderful Hospital for Injuries to Face: Mrs William Carruthers of Toronto Describes Another Feature of War Work in which Britain is Leading the World – Soldiers from Every British Dominion and Colony Benefit', *Toronto Star Weekly*, November 1917, LMA HO2/Y01/05, p. 25.

Roth, Joseph, 'Lebende Kriegsdenkmäler', *Neue Berliner Zeitung*, 31 August 1920, ed. by Klaus Westermann, *Joseph Roth, Werke: 1915–1923*, 6 vols (Köln: Kiepenheuer & Witsch, 1989), I, pp. 347–52.

——, 'Der Wiederaufbau des Menschen: Gesichtsplastik in der Charité — Kriegs- und Zivilkranke — Die Tragik der Nasen', *Neue Berliner Zeitung*, 6 June 1921, ed. by Klaus Westermann, *Joseph Roth Werke: 1915–1923*, 6 vols (Köln: Kiepenheuer & Witsch, 1989), I, pp. 580–83.

Salmon, André, [article title unknown], *La Jeune Sculpture française*, 1919, p. 74, quoted in Rivière, Anne ed., *Jane Poupelet, 1874–1932: 'La Beauté dans la Simplicité'* (Paris: Gallimard, 2005).

Tucholsky, Kurt, 'Waffe gegen den Krieg' (1926), in *Kurt Tucholsky: Gesammelte Werke*, ed. by Mary Gerold-Tucholsky and Fritz J. Raddatz, 10 vols (Reinbeck bei Hamburg: Rowohlt, 1975), IV (1925–1926), pp. 359–60.

Military and medical reports and treatises

Anon., Foreword to *Les œuvres libres*, 1, July 1921 <http://www.archive.org/stream/lesoeuvreslibres00pari/lesoeuvreslibres00pari_djvu.txt> [accessed 18 August 2015].

Anon., 'Hospitals for Facial Injuries', *The Official Journal of the British Red Cross Society*, 5, 10, 15 October 1918, p. 118.

Anon., Report on the *Centre de Prothèse Restauratrice Maxillo-dento-faciale, 8e Région, Place de Bourges*, May 1916. Paris, Musée du Service de Santé aux Armées du Val-de-Grâce, box 122.

Anon., *Report on the Work of The Queen's Hospital, Sidcup, Kent, for Sailors and Soldiers Suffering from Facial and Jaw Injuries (1917–1921)*, 1921, Wellcome Library collections.

Bryan, W.A., 'Plastic Surgery of the Face', *British Dental Journal*, 37 (1916), 229–32.

Bruhn, Christian, ed., *Die gegenwärtigen Behandlungswege der Kieferschussverletzungen* (Wiesbaden: J.F. Bergmann, 1916).

Delagenière and Lebedinsky, *Rapport sur l'Organisation et le Fonctionnement du Centre de Stomatologie et de Prothèse MF. 4e Région. Place du Mans.* Section on 'Centre de Prothèse Elementaire pour Edentés', 1–31 March 1917, p. 10. Paris, Musée du Service de Santé aux Armées du Val-de-Grâce archives, box 121.

Denuce, [first name unknown], 'Missions Etrangères', *Rapport sur le Fonctionnement du Service de Chirurgie Maxillo-Faciale et Stomatologie. Du Ier Août au 31 Août 1916 Par Monsieur le Professeur DENUCE, Médecin Principal de 2e Classe. 18e Région.* Paris, Musée du Service de Santé aux Armées du Val-de-Grâce archives, box 127.

——, *Rapport sur le Fonctionnement du Service de Chirurgie Maxillo-Faciale et Stomatologie. Septembre 1916 Par Monsieur le Professeur DENUCE, Médecin Principal de 2e Classe. 18e Région*, pp. 1–2. Paris, Musée du Service de Santé aux Armées du Val-de-Grâce archives, box 127.

——, *Rapport sur le Fonctionnement du Service de Chirurgie Maxillo-Faciale et Stomatologie. Octobre 1916, Par Monsieur le Professeur DENUCE, Médecin Principal de 2e Classe. 18e Région*, p. 2. Paris, Musée du Service de Santé aux Armées du Val-de-Grâce archives, box 127.

Dolamure, W.H., 'The Treatment in Germany of Gunshot Injuries of the Face and Jaws' (translated and shortened), *British Dental Journal: The Journal of the British Dental Association*, 37 (1916), 105–84.

Dufourmentel, Léon, and Flavien Bonnet-Roy, *Chirurgie d'Urgence des Blessures de la Face et du Cou* (Paris: A. Maloine et fils, 1918).

——, *Introduction à la Chirurgie Constructive: Essai sur l'Art et la Chirurgie* (Paris: La jeune parque, 1946).

Gelly, Georges, *Appel en Faveur du 'Foyer des Gueules Cassées'* (Etampes: Imprimerie Maurice et Cerf, 1926). Paris, Bibliothèque Inter-Universitaire de Médicine, 156766/306–16.

——, *Le Paradis des Gueules Cassées* (Etampes: Société Régionale d'Imprimerie et de Publicité, 1926).

Gillies, Harold, *Plastic Surgery of the Face Based on Selected Cases of War Injuries of the Face Including Burns, with Original Illustrations* (London: Frowde, 1920).

——, Letter to Ralph Millard, 12 September 1951 (London, Gillies Archives).

——, and D. Ralph Millard, *The Principles and Art of Plastic Surgery* (Boston: Little, Brown and Co., 1957).

Joseph, Jacques, *Nasenplastik und sonstige Gesichtsplastik: nebst einem Anhang über Mammaplastik und einige weitere Operationen aus dem Gebiete der äusseren Körperplastik ein Atlas und Lehrbuch* (Leipzig: Curt Kabitzsch, 1931).

Kazanjian, Varaztad, and John M. Converse, *Surgical Treatment of Facial Injuries* (Baltimore: Williams and Wilkins Company, 1959 [1949]).

Lebedinsky, J., and Maurice Virenque, *Prothèse et Chirurgie Cranio-maxillo-faciale* (Paris: J.-B. Baillière et fils, 1918).

Lexer, Erich, *Wiederherstellungs-Chirurgie* (Leipzig: Johann Ambrosius Barth, 1920).

Morestin, Hippolyte, 'Les Blessures de la Face', *Science et Dévouement: Le Service de Santé de la Croix-Rouge, Les Œuvres de Solidarité* (Paris: Editions d'Art Aristide Quillet, 1918), pp. 137–59.

Pickerill, Henry Percy, *Facial Surgery* (Edinburgh: E. & S. Livingstone, 1924).

Sébileau, *Hôpital Temporaire du Collège Chaptal, 73, rue de Rome, Paris. Rapport du Centre de Chirurgie maxillo-faciale. Mois de janvier 1917. Du Dr Sébileau à M. le Médecin-Inspecteur, Directeur du Service de Santé du G.M.P.* Paris, Musée du Service de Santé aux Armées du Val-de-Grâce, box 120.

Wood, Francis D., 'Masks for Facial Wounds', *The Lancet*, 189 (23 June 1917), 949–51.

Testimonies

Albee, Frederick, *A Surgeon's Fight to Rebuild Men* (London: Robert Hale, 1950).
Anon., *My Personal Experiences and Reminiscences of the Great War*, Essays 2 and 6, January 1922. Leeds, Liddle collection.
Baillaud, Hélène, testimony (14 pages), Paris, Musée du Service de Santé aux Armées du Val-de-Grâce.
Black, Catherine, *King's Nurse – Beggar's Nurse: An Autobiography* (London: Hurst & Blackett, 1939).
Braillon, Pierre-Marie, *Mémoires de Guerre d'un Poilu 14–18: Gueule Cassée le 11 Octobre 1918* (Lyon: Bellier, 2006).
Brent, Marie-Louise, Letter to Jane Poupelet, 11 September [1918?], in *Jane Poupelet, 1874–1932: 'La Beauté dans la Simplicité'*, ed. by Anne Rivière (Paris: Gallimard, 2005), pp. 48–49.
Clare, Percy, Letters (to his mother). London Imperial War Museum collection, 06/48/1 [no page number].
——, *Private papers of P. Clare*, III, written in 1918, revised in 1920, recopied in 1932 and 1935. London, Imperial War Museum, 06/48/1 [no page number].
Criqui, Eugène and Robert Bré, 'Les Aventures de ma Vie' (2), *Match: le plus grand hebdomadaire sportif*, 23 February 1932, pp. 6–7.
Danneil, Hans, 'Lebensplan von H. Danneil', Bonn, Archiv der sozialen Demokratie, Internationaler Jugendbund, Box 67.
Duhamel, Georges, *Civilisation: 1914–1917* (Paris: Mercure de France, 1918).
——, *Light On My Days: An Autobiography*, trans. by Basil Collier (London: J.M. Dent & Sons Ltd, 1948).
Galtier-Boissière, Jean, *La Fleur au Fusil* (Paris: Baudinière, 1929).
Marden, Doris, 'My First Memories of Queen Mary's' in *Queen Mary's Hospital 1929–2004: A Collection of Stories and Photographs to Commemorate the 75th Anniversary of Queen Mary's and the 30th Anniversary of the New Hospital*, compiled by Iris Presswell and Andrew Bamji, p. 5.
Muir, Ward, *The Happy Hospital* (London: Simpkin, Marshall, Hamilton, Kent & Co, 1918).
Norton-Cru, Jean, *Témoins-Essai d'Analyse et de Critique des Souvenirs de Combattants Edités en Français de 1915 à 1928 (Paris: Les Etincelles, 1929).*
Pickard, Joseph, interviewed by Peter M. Hart (1986). London, Imperial War Museum, interview 8946.
Rémi, Henriette, *Hommes Sans Visage* (Lausanne: SPES, 1942).

——, Letter to Rudolf Eucken, Verden, 31 July 1917, Vol. 1, p. 38. Jena, Thüringer Universitäts- und Landesbibliothek.
Stevens, Biddy, conversation about her father Harry Burbeck (30 March 2012), complemented by notes and photographs given by the family.

Novels

Barthélemy, Max, *Mémoires d'une 'Gueule Cassée'* (Nevers: Imprimerie de la Nièvre, 1930).
Baum, Vicki, *Grand Hotel*, trans. by Basil Creighton (London: Geoffrey Bles, 1930).
Dumas, Pierre, *L'homme qui Mourut Deux Fois* (Paris: Editions Delmas, 1943).
Galis, Henri, *Mon Visage Fait Horreur: Confession d'une Gueule Cassée* (Paris: Les œuvres libres, 1929).
Girard, Renée, *La Vie Intime d'une 'Gueule Cassée'* (Paris: Les Etincelles, 1931).
Hermann, Georg, *November 18* (Berlin: Das neue Berlin, 2000).
Remarque, Erich Maria, *All Quiet on the Western Front*, trans. by Brian Murdoch (London: Vintage, 1996), first published under the title *Im Westen nichts neues* (Berlin: Ullstein, 1929).
——, *The Road Back*, trans. by Arthur W. Wheen (London: G.P. Putnam's Sons, 1931), originally published under the title *Der Weg Zurück* (Berlin: Propyläen-Verlag, 1931).
Renaud, Jean, *Gueules Cassées* (Paris: Les Etincelles, 1929).

Photographs, paintings, drawings and films

Beckmann, Max, *Die Hölle: Der Nachhauseweg*, 1919. National Galleries of Scotland <http://www.nationalgalleries.org/object/GMA 2465 B> [accessed 18 August 2015].
Dix, Otto, *Dirne und Kriegsverletzter: Zwei Opfer des Kapitalismus*, 1923. Münster, Westfalisches Landesmuseum für Kunst und Kulturgeschichte.
——, *Die Kriegskrüppel*, 1924. New York, Museum of Modern Art.
——, *Kriegsverletzter*, 1922. London, Tate Gallery.
——, *Die Skatspieler*, 1920. Berlin, Nationalgalerie Staatliche Museen zu Berlin-Preussischer Kulturbesitz.
——, *Transplantation*, 1924. New York, Museum of Modern Art.
Freida, Raphaël, *Les Misères de la Guerre: Gueules Cassées et Mutilés* (unpublished, 1918). Musée du Service de Santé aux Armées du Val-de-Grâce, Paris, 2009.1.1–42.

Friedrich, Ernst, *War against War!* (London: The Journeyman Press, 1987).

Galtier-Boissière, Jean, *Défilé des Mutilés, 14 juillet 1919* (1919). Paris, Bibliothèque de Documentation International Contemporaine.

Gance, Abel, dir., *J'accuse* (Forrester-Parant Production, 1938) [Related publicity material: 'Pour la presse', Cinémathèque française archives, B 46–134 GANCE and Production notes, Cinémathèque française, 616–B128 and 616–B129].

Grosz, George, *Das Gesicht der herrschenden Klasse*, 1919, 28, 31. University of Iowa Libraries <http://sdrc.lib.uiowa.edu/dada/Das_Gesicht/> [accessed 18 August 2015].

——, *Die Gesundbeter, Gott mit uns* portfolio, 1916–17. New York: Museum of Modern Art.

——, *Der Held*, 1933, New York, Museum of Modern Art.

'Les Gueules Cassées?' (poster), Comité de Propagande Lyonnais [1926?]. Péronne, Historial de la Grande Guerre, 14 AFF 54.1.

Hippolyte Morestin Surrounded by Wounded Soldiers, Photograph, 1920/1950 (?) of a sculpture given by facially injured soldiers to Morestin ca. 1918, Wellcome Library no. 570434i.

Lobley, John, *The Queen's Hospital for Facial Injuries, Frognal, Sidcup: The Carpenters' Shop*, c. 1918, London, Imperial War Museum, IWM ART 3728.

——, *The Queen's Hospital for Facial Injuries, Frognal, Sidcup: The Commercial Class*, c. 1918, London, London, Imperial War Museum, IWM ART 3767.

——, *The Queen's Hospital for Facial Injuries, Frognal, Sidcup: The Dental Mechanics' Class,* c. 1918, London, Imperial War Museum, IWM ART 3757.

——, *The Queen's Hospital for Facial Injuries, Frognal, Sidcup: The Toy-Makers' Shop*, c. 1918, London, Imperial War museum, IWM ART 3756.

Nicholls, Horace, *The Development of 'Plastic Surgery', during the First World War*, official photographs, Ministry of Information, First World War Official Collection, Imperial War Museum. References Q30450, Q30452, Q 30455, Q30456, Q30457, Q30460.

Orpen, Diana, sketches (World War Two), London, BAPRAS collections, Royal College of Surgeons, references BAPRAS/DSB 1–26.

'The Photographic Collection', The Great War Archive (containing items contributed by the general public between March and June 2008, collected and digitalised by Oxford University, UK), <http://www.oucs.ox.ac.uk/ww1lit/collections/photo> [accessed 18 August 2015].

Red Cross Work on Mutilés at Paris, 1918, National Museum of Health and Medicine, Armed Forces Institute of Pathology, United States of America. Internet Archives database <http://archive.org/details/RedCrossMutiles> [accessed 18 August 2015].

'Service de Prothèse Maxillo-faciale du Docteur Pont à Lyon' (film). Part of the collections of the Etablissement de Communication et de Production Audiovisuelle de la Défense ECPAD, Paris, reference 14,18 A 910.

Tonks, Henry, pastels of facially injured soldiers treated at Queen Mary's Hospital, Sidcup (1916–1918), London, Hunterian Museum, RCSSC/P 569.1–72.

Portrait photographs of facially injured patients treated by Dr Hippolyte Morestin [no title], 91 photographs. London, Wellcome Library. References include 569937i, 570112i, 570414i, 570415i, 570434i.

Musée du Service de Santé aux Armées, Val-de-Grâce, Photographs of patients treated in various maxillofacial centres in France.

Medical records of Sidcup patients (including notes and photographs), London, Gillies archives.

Secondary sources

Alexander, Caroline, 'Faces of War', *Smithsonian Magazine*, February 2007 <http://www.smithsonianmag.com/history-archaeology/mask.html?c=y&page=2#ixzzoTRUaCcPb> [accessed 18 August 2015].

Anderson, Julie, 'Stoics: Creating Identities at St Dunstan's, 1914–1920', in Stephen McVeigh and Nicola Cooper, eds, *Men After War* (London: Routledge, 2013), pp. 79–91.

Anon., Biography of Eugène Criqui, *Le Noble Art* website <http://www.lenobleart.com/rep1/page02.php?id=25> [accessed 18 August 2015].

Anon., 'In pictures: Faces of Battle', BBC News, 2009 <http://news.bbc.co.uk/1/shared/spl/hi/picture_gallery/07/magazine_faces_of_battle/html/1.stm> [accessed 18 August 2015].

Anon., 'Les Missions Initiales', booklet edited by the *Association des Gueules Cassées* (2011), pp. 4–5.

Assmann, Jan, 'Collective Memory and Cultural Identity', trans. by John Czaplicka, *New German Critique*, 65 (1995), 125–33.

Audoin-Rouzeau, Stéphane, and Christophe Prochasson, eds, *Sortir de la Grande Guerre: Le Monde et l'Après-1918* (Paris: Tallandier, 2008).

Bamji, Andrew, 'Facial Surgery: the Patient's Experience' in Hugh Cecil and Peter H. Liddle, eds, *Facing Armageddon. The First World War Experienced* (London: Cooper, 1996), pp. 490–501.

——, 'The Macalister archive: records from the Queen's Hospital, Sidcup, 1917–1921', *Journal of Audiovisual Media and Medicine*, 16 (1993), 76–84.

——, 'The Queen's Hospital and All The King's Men', paper given at the Royal Society of Medicine's History of Medicine section meeting, in Michael Smith, 'First World War Facial Injuries', *Journal of the Royal Society of Medicine*, 88 (1995), 601–02.

——, *Queen Mary's Sidcup, 1974–1994: A Commemoration* (1994).

Barr, Niall 'The Legion that Sailed but Never Went: The British Legion and the Munich Crisis of 1938', in Julia Eichenberg and John P. Newman, eds, *The Great War and Veterans' Internationalism* (Basingstoke: Palgrave McMillan, 2013), pp. 32–52.

Bassie, Ashley, *Expressionism* (London: Parkstone Press, 2008).

Bennett, John, 'Henry Tonks and his contemporaries', *British Journal of Plastic Surgery*, 39, 1 (January 1986).

Berstein, Serge and Pierre Milza, *Histoire du XXe Siècle*, 3 vols (Paris: Hatier, 1996), i.

Biernoff, Suzannah, 'Flesh Poems: Henry Tonks and the Art of Surgery', *Visual Culture in Britain*, 11 (2010), 25–47.

——, 'The Rhetoric of Disfigurement in First World War Britain', *Social History of Medicine*, 24 (2011), 666–85.

——, and Jane Tynan, 'Making and Remaking the Civilian Soldier: The World War I Photographs of Horace Nicholls', *Journal of War and Culture Studies*, 5 (2012), 277–93.

Bingham, H.G. and C.E. Moore, 'Farewell to Queen's Hospital, Sidcup', *British Journal of Plastic Surgery*, 29 (October 1976), 297–301.

Blond-McIndoe Foundation's website <http://www.blondmcindoe.org/sir-archibald-mcindoe.html#Blond_McIndoe> [accessed 18 August 2015].

Bourke, Joanna, *Dismembering the Male: Men's Bodies, Britain and the Great War* (London: Reaktion, 1996).

——, *Shell Shock during World War One*, BBC website, available online <http://www.bbc.co.uk/history/worldwars/wwone/shellshock_01.shtml> [accessed 18 August 2015].

Bréhamet, Raymond Noël and Roubaud, Noëlle, *Le Colonel Picot et 'Les Gueules Cassées'* (Rennes: Nouvelles Editions Latines, 1960).

Brophy, John, *The Face in Western Art* (London: George G. Harrap, 1963).

Bull, Ray and Nichola Rumsey, *The Social Psychology of Facial Appearances* (New York: Springer-Verlag, 1988).

Callister, Sandy, 'Photographic Representations of Severely Wounded New-Zealand Soldiers', *Social History of Medicine*, 20, 1, 111–30.

Carden-Coyne, Ana, *Reconstructing the Body: Classicism, Modernism, and the First World War* (Oxford: Oxford University Press, 2009).

Carmichael, Jane, *First World War Photographers* (London: Routledge, 1989).

Cecil, Hugh and Peter H. Liddle, eds, *Facing Armageddon: The First World War Experienced* (London: Cooper, 1996).

Chambers, Emma, 'Fragmented Identities: Reading Subjectivity in Henry Tonks's Surgical Portraits', *Art History*, 32 (June 2009), 578–607.

Chilton, Charles, *Auntie's Charlie: An Autobiography of Charles Chilton* (Coventry: Fantom Films Limited, 2012).

Cohen, Deborah, *The War Come Home: Disabled Veterans in Britain and Germany, 1914–1939* (Berkeley: University of California Press, 2001).

——, 'Will to Work: Disabled Veterans in Britain and Germany after the First World War', in *Disabled Veterans in History*, ed. by David Gerber (Ann Arbor: University of Michigan Press, 2000), pp. 294–321.

Colas, Marie-Dominique, *Le Visage des Hommes 1914–2014: Un Face-à-Face Avec le Blessé de Guerre* (Panazol: Lavauzelle, 2014).

Connerton, Paul, *How Societies Remember* (Cambridge: Cambridge University Press, 1989, repr. 2003).

Crockett, Dennis, *German post-Expressionism: The Art of the Great Disorder, 1918–1924* (University Park, PA: Penn State University Press, 1999).

Daniel, Joseph, *Guerre et Cinéma: Grandes Illusions et Petits Soldats, 1895–1971* (Paris: Armand Colin, 1972).

Delaporte, Sophie, 'La Délégation des Gueules Cassées à Versailles, le 28 Juin 1919', *L'Histoire par l'Image*, <http://www.histoire-image.org/site/etude_comp/etude_comp_detail.php?i=112> [accessed 18 August 2015].

——, *Les Gueules Cassées: Les Blessés de la Face de la Grande Guerre* (Paris: Noêsis, 1996).

Devauchelle, Bernard, *Défigurations*, 'War and Medicine' workshop, 7 February 2004, Paris <http://www.bium.univ-paris5.fr/histmed/guerre/journee2004/x10devauchelle.pdf> [15 November 2011].

Diehl, James, 'Victors or Victims: Disabled Veterans in the Third Reich', *The Journal of Modern History*, 59 (December 1997), pp. 705–736.

Dugain, Marc, *La Chambre des Officiers* (Paris: Lattès, 1998).

Dupeyron, François, dir., *La Chambre des Officiers* (ARP Selection, 2000).

Eichenberg, Julia, and John P. Newman, eds, *The Great War and Veterans' Internationalism* (Basingstoke: Palgrave McMillan, 2013).

Elderfield, John, ed., *Dada in the Collection of the Museum of Modern Art* (New York: The Museum of Modern Art publications, 2008).

Englund, Peter, 'Remembering the First World War: Touched from a Distance', *History Today*, 61 (November 2011), pp. 3–4.

Farrand, Paul, 'Portraiture as Therapy', *Saving Faces* art project website <http://www.savingfaces.co.uk/news-media/art-project/35-art/133-dr-paul-farrand-medical-psychologist> [accessed 10 April 2014].

Fischer, Louis-Paul, et al., 'Les Gueules Cassées Représentées par de Grands Peintres (O. Dix–G. Grosz–R. Freida): La Défiguration en Histoire de l'Art', *Histoire des Sciences Médicales*, 41 (2007), 337–46.

Freeman, Julian, 'Professor Tonks: War Artist', *Burlington Magazine*, 127 (1985), 285–93.

Friedrich, Otto, *Before the Deluge: A Portrait of Berlin in the 1920s* (New York: Harper Collins Publishers, 1995).

Fumex, Jean-Pierre, *Le Docteur Albéric Pont, Sa Vie, Son Oeuvre* (PhD thesis, Lyon, 1971).

Fussell, Paul, *The Great War and Modern Memory* (Oxford: Oxford University Press, 1977).

Garcia, Stéphane, ed., *Henriette Rémi: Hommes sans visage* (Geneva: Slatkine, 2014).

Garnier, Claire, Exhibition '1917' (interview), Alsace 20, 2012 <http://www.youtube.com/watch?v=2N7VW4Dd1U0> [accessed 86 August 2015].

Gay, Peter, *Weimar Culture: The Outsider as an Insider* (London: Penguin, 1988).

Gehrhardt, Marjorie, 'Gueules Cassées: The Men Behind the Masks', *Journal of War and Culture Studies*, Special issue on Veterans' Identities, 6 (2013), 267–81.

——, 'Walking Reminders of the War: The Case of Facially Disfigured Veterans', in Jozef Niznik, ed., *Twentieth Century Wars in European Memory* (Oxford: Peter Lang, 2013), pp. 103–15.

——, 'World War One *Gueules Cassées* and the Ambiguity of Violence', in Ulrike Zitzlsperger, ed., *Gender, Violence and Agency* (Cambridge: Cambridge Scholars Publishing, 2013), pp. 151–63.

Gerber, David A., ed., *Disabled Veterans in History* (Ann Arbor: University of Michigan Press, 2000).

Gilman, Sander, *Making the Body Beautiful: A Cultural History of Aesthetic Surgery* (Princeton: Princeton University Press, 1999).

Goffman, Erving, *Stigma: Notes On the Management of the Spoiled Identity* (London: Penguin, 1963).

Guillot, Hélène, 'La Section Photographique de l'Armée et la Grande Guerre: De la Création en 1915 à la Non-dissolution', *Revue Historique des Armées*, 258 (2010), 110–17.

Hagner, Michael, 'Verwundete Gesichter, verletzte Gehirne: Zur Deformation des Kopfes im Ersten Weltkrieg' in Claudia Schmölders and Sander Gilman, eds, *Gesichter der Weimarer Republik: Eine physiognomische Kulturgeschichte* (Köln: DuMont Buchverlag, 2000).

Helmers, Marguerite, 'Iconic Images of Wounded Soldiers by Henry Tonks', *Journal of War and Culture Studies*, 3 (2010) 181–99.

Herwig, Holger, *The First World War: Germany and Austria-Hungary, 1914–1918* (London: Arnold, 1997)

Hess, Heather, *German Expressionism: Works from the Collection* (German Expressionist Digital Archive Project, 2011) <http://www.moma.org/collection_ge/object.php?object_id=63267&curated=1> [accessed 18 August 2015].

Hilbert, Jan and Johannes Hoenig, 'The Plastic Surgeon Johannes Fredericus Samuel Esser (1877 to 1946) and his Unknown Period during 1917 and 1925 in Berlin, Germany', *European Journal of Plastic Surgery*, 32 (2009), 127–30.

Hillary, Richard, *The Last Enemy* (Short Hills, NJ: Burford Books, 1997).

Hone, Joseph, *The Life of Henry Tonks* (London: Heinemann, 1939).

Julien, Elise, *Paris, Berlin: la Mémoire de la Guerre 1914–1933* (Rennes: Presses universitaires de Rennes, 2009).

Kane, Martin, *Weimar Germany and the Limits of Political Art: A Study of the Work of George Grosz and Ernst Toller* (Tayport: Hutton Press, 1987).

Kienitz, Sabine, *Beschädigte Helden: Kriegsinvalidät und Körperbilder 1914–1923* (Paderborn: Ferdinand Schöningh, 2008).

Lansdown, Richard, Nichola Rumsey, Eileen Bradbury et al., *Visibly Different: Coping with Disfigurement* (London: Hodder Arnold, 1997).

Le Breton, David, *Des Visages: Essai d'Anthropologie* (Paris: Métailié, 2003[1992]).

Lebovici, Elisabeth, 'L'art Répare les Gueules Cassées', *Libération*, 11 November 2005, <http://www.liberation.fr/culture/0101548040-l-art-repare-les-gueules-cassees> [accessed on 18 August 2015].

Leed, Eric, *No Man's Land: Combat and Identity in World War I* (Cambridge: Cambridge University Press, 1979).

Lenz, Susanne, 'Hilfe vom Nasenjoseph', *Berliner Zeitung*, 4 June 2014 <http://www.berliner-zeitung.de/kultur/gesichtsplastiken-im-ersten-weltkrieg-hilfe-vom-nasenjoseph,10809150,27347646.html> [accessed 10 December 2014].

Lloyd, David W., *Battlefield Tourism: Pilgrimage and the Commemoration of the Great War in Britain, Australia and Canada 1919–1939* (Oxford: Berg, 1998).

Long, François-Xavier, 'Les Blessés de la Face Durant la Grande Guerre: Les Origines de la Chirurgie Maxillo-faciale', *Histoire des Sciences Médicales*, 36 (2002), 175–83.

Longacre, Jacob, *Rehabilitation of the Facially Disfigured: Prevention of Irreversible Psychic Trauma by Early Reconstruction* (Springfield: Thomas, 1973).

Lubbock, Tom, 'Doing Damage', *Modern Painters*, 12 (1999), 58–62.

Lyford, Amy, *Surrealist Masculinities: Gender Anxiety and the Aesthetics of Post-World War I Reconstruction in France* (Berkeley: University of California Press, 2007).

Mayhew, Emily, *Wounded: A New History of the Western Front in World War I* (Oxford: Oxford University Press, 2014).

McVeigh, Stephen and Nicola Cooper, eds, *Men After War* (London: Routledge, 2013).

Metzger, Rainer, *Berlin, Die Zwanzigerjahre: Kunst und Kultur 1918–1933* (Vienna: Christian Brandstätter, 2006).

Monestier, Martin, *Les Gueules Cassées: Les Médecins de l'Impossible* (Paris: Le Cherche Midi, 2009).

Monségur, Guy, *Etrange et Tragique Destinée d'un Poilu – En Hommage à Jean-Victor Monségur, aux Gueules Cassées et à Tous les Combattants de 14–18* (Pau: Monhélios, 2004).

Natvig, Paul, *Jacques Joseph: Surgical Sculptor* (Philadelphia: Saunders, 1982).

Nicolson, Juliet, *The Great Silence: 1918–1920, Living in the Shadow of the Great War* (London: John Murray, 2009).

Niznik, Jozef, ed., *Twentieth Century Wars in European Memory* (Oxford: Peter Lang, 2013).

Nora, Pierre, ed., *Realms of Memory: Rethinking the French Past*, trans. by Arthur Goldhammer, 3 vols (New York: Columbia University Press, 1996–1998).

Overy, Richard, *The Morbid Age: Britain Between the Wars* (London: Penguin, 2009).

Owen, C.R., *Erich Maria Remarque: A Critical Bio-Bibliography* (Amsterdam: Rodopi, 1984).

Page, Geoffrey, *Tale of a Guinea Pig: Exploits of a World War II Fighter Pilot* (New York: Bantam Books, 1983).

Plumb, Steve, *Neue Sachlichkeit, 1918–33: Unity and Diversity of an Art Movement* (Amsterdam: Rodopi, 2006).

Poore, Carol, *Disability in Twentieth-Century German Culture* (Ann Arbor: University of Michigan Press, 2007).

Pound, Reginald, *Gillies, Surgeon Extraordinary: A Biography* (London: M. Joseph, 1964).

Prost, Antoine, *In the Wake of War: 'Les Anciens Combattants' and French Society*, trans. by Helen McPhail (Oxford: Berg, 1992).

Rankin, Marlene, and Gregory Borah, 'Perceived Functional Impact of Abnormal Facial Appearance', *Plastic and Reconstructive Surgery*, 11 (2003), 2140–46.

Reznick, Jeffrey, 'Work-Therapy and the Disabled British Soldier in Great Britain in the First World War: The Case of Shepherd's Bush Military Hospital, London', in *Disabled Veterans in History*, ed. by David Gerber (Ann Arbor: University of Michigan Press, 2000), pp. 185–203.

Riaud, Xavier, *Pionniers de la Chirurgie Maxillo-Faciale (1914–1918)* (Paris: L'Harmattan, 2010).

Rivière, Anne, ed., *Jane Poupelet, 1874–1932: 'La Beauté dans la Simplicité'* (Paris: Gallimard, 2005).

Robinson, Eileen, Nichola Rumsey and James Partridge, 'An Evaluation of the Impact of Social Interaction Skills Training for Facially Disfigured Soldiers', *British Journal of Plastic Surgery*, 49 (5), 1996), 281–89.

Rumsey, Nichola, Ray Bull and Denis Gahagan, 'A Preliminary Study of the Potential of Social Skills for Improving the Quality of Social Interaction for the Facially Disfigured', *Social Behaviour*, 1 (1986).

Rumsey, Nichola and Diana Harcourt, 'Body Image and Disfigurement: Issues and Interventions', *Body Image*, 1 (2004), 83–97.

Rumsey, Nichola and James Partridge, 'An Evaluation of the Impact of Social Interaction Skills Training for Facially Disfigured Soldiers', *British Journal of Plastic Surgery*, 49 (1996).

Schmölders, Claudia and Sander Gilman, eds, *Gesichter der Weimarer Republik: Eine physiognomische Kulturgeschichte* (Köln: Dumont, 2000).

Schubert, Dietrich, *Otto Dix* (Hamburg: Reinbek, 1980; repr. 1996).

Sontag, Susan, *On Photography* (New York: Straus and Giroux, 1977).

——, *Regarding the Pain of Others* (London: The Penguin Group, 2003).

Stibbe, Matthew, *Germany, 1914–1933: Politics, Society and Culture* (London: Pearson, 2010).

Stock, Nicola M., Katie Whale, Elizabeth Jenkinson et al., 'Young People's Perceptions of Visible Difference', *Diversity and Equality in Health and Care*, 10 (2013), 41–51.

Stone, Anna and Toby Wright, 'When Your Face Doesn't Fit: Employment Discrimination Against People with Facial Disfigurements', *Journal of Applied Social Psychology*, 43 (2013), 515–26.

Tatar, Maria, 'Entstellung im Vollzug: Das Gesicht des Krieges in der Malerei', in Claudia Schmölders and Sander Gilman, eds, *Gesichter der Weimarer Republik: Eine physiognomische Kulturgeschichte* (Köln: Dumont, 2000).

Torriero, E.A., 'Disfigured Soldiers Are War's Dark Face' *Chicago Tribune*, 26 May 2008 <http://articles.chicagotribune.com/2008-05-26/news/0805260121_1_facial-soldiers-face> [accessed 20 April 2014].

Trezise, Thomas, 'Unspeakable', *The Yale Journal of Criticism*, 14 (2001), 39–66.

Valade, Corine, *Gueules Cassées … et alors?: Sourire Quand Même* (Saint-Cyr-sur-Loire: Alan Sutton, 2004).

Véray, Laurent, 'Abel Gance, cinéaste à l'œuvre cicatricielle', *Revue 1895*, 31 (2000), p. 42.

Wallace, Antony F., *The Progress of Plastic Surgery: An Introductory History* (Oxford: Willem A. Meeuws, 1982).

Webber, C.J., 'Queen Mary's Hospital: 1915–1971', 30 November 1971. Bexleyheath, Bexley Local Archives, reference P362.11SID.

Weerda, Wilko and Wolfgang Pirsig, 'Jacques Joseph und der Patient Dr. Karl Hasbach', Jacques Joseph: 100 Jahre moderne Nasenchirurgie <http://jacquesjoseph.de/Hasbach.html> [accessed 8 December 2014].

Weston, Simon, *Walking Tall: An Autobiography* (London: Trafalgar Square Publishers, 1990).

Whalen, Robert W., *Bitter Wounds: German Victims of the Great War, 1914–1939* (Ithaca, NY: Cornell University Press, 1984).

Winter, Jay, *Remembering War: The Great War between Memory and History in the Twentieth Century* (New Haven and London: Yale University Press, 2006).

——, *Sites of Memory, Sites of Mourning: The Great War in European Cultural History* (Cambridge: Cambridge University Press, 1995, repr. 2008).

——, and Antoine Prost, eds, *The Great War in History: Debates and Controversies, 1914 to the Present* (Cambridge: Cambridge University Press, 2005).

——, and Jean-Louis Robert, eds, *Capital Cities at War: Paris, London, Berlin 1914–1919*, 3 vols (Cambridge: Cambridge University Press, 2007), ii: *A Cultural History*.

——, and Emmanuel Sivan, eds, *War and Remembrance in the Twentieth Century* (Cambridge: Cambridge University Press, 1999).

Young, Louisa, *A Great Task of Happiness: The Life of Kathleen Scott* (London: Macmillan, 1995).

——, *My Dear I Wanted to Tell You* (London: Harper and Collins, 2011).

Zitzlsperger, Ulrike, ed., *Gender, Violence and Agency* (Cambridge: Cambridge Scholars Publishing, 2013).

Index

CULTURAL HISTORY AND LITERARY IMAGINATION

EDITED BY CHRISTIAN J. EMDEN & DAVID MIDGLEY

This series promotes inquiry into the relationship between literary texts and their cultural and intellectual contexts, in theoretical, interpretative and historical perspectives. It has developed out of a research initiative of the German Department at Cambridge University, but its focus of interest is on the European tradition broadly perceived. Its purpose is to encourage comparative and interdisciplinary research into the connections between cultural history and the literary imagination generally.

The editors are especially concerned to encourage the investigation of the role of the literary imagination in cultural history and the interpretation of cultural history through the literary text. Examples of the kind of issues in which they are particularly interested include the following:

- The material conditions of culture and their representation in literature, e.g. responses to the impact of the sciences, technology, and industrialisation, the confrontation of 'high' culture with popular culture, and the impact of new media;

- The construction of cultural meaning through literary texts, e.g. responses to cultural crisis, or paradigm shifts in cultural self-perception, including the establishment of cultural 'foundation myths';

- History and cultural memory as mediated through the metaphors and models deployed in literary writing and other media;

- The intermedial and intercultural practice of authors or literary movements in specific periods;

- The methodology of cultural inquiry and the theoretical discussion of such issues as intermediality, text as a medium of cultural memory, and intercultural relations.

Both theoretical reflection on and empirical investigation of these issues are welcome. The series is intended to include monographs, editions, and collections of papers based on recent research in this area. The main language of publication is English.

Vol. 1 Christian Emden & David Midgley (eds): Cultural Memory and Historical Consciousness in the German-Speaking World Since 1500. Papers from the Conference 'The Fragile Tradition', Cambridge 2002. Vol. 1.
316 pp., 2004. ISBN 3-03910-160-9 / US-ISBN 0-8204-6970-X

Vol. 2 Christian Emden & David Midgley (eds): German Literature, History and the Nation. Papers from the Conference 'The Fragile Tradition', Cambridge 2002. Vol. 2.
393 pp., 2004. ISBN 3-03910-169-2 / US-ISBN 0-8204-6979-3

Vol. 3 Christian Emden & David Midgley (eds): Science, Technology and the German Cultural Imagination. Papers from the Conference 'The Fragile Tradition', Cambridge 2002. Vol. 3.
319 pp., 2005. ISBN 3-03910-170-6 / US-ISBN 0-8204-6980-7

Vol. 4 Anthony Fothergill: Secret Sharers. Joseph Conrad's Cultural Reception in Germany.
274 pp., 2006. ISBN 3-03910-271-0 / US-ISBN 0-8204-7200-X

Vol. 5 Silke Arnold-de Simine (ed.): Memory Traces. 1989 and the Question of German Cultural Identity.
343 pp., 2005. ISBN 3-03910-297-4 / US-ISBN 0-8204-7223-9

Vol. 6 Renata Tyszczuk: In Hope of a Better Age. Stanislas Leszczynski in Lorraine 1737-1766.
410 pp., 2007. ISBN 978-3-03910-324-9

Vol. 7 Christian Emden, Catherine Keen & David Midgley (eds): Imagining the City, Volume 1. The Art of Urban Living.
344 pp., 2006. ISBN 3-03910-532-9 / US-ISBN 0-8204-7536-X

Vol. 8 Christian Emden, Catherine Keen & David Midgley (eds): Imagining the City, Volume 2. The Politics of Urban Space.
383 pp., 2006. ISBN 3-03910-533-7 / US-ISBN 0-8204-7537-8

Vol. 9 Christian J. Emden and Gabriele Rippl (eds): ImageScapes. Studies in Intermediality.
289 pp., 2010. ISBN 978-3-03910-573-1

Vol. 10 Alasdair King: Hans Magnus Enzensberger. Writing, Media, Democracy.
357 pp., 2007. ISBN 978-3-03910-902-9

Vol. 11 Ulrike Zitzlsperger: ZeitGeschichten: Die Berliner Übergangsjahre. Zur Verortung der Stadt nach der Mauer.
241 pp., 2007. ISBN 978-3-03911-087-2

Vol. 12 Alexandra Kolb: Performing Femininity. Dance and Literature in German Modernism.
330pp., 2009. ISBN 978-3-03911-351-4

Vol. 13 Carlo Salzani: Constellations of Reading. Walter Benjamin in Figures of Actuality.
388pp., 2009. ISBN 978-3-03911-860-1

Vol. 14 Monique Rinere: Transformations of the German Novel. *Simplicissimus* in Eighteenth-Century Adaptations.
273pp., 2009. ISBN 978-3-03911-896-0

Vol. 15 Katharina Hall and Kathryn N. Jones (eds): Constructions of Conflict. Transmitting Memories of the Past in European Historiography, Culture and Media.
282pp., 2011. ISBN 978-3-03911-923-3

Vol. 16 Ingo Cornils and Sarah Waters (eds): Memories of 1968. International Perspectives.
396pp., 2010. ISBN 978-3-03911-931-8

Vol. 17 Anna O' Driscoll: Constructions of Melancholy in Contemporary German and Austrian Literature.
263pp., 2013. ISBN 978-3-0343-0733-8

Vol. 18 Martin Modlinger and Philipp Sonntag (eds): Other People's Pain. Narratives of Trauma and the Question of Ethics.
252pp., 2011. ISBN 978-3-0343-0260-9

Vol. 19 Ian Cooper and Bernhard F. Malkmus (eds): Dialectic and Paradox. Configurations of the Third in Modernity.
265pp., 2013. ISBN 978-3-0343-0714-7

Vol. 20 Kristina Mendicino and Betiel Wasihun (eds): Playing False. Representations of Betrayal.
355pp., 2013. ISBN 978-3-0343-0867-0

Vol. 21 Guy Tourlamain: *Völkisch* Writers and National Socialism. A Study of Right-Wing Political Culture in Germany, 1890–1960.
394pp., 2014. ISBN 978-3-03911-958-5

Vol. 22 Ricarda Vidal and Ingo Cornils (eds): Alternative Worlds. Blue-Sky Thinking since 1900.
343pp., 2015. ISBN 978-3-0343-1787-0

Lightning Source UK Ltd.
Milton Keynes UK
UKHW021252170722
405967UK00006B/45

9 783034 318693